EYE AND VISION RESEARCH DEVELOPMENTS SERIES

EYE RESEARCH DEVELOPMENTS: GLAUCOMA, CORNEAL TRANSPLANTATION, AND BACTERIAL EYE INFECTIONS

Eye and Vision Research Developments Series

Eye Cancer Research Progress
Edwin B. Bospene (Editor)
2008. ISBN: 978-1-60456-045-9

Non-Age Related Macular Degeneration
Enzo B. Mercier
2008. ISBN: 978-1-60456-305-4

Optic Nerve Disease Research Perspectives
Benjamin D. Lewis and Charlie James Davies (Editors)
2008. ISBN: 978-1-60456-490-7

New Topics in Eye Research
Lauri Korhonen and Elias Laine (Editors)
2009. ISBN: 978-1-60456-510-2

Eye Infections, Blindness and Myopia
Jeffrey Higgins and Dominique Truax (Editors)
2009. ISBN: 978-1-60692-630-7

Retinal Degeneration: Causes, Diagnosis and Treatment
Robert B. Catlin (Editor)
2009. 978-1-60741-007-2

Eye Research Developments:
Glaucoma, Corneal Transplantation, and Bacterial Eye Infections
Alan N. Westerhouse (Editor)
2009.ISBN: 978-1-60741-1772

EYE AND VISION RESEARCH DEVELOPMENTS SERIES

EYE RESEARCH DEVELOPMENTS: GLAUCOMA, CORNEAL TRANSPLANTATION, AND BACTERIAL EYE INFECTIONS

ALAN N. WESTERHOUSE
EDITOR

Nova Biomedical Books
New York

For permission to use material from this book please contact us:
Telephone 631-231-7269; Fax 631-231-8175
Web Site: http://www.novapublishers.com

Library of Congress Cataloging-in-Publication Data

Eye research developments : glaucoma, corneal transplantation, and bacterial eye infections / editor, Alan N. Westerhouse.

p. ; cm.

Includes bibliographical references and index.

ISBN 978-1-60741-177-2 (hardcover)

1. Glaucoma. 2. Cornea--Transplantation. 3. Eye--Infections. I. Westerhouse, Alan N.

[DNLM: 1. Glaucoma. 2. Corneal Transplantation. 3. Eye Infections, Bacterial. WW 290 E97 2009]

RE871.E973 2009

617.7'41--dc22

2009021699

Published by Nova Science Publishers, Inc. ✝ New York

Contents

Preface

The consequences of aging populations combined with the strain to the human eye caused by computers and widespred poor nutritional pratices has resulted in an upsurge of research dealing with vision. This new book presents leading-edge research in this field focusing on glaucoma, corneal transplantation and bacterial eye infections.

Chapter I - Trabeculectomy has been a standard procedure for medically uncontrollable glaucoma. Combined phacoemulsification and trabeculectomy (phacotrabeculectomy) has been reported to provide less intraocular pressure reduction and smaller success rate compared with trabeculectomy alone. To prevent serious complications of trabeculectomy and phacotrabeculectomy, some medications, including viscocanalostomy, have been proposed. Combined phacoemulsification and viscocanalostomy (phacoviscocanalostomy) produced a better hypotensive effect than that of viscocanalostomy alone.

Chapter II - Glaucoma is an optic neuropathy, considered as the second leading cause of blindness worldwide. Glaucoma is characterized by selective death of retinal ganglion cells (RGC) and a progressive loss of vision.

Chapter III - Decades of epidemiologic research into glaucoma have elucidated several risk factors related in some way to the disease. Moreover, limited data indicate that marked geographical variations have been demonstrated regarding mainly the pseudo-exfoliation glaucoma (XFG). Currently, the best-known causative risk factor is raised intraocular pressure. Among other risk factors, age, ischemia, increased homocysteine levels, changes in endothelium-dependent vascular regulation, impaired blood-brain barrier and ocular blood flow and cytokines have been implicated in the mechanisms underlying glaucoma. Although degenerative diseases, including glaucoma, have an increasingly high impact on aged population, their association with *Helicobacter pylori* (*H. pylori*) infection has not been thoroughly researched. This issue has only recently been addressed by Kountouras et al. who documented: a high prevalence of *H. pylori* infection in Greek patients with primary open-angle glaucoma (POAG) and XFG, a beneficial effect of eradication of *H. pylori* on glaucoma progression, suggesting a possible causal link between the bacterium and POAG and an increased *H. pylori*-specific IgG antibody concentration in the aqueous humor of patients with glaucoma the titer of which correlated with the degree of vertical cupping, possibly indicating the severity of glaucomatous damage. A positive association between *H. pylori* infection serology and glaucoma was also reported by three studies from Turkey,

China, and India. An elevation in aqueous humor anti-*H. pylori* IgG antibodies in XFG was further reported by an Iranian study. Conversely, two ~~other~~ studies from Canada and Israel found no association between *H. pylori* infection and POAG. Apart from a brief description of the potential underlying pathogenetic mechanisms, the data of these studies are herein analyzed according to their geographical similarities and diversities, and the methodological flaws and weaknesses are highlighted, emphasizing the need for larger, randomized, multicenter studies.

Chapter IV - Multiple drug therapy is used to treat glaucoma when monotherapy is not effective or sufficient. A combination of several drugs, including prostaglandin analogues, β-blockers, cholinergic agonists, adrenergic agonists, α_2-stimulants, α_1-blockers, and carbonic anhydrase inhibitors has been reported to be effective. These studies are carried out at the time when additional drugs were first administered in patients already receiving one drug. Efficacy of each drug in the patients who continue to administer two or more drugs was unknown. In this study, we studied the efficacy of each drug in these patients with its discontinuation.

Chapter V - Glaucoma, a leading cause of blindness worldwide, is a progressive optic neuropathy with characteristic structural changes in the optic nerve head and concomitant visual field defects. Ocular hypertension (i.e. elevated intraocular pressure without glaucoma) is the most important risk factor to develop glaucoma. Even though a number of variables, including various optic disc and visual field parameters, have been used in order to identify early glaucomatous damage, there is a need for computer-based methods that can detect early glaucomatous progression so that treatment to prevent further progression can be initiated. The chapter is mainly focused on the analytical description of a computer-based system that consists of two modules: a) the module for the calculation of quantitative parameters to define vessel deformation in glaucomatous images and the classification of subjects based on these parameters, and b) the module for visualizing ophthalmologic data. Qualitative and quantitative results are presented to verify the usefulness of the developed computer-based system towards the discrimination of patients with ocular hypertension who developed glaucomatous damage and patients with ocular hypertension who remain stable.

Chapter VI - Good vision requires a perfect corneal transparency which is largely supported by endothelial cells (EC). Secondary endothelial failure is a common cause of vision loss and the major cause of corneal graft failure. Any corneal graft is exposed to metabolic stress from the day of the initial keratoplasty surgery to the cumulative consequences of graft ageing. Additionally, during the graft rejection process, an acute cell stress occurs, leading to EC death through both necrosis and apoptosis. Oxidative and nitrosative reactions combine to release highly reactive substances that are toxic to the biological microenvironment. As a consequence, ECs either engage cytoplasm cell defense mechanisms or initiate apoptosis cascade. We observed in animal models that inducible Nitric Oxide Synthase (iNOS) was overproduced during the rejection process in the corneal graft endothelium and that nitrosative EC stress could be caused by in situ formed peroxynitrite. To counterbalance this phenomenon, EC are overproducing anti-apoptotic proteins that can convert into proapoptotic proteins once the defense mechanisms are overwhelmed. Highly specific iNOS inhibitors have been tested in animal models to lower the graft's oxidative reactions and therefore protect graft ECs during acute rejection with encouraging results. Validation of these mechanisms remains to be confirmed in human. In the future however, new therapeutic perspectives could be further investigated to protect metabolically stressed corneal ECs, using focused anti-oxidative or anti-apoptotic drugs.

Chapter VII - This chapter considers boundary control problem for the wave equation with boundary conditions of Dirichlet type, and control actions from L^2. To get numerical solutions to these problems we apply the stable variational method proposed earlier by the author. This method works well when original continuous system is controllable. Controllability property has a usual form $T > T^*$ and is supposed to be satisfied. We provide a detailed outline of the computational algorithm and give several numerical results obtained for data of varying smoothness and difference grids of varying densities. These results are compared with results of direct finite-difference approximation of initial continuous control problem via system of linear equations of high dimensionality.

Chapter VIII - In the last years, Deep Anterior Lamellar Keratoplasty (DALK) has emerged as the standard surgical technique for the treatment of advanced keratoconus and anterior corneal dystrophies. DALK has several advantages over penetrating keratoplasty (PKP): it preserves the recipient endothelium, it is an external procedure, it has an extremely low rejection rate, and the rejection is only directed toward the stroma and is therefore well controllable.

The most popular method for DALK is the Big-Bubble technique, by which air, forcefully injected into the stroma, separates the Descemet's membrane from the recipient stromal tissue, creating a smooth interface for the donor stroma.

Chapter IX - Eales' disease is an idiopathic retinal periphlebitis that primarily affects the peripheral retina in young adults. Eales' disease is characterized by retinal periphlebitis, peripheral retinal ischemia, and neovascularization. Visual loss is characteristically caused by recurrent vitreous haemorrhage. Eales' disease appears to be an immunologic reaction that may be triggered by an exogenous exposure. Eales' disease is distinctively characterized both by stage of inflammation as well as stage of proliferation. Hypoxia-induced expression of vascular endothelial growth factor is only one aspect of the complicated processes in intraocular neovascularization. The increased expression of VEGF, when compared to other conditions inducing neovascularization, might explain the severity of neovascular growth and the propensity of repeated vitreous hemorrhage in Eales' disease. Photocoagulation is the mainstay of therapy in proliferative stage of the disease. Chemokines have also been found to play a role in the intraocular neovascularization. Anti-cytokine therapeutic agents may prove to be beneficial.

Chapter X - Determine whether IOP-lowering medications reduce the risk of retinal arterial occlusions or retinal venous occlusions

Chapter XI - To compare the incidence of perioperative complications, microbiological contamination of the anterior chamber and postoperative outcomes after two standard methods of implantation of the hydrophilic acrylic intraocular lens (IOL)

Chapter XII - Glaucoma refers to a specific pattern of optic nerve damage and visual field loss caused by a number of different eye pathologies that affect the optic nerve, the retina and the vascular network. It is the second leading cause of blindness worldwide. About 60 millions people will be affected by this disease in the year 2010 [1]. Most, but not all, of these conditions are characterized by elevated intraocular pressure (IOP), which is not the disease itself, but the most important risk factor for the development of glaucoma. It has been suggested that high values of IOP produce direct mechanical damage to the axons of the optic nerve by interfering with the axonal cytoplasm flow and create gradual ischemia of the retina by mechanical compression of the vascular network of the retina. These processes can generate a chain of metabolic events that lead to slow axonal degeneration of retinal ganglion cells (RGC) and ultimately to apoptotic death of these cells [2].

Chapter XIII - Whereas intraocular pressure (IOP) is considered a major risk factor in glaucoma, growing evidence now indicates that it is not the only one.

There is increasing evidence that ocular ischemia plays a major role not only in the pathogenesis but also in the progression of the glaucomatous damage.

By virtue of this and because many existing techniques are able to evaluate the blood supply in the different vascular beds, it is essential that current and future investigations for glaucoma evaluate the role of ischemia on the progression of the glaucomatous optic neuropathy.

During the last decade, the study of haemodynamics in ocular tissues has been increasing interest and we observed exceptional advances in the development of new devices.

Chapter XIV - To evaluate the efficacy and safety of the Ahmed glaucoma valve implant in children with refractory glaucoma in the early, intermediate and long term follows up period.

In: Eye Research Developments
Editor: Alan N. Westerhouse

ISBN: 978-1-60741-177-2

Chapter I

New Management of Concurrent Glaucoma and Cataract: Phacoviscoanalostomy Versus Phacotrabeculectomy

Hiroshi Kobayashi [*] ***and Kaori Kobayashi***
[1] Department of Ophthalmology, Kokura Memorial Hospital, Kitakyusyu,
[2] Department of Ophthalmology, Kurashiki Central Hospital, Kurashiki, Japan.

Abstract

Trabeculectomy has been a standard procedure for medically uncontrollable glaucoma. Combined phacoemulsification and trabeculectomy (phacotrabeculectomy) has been reported to provide less intraocular pressure reduction and smaller success rate compared with trabeculectomy alone. To prevent serious complications of trabeculectomy and phacotrabeculectomy, some medications, including viscocanalostomy, have been proposed. Combined phacoemulsification and viscocanalostomy (phacoviscocanalostomy) produced a better hypotensive effect than that of viscocanalostomy alone.

In a randomized study, the hypotensive effects of phacoviscocanalostomy and phacotrabeculectomy were studied in eyes with primary open angle glaucoma. Eighty eyes of 80 Japanese patients who had visually significant cataract and primary open angle glaucoma were studied. All patients enrolled in the study had intraocular pressure of greater than or equal to 22 mmHg despite medical therapeutic interventions. These patients were prospectively randomized to receive either trabeculectomy or viscocanalostomy in combination with phacoemulsification. The conditions of all patients were followed for 24 months. Significant reductions in the intraocular pressure were found in both procedures at any visit. No significant differences were found between the two groups at any of the follow-up examinations after 1 month postoperatively for either the intraocular pressure or the intraocular pressure reductions. There was significantly less hypotony and choroidal

* Address for correspondence: To Hiroshi Kobayashi MD, PhD, Department of Ophthalmology, Kokura Memorial Hospital, 1-1 Kifune-machi, Kokurakita-ku, Kitakyusyu 802-8555, Japan. PHONE: 093-921-2231, FAX: 093-921-8497; E-mail: kobi@earth.ocn.ne.jp

detachment in the viscocanalostomy group. In the trabeculectomy group, 7 eyes (17.5%) exhibited hypotony in contrast to the viscocanalostomy group, in which none of the eyes were affected. There was no significant difference in the visual improvement between the two groups.

Multiple regression analysis showed a significant correlation between the postoperative intraocular pressure and a combination of preoperative intraocular pressure and age in the viscocanalostomy group. There was a significant increase in the postoperative intraocular pressure in relation to the increase for the preoperative pressure. No significant correlation was found between the preoperative and postoperative intraocular pressure in the phacotrabeculectomy group.

In conclusion, there were no significant differences in hypotensive effects between phacoviscocanalostomy- and phacotrabeculectomy-treated eye. There was a significant correlation between the preoperative and postoperative intraocular pressure in phacoviscocanalostomy-treated but not phacotrabeculectomy- treated eyes.

Introduction

Patients with glaucoma and a visually significant cataract requiring cataract surgery present a challenge to the ophthalmic surgeon. Development of new therapies and techniques, including small-incision phacoemulsification and foldable intraocular lens (IOL), has evolved the management of concurrent glaucoma and cataract [1-3]. Combined surgery to remove a cataract and control glaucoma is becoming more common in glaucomatous eyes with visually significant cataract because only one operation is required.

Trabeculectomy has been a standard procedure for medically uncontrollable glaucoma [4]. Friedman et al. reported the superior hypotensive effect of combined trabeculectomy and phacoemusification (phacotrabeculectomy) in comparison with cataract surgery alone [5]. However, several investigators reported that phacotrabeculectomy provided less intraocular pressure reduction, higher postoperative intraocular pressure, and smaller success rates compared with trabeculectomy alone [6-8]. Serious postoperative complications are not infrequently associated with trabeculectomy and also phacotrabeculectomy [9-14].These include intraoperative and postoperative bleeding, flat anterior chamber and hypotony caused by overfiltration, choroidal detachment, and long-term complications, including bleb-related endophthalmitis and cataract progression. Therefore, several modifications of trabeculectomy have been proposed and recent among them is the non-penetrating approach, including non-filtering glaucoma surgery [15-19].

Viscocanalostomy, one of the non-filtering glaucoma surgery, provides a significant intraocular pressure reduction, although the reduction is less than that seen with trabeculectomy [20-25]. Wishart et al. demonstrated that combined viscocanalostomy and phacoemulsification (phacoviscocanalostomy) produced better hypotensive effect in comparison with viscocanalostomy alone [26,27]. The aim of this study is to compare the hypotensive effect and safety of phacoviscocanalostomy and phacotrabeculectomy with mitomycin C in eyes with primary open-angle glaucoma.

Materials and Methods

Patients

We studied 80 eyes of 80 Japanese patients with visually significant cataracts and chronic primary open-angle glaucoma with an intraocular pressure of greater than or equal to 22 mmHg despite medical therapy. A diagnosis of glaucoma was based on the appearance of the optic nerve head cupping, gonioscopy results, and visual field alteration according to the Japan Glaucoma Society guideline for glaucoma [28]. Excluded were patients with angle closure glaucoma or post-traumatic, uveitic, neovascular, or dysgenetic glaucoma, as well as patients with a known life-threatening disease. The study protocol and consent forms were approved by the Human Subjects Committee. Patients were informed of the purpose of our study and they provided written informed consent. The patients were prospectively randomized to receive trabeculectomy or viscocanalostomy, with only one eye of a patient to be randomized. When both eyes were eligible, the right eye became the study eye. Within 24 hours after enrollment, the patients were randomized using an envelope method. In brief, we prepared each 40 envelopes which contained a card which showed either viscocanalostomy group or trabeculectomy group. Within 24 hours after enrollment, an envelope was picked-up and the inside card showed the way to treat the patient, viscocanalostomy or trabeculectomy. Forty patients underwent trabeculectomy and the remaining 40 patients underwent viscocanalostomy. Treatment began within a week after these random assignments.

Surgical Procedure

All surgeries were performed by a single surgeon (HK). Phacoemulsification and intraocular lens implantation was performed through a temporal corneal incision separate from the viscocanalostomy site or trabeculectomy site. A standard phacoemulsification technique was used. In all cases, a three-piece hydrophobic acrylic intraocular lens (AcrySof™ MA30BM; Alcon, Fort Worth, TX, USA) was implanted. Sodium hyaluronate 1% (Healon, AMO, Santana, CA, USA) was used as viscoelastics. All residual viscoelastics in the anterior chamber was attempted to be removed.

Viscocanalostomy (figure 1)

Viscocanalostomy was performed according to Stegmann's technique with some modifications [18]. A 5 x 5 x 5-mm limbal-based parabolic half-thickness scleral flap was dissected deeply into clear cornea, 1.5 mm from the limbus. A second, deep scleral flap was dissected close to the ciliary body. The Schlemm's canal was unroofed by gently pulling on the scleral flap; the membrane was then cleaved from the cornea, creating a corneal "window." Afterwards, the inner scleral flap was excised.

After a 150-μm cannula (Visco Canalostomy Cannula, 149.40; Grieshaber & Co., AG, Schaffhausen, Switzerland) was inserted and correctly positioned, the proximal ends of the

Schlemm canal, as well as the intrascleral space, were filled with sodium hyaluronate. Afterwards, the inner flap was cut off and the superficial flap was closed tightly with 10-0 nylon sutures. To prevent early postoperative scarring, sodium hyaluranate was injected underneath the flap. The conjunctival flap was closed with 10-0 nylon sutures.

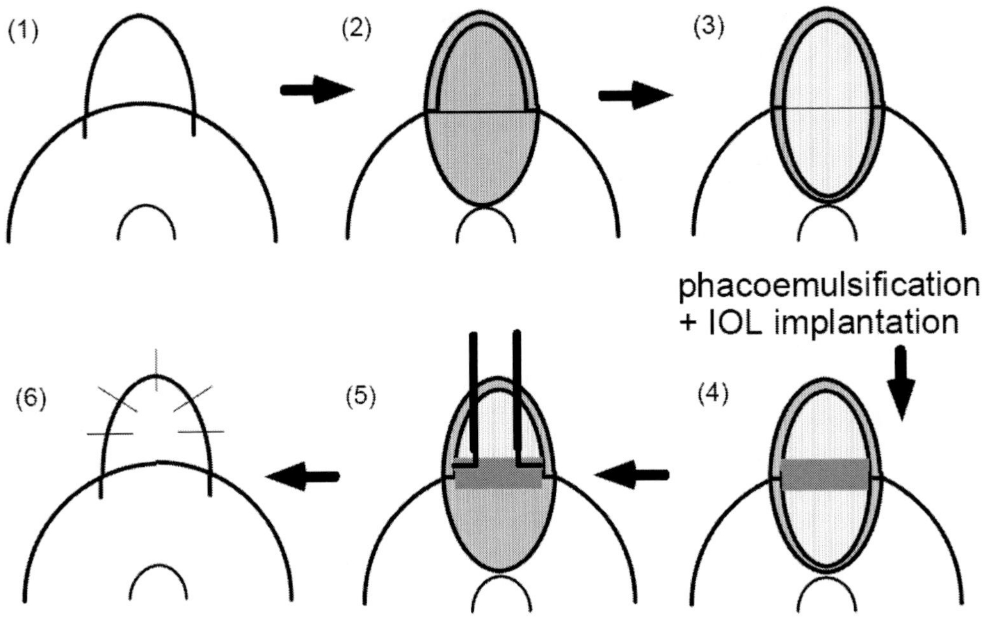

Figure 1. Surgical procedure of viscocanalostomy. (1) Following peritomy over 120°, a 5 x 5 x 5-mm parabolic half-thickness scleral flap was dissected deeply into clear cornea, 1.5 mm from the limbus. (2) A second, deep scleral flap was dissected close to the ciliary body inside the edge of the superficial flap. (3) The Schlemm's canal was unroofed, and the fibrotic was peeled from the bottom of the canal and the juxtacanalicular trabecular meshwork. (4) The membrane was cleaved from the cornea, creating a corneal "window." (5) After the inner flap was excised, the proximal ends of Schlemm's canal was filled with sodium hyaluronate. (6) The superficial flap was closed tightly with 10-0 nylon sutures, and sodium hyaluronate was injected underneath the flap.

Trabeculectomy

A modified Cairns-type technique was performed [4]. After making a fornix-based conjunctival flap and dissecting a limbus-based 4 x 4-mm scleral flap, mitomycin C 0.04%-soaked sponges were placed underneath the conjunctival flap for 3 minutes. Afterwards, 250 ml of balanced salt solution (Balanced Salt Solution Plus™; Alcon, Fort Worth, TX, USA) was used to wash the surgical area. Paracentesis was carried out, but a peripheral iridectomy was not performed [29]. The scleral flap was closed with 10-0 nylon sutures adjusted to allow minimal leakage during reformation of the anterior chamber. Finally, Tenon's capsule and the conjunctiva were separately closed with 10-0 nylon suture.

Postoperative Interventions

All glaucoma medications were discontinued after surgery. In both groups, all patients were given topical Levofloxacin, dexamethazone and diclofenac three times daily during the first 2 weeks, tapered over the next 3 months. Diclofenac, a nonsteroidal anti-inflammatory drug, was used to reduce inflammation and cystoid macular edema [30].

In the viscocanalostomy group, goniopuncture was performed after surgery if the surgeon felt that the intraocular pressure was not low enough. With a gonioscopy contact lens, the aiming beam was focused on the semi-transparent trabeculo-descemetic membrane [31]. In the free running Q-switched mode with a power of 4-8 mJ, 4 to 15 shots were applied.

In the trabeculectomy group, laser suture lysis was performed if the bleb was flat or the intraocular pressure was not low enough [32].

Evaluation of Outcomes

All recruited patients underwent a detailed ophthalmic examination, including Humphrey visual field analysis, gonioscopy, and confocal scanning laser tomography. Patient progress was reviewed at 1 and 3 days, 1 and 2 weeks, and 1, 2, 3, 4, 5, 6, 9, 12, 15, 18, 21 and 24months after surgery, and intraocular pressure was studied. A single observer (KK) took intraocular pressure measurements in all eyes. Intraocular pressure was measured with Goldman applanation tonometer. Three measurements were recorded in each eye at the same time (±1:00), the mean of which was used in the calculations. The optic nerve was examined with a Goldman three-mirror lens and measurements were taken of the size of the disk, the vertical and horizontal cup/disk ratios, the presence of rim notching or splinter hemorrhage, and the presence of peripapillary atrophy. Visual field testing with a Humphrey visual field analyzer (Humphrey-Zeiss, Dublin, CA), Program 30-2 SITA STANDARD™ testing was carried out before surgery and 6, 12, 18 and 24 months after surgery. Best-corrected visual acuity was measured at the 1-, 2-, 3-, 4-, 5-, 6-, 9-, 12-, 15-, 18-, 21- and 24-month visits, and the log of the minimum angle of resolution (logMAR) was calculated and used for all statistical analyses. An increase or decrease in visual acuity was defined as a change of greater than 0.2 in logMAR visual acuity.

The presence of complications was determined intraoperatively and at every postoperative visit. Hypotony was defined as an intraocular pressure of less than 4 mmHg after surgery. A shallow anterior chamber was defined as reported by Teehasaenee and Ritch [34]. An intraocular pressure spike was defined as an intraocular pressure on the first postoperative day of greater than or equal to 3 mmHg higher than the preoperative level.

The surgery was considered a complete success with an intraocular pressure between 6 and 20 mmHg and an intraocular pressure reduction of greater than or equal to 30% without glaucoma medication or additional surgery, compared to the preoperative level with medical therapy. A qualified success was defined as an intraocular pressure between 6 and 20 mmHg with glaucoma medication or an intraocular pressure reduction of less than 30% compared to the preoperative level with medical therapy. A failure was defined when an eye required further glaucoma surgery or lost visual function.

In case of postoperative intraocular pressure measurements greater than 21 mm Hg, despite all procedures including laser suture lysis, 5-fluorouracil injection and needling in the trabeculectomy group and goniopuncture in the viscocanalostomy group, intraocular pressure-lowering medication was added. In case of complications requiring surgery or still inadequate intraocular pressure control, additional procedures could be performed as required.

Study End

All patients were meant to reach a 24-month follow-up, but the following were considered as endpoints: (1) the need for any further surgical procedure (except laser suture lysis, 5-fluorouracil injection and needling in the trabeculectomy group, goniopuncture in the viscocanalostomy group); (2) an intraocular pressure of greater than 21 mmHg on two consecutive visits; and (3) patient failure to attend scheduled visits, allowing for a margin of tolerance. If the study was ended before month 24, the last values obtained in the trial were considered as the final data.

Statistical Analysis

The sample size was chosen to assure a power of at least 90% in detecting at least a 3-mm Hg difference between groups with a standard deviation of 3 mmHg with a two-sided α error of 5%.

Evaluation of continuous variables was achieved using the Student's *t*-test. To evaluate the difference in intraocular pressures between follow-up intervals, the paired *t*-test was used. All *t*-tests were two-tailed. Categoric variables were evaluated with the chi-square test, the Fisher exact test, or the Spearman rank correlation as appropriate. A level of $P < 0.05$ was accepted as statistically significant. Each potential confounding variable was screened for association with the outcome. Only those confounding variables that were statistically associated were eligible to be incorporated into the potential final multivariate model.

For the pairing of groups, the age, sex, best-corrected visual acuity, dimensions of disc and cupping at baseline were used for matching. We studied a correlation between the paired observations. If observations were correlated, the F-test was used to study two population variances.

Because a representation of mean intraocular pressure over time could be misleading because of exclusion of cases after failure, the mean intraocular pressure was recalculated by carrying forward the last intraocular pressure reading before repeat surgery. The proportion of surgical failures and adverse events in each treatment group was compared. Success was evaluated on basis of Kaplan-Meier cumulative probability (log rank test).

Results

Baseline

Forty patients in the viscocanalostomy group and 40 patients in the trabeculectomy were enrolled in the study. Patient demographics are summarized in table 1. Mean age was 71.7 ± 8.7 years in the viscocanalostomy group and 71.2 ± 7.8 years in the trabeculectomy group. No significant difference was found in age, sex, and number of preoperative hypotensive agents between groups.

Table 1. Demographics of Patients

	Viscocanalostomy group	Trabeculectomy group	P
No. of patients	40	40	-
men women	23 (57.5 %) 17 (42.5 %)	20 (50 %) 20 (50 %)	0.5
Age (years)	71.7 ± 8.7 (47 to 83)	71.2 ± 7.8 (53 to 82)	0.8
RE LE	22 (55 %) 18 (45 %)	21 (52.5%) 19 (47.5%)	0.8
Mean	0.210 (20/95.2)	0.227 (20/88.1)	-
Mean ± SD (LogMAR)	0.678 ± 0.296	0.643 ± 0.288	0.6
Mean deviation at Humphrey visual field analyzer (dB)	-19.89 ± 6.67 (-28.83 to -7.27)	-18.50 ± 5.40 (-28.31 to -6.34)	0.3
Cupping/Disk ratio	0.72 ± 0.26 (0.4 to 1.0)	0.70 ± 0.26 (0.4 to 1.0)	0.7
Nuclear sclerosis	1.9 ± 0.9	1.9 ± 0.8	1.0
Intraocular pressure	24.0 ± 2.0 (22 to 30)	23.7 ± 2.6 (22 to 32)	0.6
No. of anti-glaucomatous drugs	2.8 ± 0.8 (2 to 4)	2.6 ± 0.9 (2 to 4)	0.3

Change in Intraocular Pressure

All patients were completely followed-up (table 2). Baseline mean intraocular pressure was 24.0 ± 2.0 mmHg (range, 22 to 30 mmHg) in the viscocanalostomy group and 23.7 ± 2.6 mmHg (range, 22 to 32 mmHg) in the trabeculectomy group ($P = 0.6$) (table 2). In both groups, significant reductions ($P < 0.01$) in intraocular pressure were obtained at all visits (figure 2). Mean intraocular pressure was 12.5 ± 2.2 mmHg at 1 month, 13.7 ± 2.6 mmHg at 3 months, 14.8 ± 3.4 mmHg at 6 months, 14.9 ± 3.0 mmHg at 12 months, and 15.3 ± 2.9 mmHg at 24 months in the viscocanalostomy group and 11.3 ± 3.2 mmHg at 1 month, 12.4 ± 3.9 mmHg at 3 months, 13.9 ± 4.7 mmHg at 6 months, 14.1 ± 4.4 mmHg at 12 months, and 14.7 ± 4.0 mmHg at 24 months in the trabeculectomy group (figure 2). There was no significant difference in mean intraocular pressure between the viscocanalostomy group and the trabeculectomy group at any visit 1month after surgery, although the intraocular pressure was lower in the trabeculectomy group at every visit (table 2).

Mean intraocular pressure reduction was -35.4 ± 14.1 % (range, -60.0 to 0 %) in the viscocanalostomy group and -38.1 ± 16.2 % (range, -60.0 to +9.1%) in the trabeculectomy group at 24 months (table 2, figure 3). Thirty-seven eyes (92.5%) in the viscocanalostomy group and 35 eyes (87.5%) in the trabeculectomy group were considered to be a success (P = 0.5), whereas 33 eyes (82.5%) in the viscocanalostomy group and 31 eyes (77.5%) in the trabeculectomy group were considered to be a complete success (P = 0.6) (table 3, figure 4). At 24 months, the probability of obtaining an intraocular pressure of less than or equal to 16 mmHg without medical treatment was 60% (24 eyes) in the viscocanalostomy group and 55% (22 eyes) in the trabeculectomy group (P = 0.7) (figure 4).

Table 2. Change of Intraocular Pressure

	Viscocanalostomy group	Trabeculectomy group	P
Intraocular pressure (mmHg)			
Baseline	24.0 ± 2.0 (22 to 30)	23.7 ± 2.6 (22 to 32)	0.6
1 week	12.0 ± 2.2 (8 to 16)	9.7 ± 3.0 (4 to 16)	0.0002
2 weeks	12.6 ± 1.7 (8 to 16)	10.4 ± 2.8 (6 to 16)	0.0001
1 month	12.5 ± 2.2 (8 to 16)	11.3 ± 3.2 (6 to 18)	0.1
2 months	13.1 ± 2.3 (8 to 17)	11.9 ± 3.9 (6 to 21)	0.1
3 months	13.7 ± 2.6 (10 to 21)	12.4 ± 3.9 (6 to 22)	0.1
6 months	14.8 ± 3.4 (10 to 23)	13.9 ± 4.7 (6 to 24)	0.3
9 months	14.8 ± 3.0 (11 to 23)	13.7 ± 3.1 (7 to 24)	0.1
12 months	14.9 ± 3.0 (11 to 23)	14.1 ± 4.4 (8 to 24)	0.3
18 months	15.2 ± 3.2 (11 to 23)	14.4 ± 4.5 (8 to 24)	0.4
24 months	15.3 ± 2.9 (11 to 23)	14.7 ± 4.0 (10 to 24)	0.4
Change of intraocular pressure (mmHg)			
1 week	-13.0 ± 3.0 (-19 to -6)	-14.1 ± 4.6 (-25 to -9)	0.1
2 weeks	-11.5 ± 2.7 (-17 to -7)	-13.4 ± 4.2 (-22 to -6)	0.0184
1 month	-11.5 ± 3.2 (-20 to -6)	-12.4 ± 3.8 (-20 to -4)	0.2
2 months	-10.9 ± 3.8 (-20 to -6)	-12.2 ± 5.0 (-20 to -3)	0.4
3 months	-10.4 ± 3.6 (-18 to -6)	-11.6 ± 4.9 (-18 to 0)	0.2
6 months	-10.3 ± 4.9 (-23 to 0)	-9.9 ± 4.4 (-17 to +2)	0.7
9 months	-9.3 ± 3.9 (-18 to 0)	-10.0 ± 4.2 (-18 to +2)	0.4
12 months	-9.1 ± 3.4 (-18 to 0)	-9.6 ± 4.2 (-17 to +2)	0.6
18 months	-8.9 ± 4.1 (-18 to 0)	-9.4 ± 4.3 (-17 to +2)	0.6
24 months	-8.7 ± 3.9 (-18 to 0)	-9.1 ± 3.9 (-15 to +2)	0.7
Change of intraocular pressure (%)			
1 week	-49.7 ± 10.2 (-65.2 to -27.3)	-58.8 ± 13.3 (-81.8 to -36.0)	0.0001
2 weeks	-47.4 ± 8.7 (-65.2 to -30.4)	-55.9 ± 12.8 (-73.3 to -27.3)	0.0008
1 month	-47.5 ± 10.7 (-66.7 to -27.3)	-52.1 ± 13.6 (-72.7 to -18.2)	0.1
2 months	-45.0 ± 11.0 (-66.7 to -26.1)	-51.2 ± 17.5 (-72.7 to -13.6)	0.1
3 months	-42.7 ± 12.5 (-60.0 to -8.7)	-48.8 ± 17.1 (-72.7 to 0)	0.1
6 months	-37.3 ± 16.7 (-60.0 to 0)	-41.5 ± 18.2 (-76.0 to +9.1)	0.3
9 months	-38.5 ± 13.9 (-60.0 to 0)	-42.2 ± 17.9 (-72.0 to +9.1)	0.3
12 months	-37.9 ± 12.0 (-60.0 to 0)	-40.4 ± 17.7 (-68.0 to +9.1)	0.5
18 months	-36.3 ± 15.1 (-60.0 to 0)	-39.3 ± 18.2 (-68.0 to +9.1)	0.4
24 months	-35.4 ± 14.1 (-60.0 to 0)	-38.1 ± 16.2 (-60.0 to +9.1)	0.4

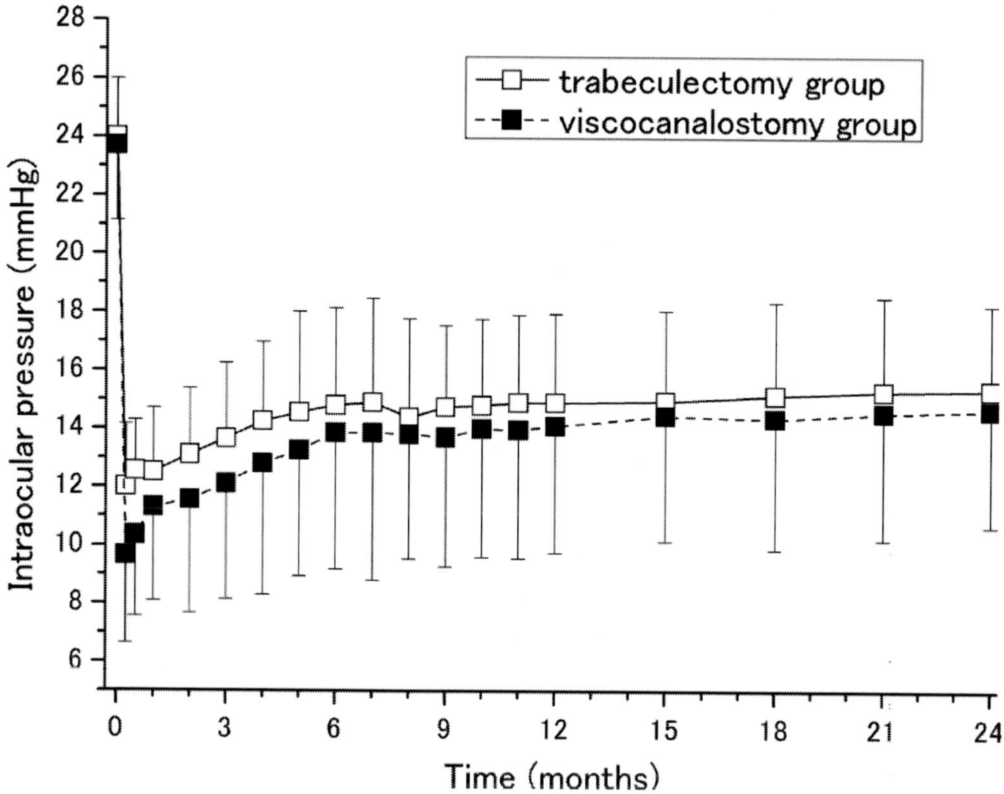

Figure 2. Intraocular pressure. Open square and solid line indicates the viscocanalostomy group and solid square and broken line indicates the trabeculectomy group.

Table 3. Surgical outcome at 12 months for each patient

	Viscocanalostomy group	Trabeculectomy group	P
No. of patients	40	20	
Overall success	37 (92.5%)	35 (87.5%)	0.5
Complete success	33 (82.5%)	31 (77.5%)	0.6
Qualified success	4 (10%)	4 (10%)	1.0
Failure	3 (7.5%)	5 (12.5%)	0.5
≤16 mmHg without medication	24 (60%)	22 (55%)	0.7
≥ 30% reduction without medication	28 (70%)	28 (70%)	1.0
Number of anti-glaucomatous medication	0.2 ± 0.5 (0 to 2)	0.2 ± 0.3 (0 to 1)	1.0

Note: Success and failure rate are defined according to the following criteria: complete success: intraocular pressure ≤ 20mmHg and intraocular pressure reduction ≥ 30% without additional medical or surgical treatment. Qualified success: intraocular pressure ≤ 20mmHg with medical treatment or intraocular pressure reduction < 30%. Qualified failure: intraocular pressure > 20mmHg despite medical treatment. Failure: new filtering surgery required.[10]

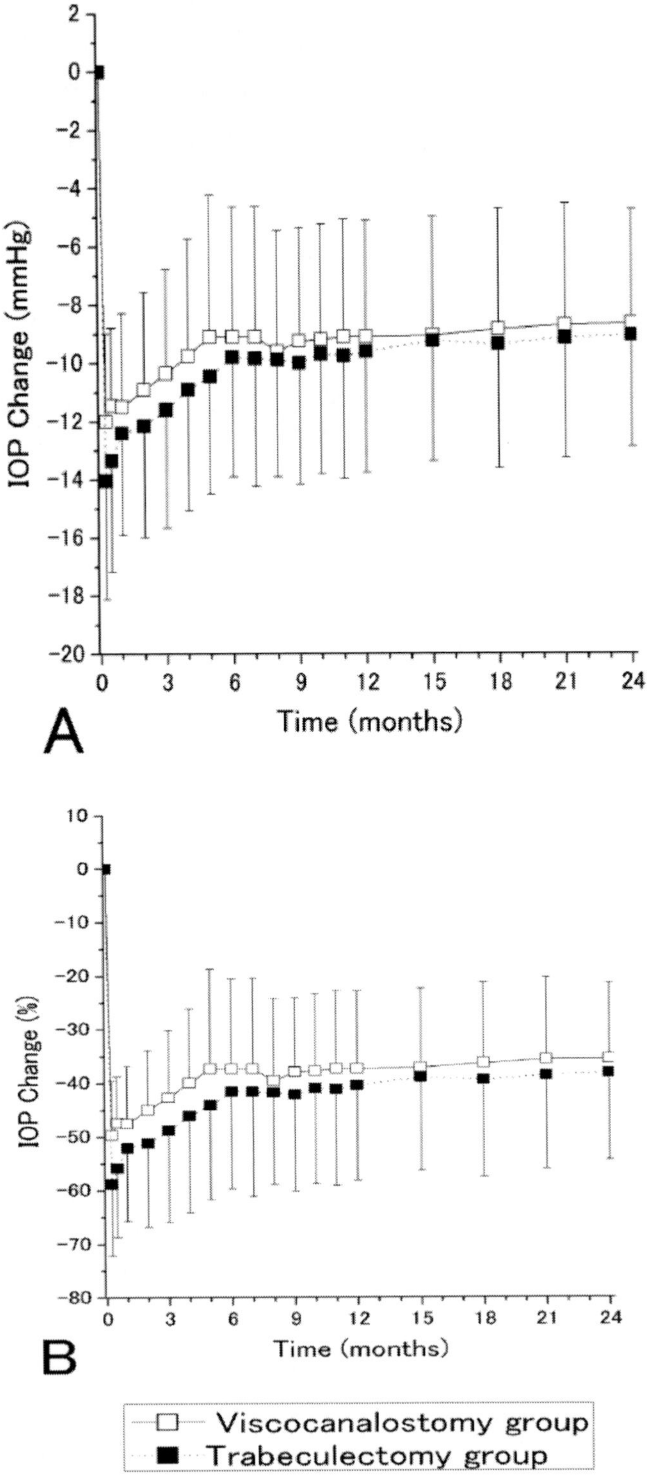

Figure 3. A change of intraocular pressure in mmHg (A) and % (B). Open square and solid line indicates the viscocanalostomy group and solid square and broken line indicates the trabeculectomy group.

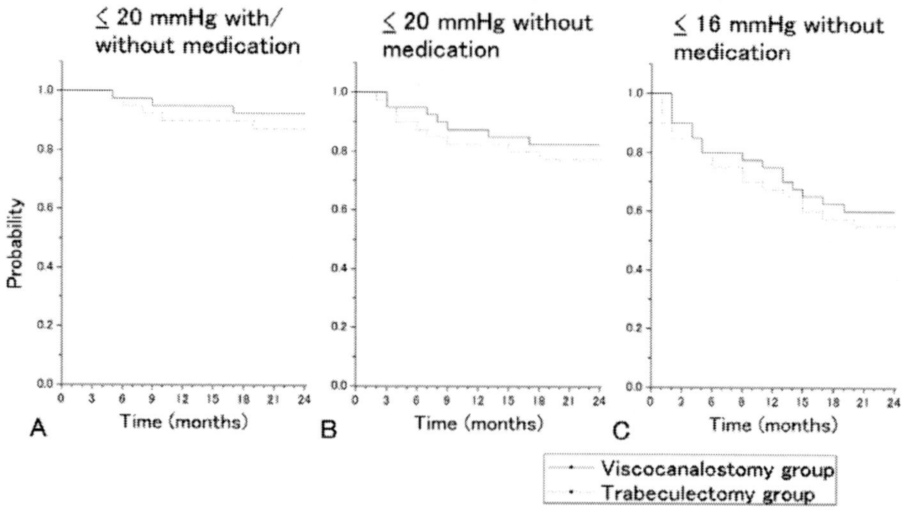

Figure 4. A.Cumulative probability of overall success, defined as an intraocular pressure of less than or equal to 20 mmHg and an intraocular pressure reduction greater than or equal to 30% with or without glaucoma medication, compared with preoperative level with medical therapy. B. Cumulative probability of complete success, defined as an intraocular pressure of less than or equal to 20 mmHg and an intraocular pressure reduction greater than or equal to 30% without glaucoma medication, compared with preoperative level with medical therapy. C. Cumulative probability of success, defined as an intraocular pressure of less than or equal to 16 mmHg without medical treatment. Solid line indicates the viscocanalostomy group and broken line indicates the trabeculectomy group.

Table 4. Change of Best-Corrected Visual Acuity and Visual Field

		Viscocanalostomy group	Trabeculectomy group	
Best-corrected visual acuity				
Baseline	Mean	0.210 (20/95.2)	0.227 (20/88.1)	
	Mean LogMAR ± SD	0.678 ± 0.296	0.643 ± 0.288	0.6
6 months	Mean	0.943 (20/21.2)	0.896 (20/22.3)	
	Mean LogMAR ± SD	0.025 ± 0.053	0.048 ± 0.066	0.9
12 months	Mean	0.943 (20/21.2)	0.907 (20/22.1)	
	Mean LogMAR ± SD	0.026 ± 0.058	0.043 ± 0.062	0.3
24 months	Mean	0.923 (20/21.7)	0.894 (20/22.4)	
	Mean LogMAR ± SD	0.034 ± 0.093	0.049 ± 0.073	0.4
Mean deviation at Humphrey visual field analyzer (dB)				
Baseline		-19.89 ± 6.67 (-28.83 to -7.27)	-18.50 ± 5.40 (-28.31 to -6.34)	0.3
6 months		-16.39 ± 6.08 (-26.02 to -5.23)	-16.01 ± 5.25 (-26.93 to -5.21)	0.8
12 months		-16.48 ± 6.11 (-26.33 to -4.91)	-16.21 ± 5.34 (-27.48 to -4.88)	0.8
18 months		-16.72 ± 6.33 (-27.31 to -3.53)	-16.42 ± 5.55 (-27.21 to -4.46)	0.8
24 months		-16.81 ± 6.07 (-26.53 to -5.34)	-16.64 ± 5.53 (-26.88 to -5.03)	0.9

Mean LogMAR ± SD: Mean log of the minimum angle of resolution ± standard deviation.

Table 5. Incidence of complications and adverse events

	Viscocanalostomy group	Trabeculectomy group	P
No. of patients	40	40	
Perforation of Descemet's membrane	4 (10%)	—	—
Choroidal deroofing	3 (7.5%)	—	—
Hypotony	0 (0%)	7 (17.5%)	0.0056
Flat/shallow anterior chamber	0 (0%)	3 (7.5%)	0.0402
Choroidal detachment	0 (0%)	4 (12.5%)	0.0402
Hypotension maculopathy	0 (0%)	0 (0%)	1.0
IOP spike	4 (10%)	0 (0%)	0.0402
Hyphema	0 (0%)	1 (2.5%)	0.2
Peripheral anterior synechia	6 (15%)	9 (22.5%)	0.1
Posterior synechia	0 (0%)	0 (0%)	1.0
Failed bleb	—	4 (10%)	—
Bleb formation	10 (25%)	—	—
Rupture of posterior lens capsule	0 (0%)	0 (0%)	1.0
Vitreous loss	0 (0%)	0 (0%)	1.0

Age, sex, ocular laterality, and pretreatment medications were evaluated as potential confounding variables at 24 months and were not found to be significantly associated with any confounder.

Change of Visual Acuity and Field

In both the viscocanalostomy group and trabeculectomy group, all eyes showed an increase of greater than 0.2 in logMAR best-corrected visual acuity at 24 months compared with the preoperative level (table 4). At 24 months, the mean best-corrected visual acuity in the viscocanalostomy group was better than that in the trabeculectomy group, but this improvement was not statistically significant.

Mean deviation at Humphrey visual field analyzer testing at baseline was -19.89 ± 6.67 dB in the viscocanalostomy group and -18.50 ± 5.40 dB in the trabeculectomy group (P = 0.3). Improvement of mean deviation was +3.41 ± 1.72 dB at 12 months and 3.08 ± 1.68 dB at 24 months in the viscocanalostomy group and +2.30 ± 1.84 dB at 12 months and 1.96 ± 1.68 dB at 24 months in the trabeculectomy group.

Incidence of Complications and Adverse Events

Complications are listed in table 5. During the viscocanalostomy, microperforation of the trabeculo-descemetic membrane was noted without iris prolapse or shallowing of the anterior chamber in 4 eyes (10%), and the procedures were completed as a viscocanalostomy with a successful postoperative outcome that did not require further intervention.

There was less hypotony and choroidal detachment in the viscocanalostomy group than in the trabeculectomy group; hypotony was found in none of the eyes (0%) in the viscocanalostomy group and in 7 eyes (17.5%) in the trabeculectomy group (P = 0.0056).

Postoperative intraocular pressure spike was found in 4 eyes (10%) in the viscocanalostomy group and no eye (0%) in the trabeculectomy group (P = 0.0402).

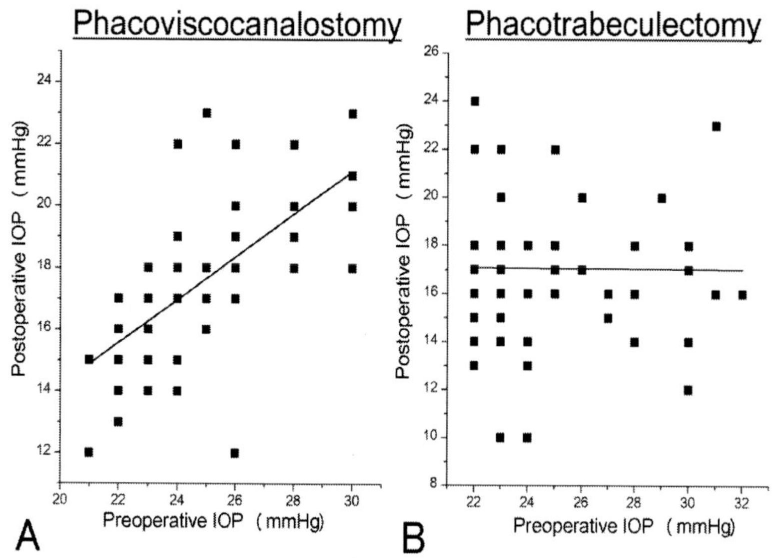

Figure 5. Effect of combined phacoemulsification on trabeculectomy and viscocanalostomy. Phacoviscocanalostomy and phacotrabeculectomy provided mean intraocular pressure reduction of -8.7 ± 3.9 mmHg and -9.1 ± 3.9 mmHg at 24 months, respectively. In our previous study, viscocanalostomy alone produced intraocular pressure reduction of -7.6 ± 3.1 mmHg at 24 months, whereas trabeculectomy alone decreased intraocular pressure of -11.8 ± 4.5 mmHg. Therefore, trabeculectomy appeared to be compromised the intraocular pressure-lowering effect when combined with phacoemulsification, although phacoviscocanalostomy may produce provide an additional reduction compared with the results of viscocanalostomy alone.

In contrast to the phacoviscocanalostomy, there were no significant correlations noted between the preoperative and postoperative intraocular pressure in the phacotrabeculectomy group (figure 6).

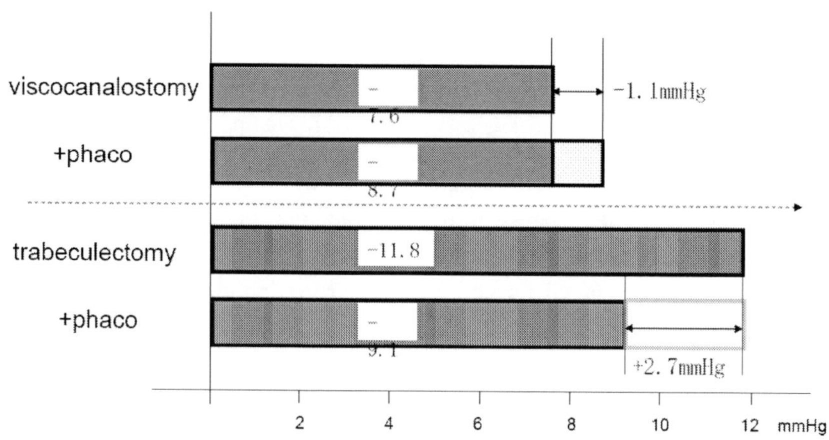

Figure 6.

In the viscocanalostomy group, bleb formation lasting longer than 14 days occurred in 10 eyes (25%) and subsided within 2 months. All blebs were flat and localized. The significant reduction of intraocular pressure continued after resolution of the bleb.

Relationship between Preoperative and Postoperative Intraocular Pressure

Multiple regression analysis showed a significant correlation between the postoperative intraocular pressure and a combination of preoperative intraocular pressure and age in the viscocanalostomy group. There was a significant increase in the postoperative intraocular pressure in relation to the increase for the preoperative pressure ($r = 0.691$, $P = 0.0001$) (figure 5). The postoperative intraocular pressure could be calculated from the preoperative pressure with using of the correlation equation as follows (table 6);

[Postoperative IOP] = 0.703 x [preoperative IOP]-1.668

Table 6. Projected postoperative intraocular pressure calculated from preoperative intraocular pressure

Preoperative IOP	Projected postoperative IOP
20	12.3
22	13.6
25	15.8
30	19.3
30.8	20
35	22.8

Discussion

In the current study, 37 eyes (92.5%) in the viscocanalostomy group and 35 eyes (87.5%) in the trabeculectomy group were considered to be a success, whereas 33 eyes (82.5%) in the viscocanalostomy group and 16 eyes (77.5%) in the trabeculectomy group were considered to be a complete success. Mean intraocular pressure reduction was -8.7 ± 3.9 mmHg in the viscocanalostomy group and -9.1 ± 3.9 mmHg in the trabeculectomy group at 24 months. In combination with phacoemulsification and intraocular lens implantation, there was no significant difference in the success rate or intraocular pressure reduction between the viscocanalostomy group and the trabeculectomy group. In our previous study, viscocanalostomy alone produced intraocular pressure reduction of -7.6 ± 3.1 mmHg at 24 months, whereas trabeculectomy alone decreased intraocular pressure of -11.8 ± 4.5 mmHg [25]. Therefore, trabeculectomy appeared to be compromised the intraocular pressure-lowering effect when combined with phacoemulsification, although phacoviscocanalostomy may produce provide an additional reduction compared with the results of viscocanalostomy alone (figure 6).

Intraocular Pressure-Lowering Effect of Cataract Surgery

Cataract surgery offers an opportunity for patients with angle closure glaucoma to significantly improve intraocular pressure regulation [34]. Early phacoemulsification can be considered as a definitive treatment to prevent IOP rise rather than laser peripheral iridotomy in patients after abortion of acute primary angle closure [35]. Even in patients with primary open angle glaucoma, cataract surgery and intraocular lens implantation has been demonstrated to result in a long-term reduction of intraocular pressure between 1 and 5 mm Hg as well as healthy individuals [36-43]. Friedman, in an evidence-based review, confirmed that cataract surgery alone provided a long-term intraocular pressure reduction of 2 to 4 mm Hg [5]. The decrease in the intraocular pressure was more pronounced in eyes with a higher preoperative pressure in both the glaucoma and control groups [41]. In a study of Shingleton et al, after 5 years, 76% in patients with glaucoma, 79%, in glaucoma suspects and 85% in patients without with glaucoma had intraocular pressure of less than or equal to their preoperative pressure [41]. Hayashi et al. demonstrated a mean pressure reduction of 5 mm Hg at 2 years after phacoemulsification in patients with primary open angle glaucoma, which is the greatest reported hypotensive effect of cataract surgery [39]. They reported that by 2 years postoperatively, 5 of 68 patients (7%) needed glaucoma-filtering surgery.

Pseudoexfoliative Glaucoma and Syndrome

Intraocular pressure decreased in patients with pseudoexfoliative syndrome after cataract surgery compared with those without pseudoexfoliative syndrome [42,43]. This effect is more pronounced in glaucoma patients (-1.85 mm Hg) compared with those without glaucoma (-0.62 mm Hg). Cimetta et al. showed that phacoemulsification with anterior capsule exfoliation material aspiration significantly reduced the mean diurnal intraocular pressure lasting 1 year postoperatively [44].

Intraoperative and Postoperative Complications

1) Vitreous Loss

Vitreous loss during cataract surgery in glaucoma patients adversely affected intraocular pressure control in the long term [45]. This study suggested that uneventful cataract surgery in glaucoma patients improves intraocular pressure control.

2) Intraocular Pressure Spike

This is a common complication after cataract surgery. Medically well-controlled glaucoma patients and patients with exfoliation syndrome may experience intraocular pressure elevation shortly after cataract surgery, which has been reported to occur with a frequency of 10 to 37% [46-50]. Levkovitch-Verbin et al. compared intraocular pressure change after phacoemulsification in eyes with glaucoma, exfoliation syndrome without glaucoma and normal eyes [50]. Most pressure elevation occurred at 4hours. The changes in intraocular pressure over time differed between glaucoma, exfoliation syndrome and normal. An increase of intraocular pressure over 25 mmHg did not occur in normal eyes, whereas the increase over 25 mm and 30mmHg occurred in 55% and 28% of glaucoma patients, respectively, and 27% and 11% of exfoliation syndrome. Other studies showed that, at 6 hours postoperatively, even in nonglaucomatous eyes, the frequency of relevant intraocular pressure spikes (>30 mm Hg) is greater than 10% without use of intraocular pressure-lowering topical medication at the end of surgery [46-49]. Instillation of timolol maleate 0.5%, bimatoprost or dorzolamide at the end of the procedure in this series eliminated intraocular pressure over 30 mmHg, but pressure elevation below that level can still occur.[46-49]

3) Nd:YAG Laser Posterior Capsulotomy

Lin et al. demonstrated that gradual intraocular pressure elevation or a need for more aggressive therapy is common in glaucoma patients following Nd:YAG laser posterior capsulotomy [51].The rate of "glaucoma progression" was 38.1% at 12 months, 46.1% at 24 months, 52.1% at 36 months and 52.1% at 47 months following the capsulotomy. It is unclear whether this progression is related directly to the Nd:YAG laser procedure or whether it is an independent progression of the patient's glaucoma unrelated to the Nd:YAG laser procedure.

Phacotrabeculectomy

Although, as mentioned before, combined cataract surgery and trabeculectomy provided significantly greater reduction when compared with cataract surgery alone [5], the combined procedures provided less pressure reduction, higher postoperative intraocular pressure, or smaller success rates than that seen in trabeculectomy alone [6-8]. Even with the use of antimebolites, a combined procedure a worse hypotensive effect and a significantly smaller success rate compared with trabeculectomy alone [52-56]. The reason for the poorer IOP-lowering effect of combined phacotrabeculectomy is unclear. Phacoemulsification may provide a significantly longer lasting breakdown of the blood aqueous barrier and higher levels of growth factors [57-59], including transforming growth factor-beta, which has been reported to last for 2 weeks [60]. This may lead to aggressive healing [61,62]. Phacoemulsification could also increase damage to the wound and need more time, resulting the longer exposition to the wound. Therefore, two-site surgery (separation of the two incisions for cataract surgery and for trabeculectomy) has been proposed. Seven randomized controlled trials were carried out, but all of them failed to show superiority of two-site compared with one-site surgery [63-69]. One study showed that corneal endothelial cell loss was significantly lower in the two-site surgery, although two-site surgery took significantly more time [69]. Jampel et al., in an evidence-based review, showed weak evidence of a small positive effect of the two-site surgery and the pressure reduction archieved by the surgery was 1 to 2 mmHg [70]. Li and Kasner recommended that early needle revision and antimetabolites may improve outcomes of combined cataract and glaucoma surgery [71].

Intraoperative Modification

1) Microincision Phacoemulsication

Development of phacoemulsification technique, including microincision coaxial and bimanual phacoemulsifcation, foldable IOL and microtrabeculectomy allowed the reduction of inflammation. Studies using these techniques were carried out in a small case series, and the results of efficacy have been awaited [3,72-75].

2) Anterior Lens Capsule Autotransplantation

Lu et al. reported that autotransplantation of human anterior lens capsule in the trabeculectomy site (application of the anterior lens capsule under scleral tunnel) provided comparable hypotensive effect as mitomycin-C in phacoemulsification with few complications [76]. A large-scale study is awaited.

Association between Long-Term Intraocular Pressure Fluctuation and Visual Field Deterioration

Hong et al. demonstrated that patients with greater than 2 mmHg of intraocular pressure standard deviation experienced a faster progression of visual field deterioration compared with those with less than or equal to 2 mmHg even though both groups kept low intraocular pressure after the triple procedure. Long-term intraocular pressure fluctuation was significantly correlated with visual field deterioration [77,78]. Therefore, to prevent visual field deterioration, surgical interventions not only to decrease intraocular pressure itself but also to reduce its fluctuation may be necessary.

Phacoemulsification Combined with Non-Penetrating Glaucoma Surgery

The main concern of trabeculectomy and also phacotrabeculectomy is the risk of ocular hypotony and its consequences [10-14]. The newer types of nonpenetrating filtering surgery, deep sclerectomy and viscocanalostomy, promise increased safety regarding postoperative complications [19]. Regarding the intraocular pressure-lowering effect, recent randomized controlled trials have demonstrated a higher efficacy of trabeculectomy compared with viscocanalostomy [20-25] and deep sclerectomy [79,80].

Prospective Randomized Trials Comparing Viscocanalostomy and Trabeculectomy

Several randomized studies comparing viscocanalostomy and trabeculectomy were carried-out [21-26,81,82]. Jonescu-Cuypers et al. conducted a randomized trial on 20 patients, but intraocular pressure less than or equal to 20 mm Hg without medication was achieved in none of the 10 eyes of the viscocanalostomy group and in 50% of the 10 eyes in the trabeculectomy group at a follow-up of 6 months, a rather discouraging finding for both techniques [82]. The same group, with threefold the sample size, reported intraocular pressure of less than 22 mm Hg in 30% in the viscocanalostomy group and 56.7% in the trabeculectomy group [21]. Some authors pointed out that some bias in the surgical technique may account for these results [21], because, in a histologic study conducted on the excised inner flap, the same authors reported a 64% rate of improper Schlemm's canal dissection in their cases [83]. Carassa et al. conducted a 12 month prospective trial, and mean initial and final IOP were 24.6 ± 10.6 and 14.0 ± 2.6 mm Hg in the trabeculectomy group and 22.3 ± 7.4 and 13.3 ± 3.8 mm Hg in the viscocanalostomy group, respectively, and hypotensive effects were comparable in the two groups [81]. The same author group also reported a 2-year randomized study on 50 patients with open-angle glaucoma, and, at 24 months, intraocular pressure of 21 mm Hg or less and greater than 6 mm Hg was achieved in 76% in the viscocanalostomy group and in 80% in the trabeculectomy group; and an intraocular pressure between 6 and 16 mm Hg was obtained in 56 % in the viscocanalostomy group and in 72% in the trabeculectomy group; trabeculectomy provides lower intraocular pressure, but this is not significant [23].

Phacoviscocanalostomy

Interestingly, contrary to trabeculectomy, nonpenetrating filtering surgery does not appear to be compromised in its intraocular pressure-lowering efficacy when combined with phacoemulsification and intraocular lens implantation. Combined viscocanalostomy and cataract surgery have been reported to provide a significant reduction in intraocular pressure [84-88]. Gimbel et al. reported a retrospective series of 83 eyes undergoing combined viscocanalostomy, phacoemulsification and intraocular lens implantation, and the surgical procedure produced mean reduction of 5.2 mm Hg at 6 months [84]. Hassan and Awadalla showed an excellent hypotensive effect in patients with exfoliation glaucoma as well as primary open angle glaucoma [85]. In a nonrandomized study, Shoji et al. showed that the success probabilities of the phacoviscocanalostomy group achieving 20% and 30% intraocular pressure reductions were 58 %and 28 % at 48 months, which were significantly better than the probabilities in the cataract surgery only group, which were 16 % and 6 % [87]. The same author group demonstrated that the success rate at 3 years ($\leq$ 21 mmHg) in the phacoviscocanalostomy group significantly better than those of the phacotrabeculotomy group [88,89]. Postoperative hyphema and intraocular pressure spikes occurred significantly less in the phacoviscocanalostomy group compared with phacotrabeculotomy group. Wishart et al.demonstrated a long-term intraocular pressure-lowering effect of phacoviscocanalostomy [90]; there was a statistically significant decrease in the intraocular pressure from 24.1 ± 5.1 mm Hg preoperatively to 16.0 ± 4.1 mm Hg at 5 years ($P<0.001$). The percentage fall in intraocular pressure was linearly related to the preoperative pressure level ($P<0.001$).

Combined Phacoemulsification and Deep Sclerectomy

Phacoemulsification may not impair the hypotensive effect of the simultaneous deep sclerctomy [91]. One of the reasons is that there was less inflammation following deep sclerectomy compared with trabeculectomy [92]. There was only one report regarding the difference between the combined procedures versus the deep sclerectomy alone [93]. D'Eliseo et al.conducted a randomized trial to compare the hypotensive effect of combined phacoemulsification and deep sclerectomy and deep sclerectomy alone. The combined group showed significant better intraocular pressure regulation (13.1 mmHg versus 15.2 mm Hg) and higher success rates (90% versus 62%) compared with deep sclerectomy alone. Only a few studies have been published comparing deep sclerectomy, viscocanalostomy and trabeculectomy in conjunction with phacoemulsification [94-96]. There was no significant difference in the final outcome after phacoviscocanalostomy compared with phacoemulsification and deep sclerectomy. Wishart et al. conducted a non-randomized prospective trial of 192 eyes comparing viscocanalostomy and deep sclerectomy [95]. After mean follow-up of 36 months, the success rate ($\leq$ 21 mm Hg without medication) was 96% for the phacoviscocanalostomy group and 94% for the phaco-deep sclerectomy group. Both groups showed excellent efficacy, but it should be noted that their study was nonrandomized and included patients with angle closure glaucoma. Gianoli et al. showed, in a randomized prospective study, no significant differences in success rates or postoperative intraocular pressure between combined phacoemulsification and deep sclerectomy and phacotrabeculectomy [94]. With use of deep sclerectomy with trabeculotomy, Luke et al demonstrated the better success rate (<18 mmHg without medication) of the phaco-deep sclerectomy group compared with the phacotrabeculectomy group (50% versus 20%) [96].

Non-Penetrating Surgery-Specific Complication-Descemet's Membrane Detachment

In spite of a low incidence of overfiltration-related complications, there was a serous complication specific to non-penetrating surgery, including Descemet's membrane detachment. Eleven cases of partial detachment of Descemet's membrane, including 3 cases of hemorrhagic detachment, have been reported [97-102]. After viscocanalostomy, the detachment was generally noticed shortly after the procedure and the cornea maintained its clarity, whereas, after deep sclerectomy, it developed weeks to months postoperatively with adjacent corneal edema [101]. This unusual complication is likely to be more common after nonpenetrating filtering surgery than after trabeculectomy. Some authors advocated that, if a hemorrhagic detachment is sufficiently extensive to cover the pupillary area, a descetmetopexy should be performed immediately [102].

Other Options

1. Trabeculotomy

Phacotrabeculotomy provided a significantly better IOP-lowering effect compared with phacoemulsification alone [103-105]. The additional IOP reduction lasts for at least 2 years and amounts to 3 to 4 mm Hg. Phacoemulsification might not compromise the effect of trabeculotomy. Only one nonrandomized trial, conducted by Hoffmann et al. to compare hypotensive effect of phacotrabeculotomy, phacotrabeculectomy, and a combination of both. The study failed to show the superiority in the hypertensive effect of any of the three groups [106].

The advantage of trabeculotomy over trabeculectomy is its safety even in combination of phacoemulsification [107,108]. Common complications were hyphema (20-30%) and early postoperative intraocular pressure elevation (intraocular spike, 10-20%), which self-limited and do not need surgical interventions. Postoperative hypotony, which was found in 10% of patients, may usually show spontaneous resolution without further complications within a few days.

2. Shunt Operation

2-1. Conventional Shunt Operation

In a retrospective case series, phacoemulsification and Ahmed valve implantation reduced mean IOP from 28.2 ± 3.1 to 16.8 ± 2.1 mmHg at 12 months [109]. Large lprospective studies with long-term follow-up are needed.

2-2. Miniature Shunt

2-2-1. Ex-PRESS Miniature Implant

Ex-PRESS R-50 miniature glaucoma implant insertion under the conjunctiva combined with cataract extraction decreased from 19.3 ± 6.3 mmHg to 13.3 ± 2.0 mm Hg at 48 months [110], but a relatively high incidence of complication were found, including conjuctival erosion, which might lead to endophthalmitis and failure from fibrosis [111]. As a consequence, the implant site was changed to under a scleral flap, and its implantation showed similar intraocular-lowering efficacy with a lower rate of early hypotony compared with trabeculectomy [112].

2-2-2. Eyepass Shunt Implantation

(GMP Vision Solutions, Inc.) An application of thisY-shaped Eyepass glaucoma implant decreased an intraocular pressure from 30.4 ± 7.5 to 18.3 ± 4.5 mm Hg at the end of the follow-up (mean 7.1 months) [113].

2-2-3. Gold Micro Shunt (SOLX, Waltham, MA)

A gold micro-shunt, 5.2mm long and 3.2 mm wide shunt device containing internal micro-channels to direct aqueous humor from the anterior chamber to the suprachoroidal space [114]. At 12 months, an intraocular pressure was reduced by 31% from baseline. One patients experienced retinal detachment although 28% of patients showed mild complications.

3. Endoscopic Cyclophotocoagulation

Endoscopic cyclophotocoagulation combined with cataract surgery provided a good IOP-lowering effect, whereas it has previously been in difficult, refractory cases [115,116].

Complication rates are relatively low with endoscopic cyclophotocoagulation. It is promising, but large studies with long-term follow-up are needed..

4. Others

1) Phacosclerothalamotomy

(4 ab interno sclerostomy with high frequency diathermic probe) [117]

2) Canalostomy

(Circumferential viscodilation and tensioning of Schlemm canal)

In 54 patients with OAG, canalostomy reduced mean baseline of 24.4±6.1mmHg to 13.7±4.4 mm Hg at 12 months after surgery [118].

Relationship between Preoperative and Postoperative Intraocular Pressure in Phacoviscocanalostomy and Phacotrabeculectomy

In this study, there was a significant correlation between the postoperative intraocular pressure and a combination of preoperative intraocular pressure and age in the viscocanalostomy group. In eyes undergoing combined phacoemulsification and trabeculotomy, other type of non-filtering surgery, the success rate of phacotrabeculotomy was better in older patients [119]. Also, the IOP reduction of both phacotrabeculotomy and phacoemulsification alone was 1 to 2 mm Hg larger in patients older than 70 years

There was a significant increase in the postoperative intraocular pressure in relation to the increase for the preoperative pressure. Wishart et al. also demonstrated this correlation in the phacoviscocanalostomy-treated eyes [90]. The postoperative intraocular pressure could be calculated from the preoperative pressure as shown in table 6. If the aim of the target postoperative pressure is 20 mmHg, the preoperative intraocular pressure needs to be 27 mmHg or lower. In contrast to the phacoviscocanalostomy, there were no significant correlations noted between the preoperative and postoperative intraocular pressure in the phacotrabeculectomy-treated eyes. This procedure can be employed in all patients regardless of their preoperative intraocular pressure. Indication for each of these methodologies should be carefully considered prior to any surgical interventions.

Conclusion

Although the sample size in each group was small, the current study demonstrated that (1) in a randomized study, there was no significant difference in intraocular pressure-lowering effect between phacoviscocanalostomy- and phacotrabeculectomy- treated eyes, (2) phatoviscocanalostomy-treated eyes had a significantly lower incidence of complications than phacotrabeculectomy-treated eyes, and (3) There was a significant correlation between preoperative and postoperative intraocular pressure in the phacoviscocanalostomy- treated but not phacotrabeculectomy-treated eyes. Future study of a large population is needed to verify this observation. However, this information may be clinically valuable when treating primary open angle glaucoma.

References

[1] Storr-Paulsen A, Bernth-Petersen. Combined cataract and glaucoma surgery. *Curr. Opin. Ophthalmol.* 2001;12:41-46.

[2] Vass C, Menapace R. Surgical strategies in patients with combined cataract and glaucoma. *Curr. Opin. Ophthalmol.* 2004;15:61-66.

[3] Verges C, Cazal J, Lavin C. Surgical strategies in patients with combined cataract and glaucoma. *Curr. Opin. Ophthalmol.* 2004;15:61-66.

[4] Cairns DE. Trabeculectomy – a preliminary report of a new method. *Am. J. Ophthalmol.* 1968;66:673-679.

[5] Friedman DS, Jampel HD, Lubomski LH, et al.: Surgical strategies for coexisting glaucoma and cataract: an evidence-based update. *Ophthalmology.* 2002;109:1902-1913.

[6] Derick RJ, Evans J, Baker ND: Combined phacoemulsification and trabeculectomy versus trabeculectomy alone: a comparison study using mitomycin-C. *Ophthalmic Surg. Lasers.* 1998, 29:707-713.

[7] Kleinmann G, Katz H, Pollack A, et al.: Comparison of trabeculectomy with mitomycin C with or without phacoemulsification and lens implantation. *Ophthalmic Surg. Lasers.* 2002, 33:102-108.

[8] Lochhead J, Casson RJ, Salmon JF: Long term effect on intraocular pressure of phacotrabeculectomy compared to trabeculectomy. Br J Ophthalmol 2003, 87:850-852.

[9] Costa VP, Smith M, Spaeth GL, et al. Loss of visual acuity after trabeculectomy. *Ophthalmology.* 1993;100:599-612.

[10] Bellucci R, Perfetti S, Babighian S, et al.: Filtration and complications after trabeculectomy and after phaco-trabeculectomy. *Acta Ophthalmol. Scand.* 1997:Suppl:44-45.

[11] Lehmann OJ, Bunce C, Matheson MM, et al. Risk factors for development of post-trabeculectomy endophthalmitis. *Br. J. Ophthalmol.* 2000;84:1349-1353.

[12] Poulsen EJ, Allingham RR. Characteristics and risk factors of infections after glaucoma filtering surgery. *J. Glaucoma.* 2000;9:438-443.

[13] DeBry PW, Perkins TW, Heatley G, Kaufman P, Brumback LC. Incidence of late-onset bleb-related complications following trabeculectomy with mitomycin. *Arch. Ophthalmol.* 2002;120:297-300.

[14] Rothman RF, Liebmann , Ritch R. Low-dose 5-fluorouracil trabeculectomy as initial surgery in uncomplicated glaucoma: long-term follow-up. *Ophthalmology.* 2000;107:1184-1190.

[15] Krasnov MM. Sinusotomy: foundations, results, prospects. *Trans. Am. Ophthalmol. Otolaryngol.* 1972;76:369-372.

[16] Zimmerman TJ, Kooner KS, Ford VJ, et al. Effectiveness of nonpenetrating trabeculectomy in aphakic patients with glaucoma. *Ophthalmic Surg.* 1984;15:332-336.
[17] Zimmerman TJ, Kooner KS, Ford VJ, et al. Trabeculectomy vs. nonpenetrating trabeculectomy: a retrospective study of two procedures in phakic patients with glaucoma. *Ophthalmic Surg.* 1984;15:734-740.
[18] Stegmann R, Pienaar A, Miller D. Viscocanalostomy for open-angle glaucoma in black African patients. *J. Cataract. Refract. Surg.* 1999;25:316-22.
[19] Lachkar Y. Nonpenetrating glaucoma surgery. *Curr. Opin. Ophthalmol.* 2002;13:
[20] Lachkar Y. Nonpenetrating deep sclerectomy with external trabeculectomy vs trabeculectomy, *Invest. Ophthalmol. Vis. Sci.* 2001;42:s67.
[21] Luke C, Dietlein TS, Jacobi PC, Konen W, Krieglstein GK. A prospective randomized trial of viscocanalostomy versus trabeculectomy in open-angle glaucoma: a 1-year follow-up study. *J. Glaucoma.* 2002; 11: 294-299.
[22] O'Brart DP, Rowlands E, Islam N, Noury AM. A randomised, prospective study comparing trabeculectomy augmented with antimetabolites with a viscocanalostomy technique for the management of open angle glaucoma uncontrolled by medical therapy. *Br. J. Ophthalmol.* 2002;86:748-754.
[23] Carassa RG, Bettin P, Fiori M, Brancato R. Viscocanalostomy versus trabeculectomy in white adults affected by open-angle glaucoma. A 2-year randomized, controlled trial. *Ophthalmology.* 2003;110:882-887.
[24] Kobayashi H, Kobayashi K, Okinami S. A comparison of the intraocular pressure-lowering effect and safety of viscocanalostomy and trabeculectomy with mitomycin C I bilateral open-angle glaucoma. *Graefe's Arch. Clin. Exp. Ophthalmol.* 2003;241:359-366.
[25] Kobayashi H, Kobayashi K. Viscocanalostomy versus Trabeculectomy Augmented with Mitomycin C *A 2-year randomized clinical trial.* Trends in Glaucoma Research (ed. Reece SM), pp111-137, Nova Science Publishers, New York, 2005.
[26] Wishart MS, Shergill T, Porooshani H. Viscocanalostomy and phacoviscocanalostomy: long-term results. *J. Cataract. Refract. Surg.* 2002;28:746-751.
[27] Wishart PK, Wishart MS, Porooshani H. Viscocanalostomy and deep sclerectomy for the surgical treatment of glaucoma: a longterm follow-up. *Acta Ophthalmol.* 2003;81:343-348.
[28] The Japan Glaucoma Society guidelines for glaucoma (2nd edition). *Nippon Ganka Gakkai Zasshi.* 2006;110:777-815.
[29] de Barros DS, Da Silva RS, Siam GA, et al. Should an siridectomy be routinely performed as a part of trabeculectomy? Two surgeons' clinical experience. *Eye.* 2007;Nov 9 [epub].
[30] Miyake K, Ibaraki N. Prostaglandins and cystoid macular edema. *Surv. Ophthalmol.* 2002;47(suppl 1):s203-230.
[31] Mermoud A, Karlen ME, Schnyder CC, et al. Nd:Yag goniopuncture after deep sclerectomy with collagen implant. *Ophthalmic Surg. Lasers.* 1999;30:120-125.
[32] Savege JA, Condon GP, Lytle RA, et al. Laser suture lysis after trabeculectomy. *Ophthalmology.* 1988;95:1631-1638.

[33] Teehasaenee C, Ritch R. The use of PhEA 34c in trabeculectomy. *Ophthalmology.* 1986;93:487-490.
[34] Lai JS, Tham CC, Chan JC. The clinical outcomes of cataract extraction by phacoemulsification in eyes with primary angle-closure glaucoma (PACG) and co-existing cataract: a prospective case series. *J. Glaucoma.* 2006;15:47-52.
[35] Lam DS, Leung DY, Tham CC, et al. Randomized trial of early phacoemulsification versus peripheral iridotomy to prevent intraocular pressure rise after acute primary angle closure. *Ophthalmology.* 2008;115:1134-40.
[36] Matsumura M, Mizoguchi T, Kuroda S, Terauchi H, Nagata M. Intraocular pressure decrease after phacoemulsification-aspiration+ intraocular lens implantation in primary open angle glaucoma eyes. *Nippon Ganka Gakkai Zasshi.* 1996;100:885-9.
[37] Shingleton BJ, Gamell LS, O'Donoghue MW, Baylus SL, King R. Long-term changes in intraocular pressure after clear corneal phacoemulsification: Normal patients versus glaucoma suspect and glaucoma patients. *J. Cataract. Refract. Surg.* 1999;25:885-890.
[38] Pohjalainen T, Vesti E, Uusitalo RJ, et al.: Phacoemulsification and intraocular lens implantation in eyes with open-angle glaucoma. *Acta Ophthalmol. Scand.* 2001;79:313-316.
[39] Hayashi K, Hayashi H, Nakao F, et al.: Effect of cataract surgery on intraocular pressure control in glaucoma patients. *J. Cataract. Refract. Surg.* 2001;27:1779-1786.
[40] Mathalone N, Hyams M, Neiman S, et al. Long-term intraocular pressure control after clear corneal phacoemulsification in glaucoma patients. *J. Cataract. Refract. Surg.* 2005;3:479-83.
[41] Shingleton BJ, Pasternack JJ, Hung JW, O'Donoghue MW. Three and five year changes in intraocular pressures after clear corneal phacoemulsification in open angle glaucoma patients, glaucoma suspects, and normal patients. *J. Glaucoma.* 2006;15:494-8.
[42] Merkur A, Damji KF, Mintsioulis G, et al.: Intraocular pressure decrease after phacoemulsification in patients with pseudoexfoliation syndrome. *J. Cataract. Refract.* Surg 2001;27:528–532.
[43] Damji KF, Konstas AG, Liebmann JM et al. Intraocular pressure following phacoemulsification in patients with and without exfoliation syndrome: a 2 year prospective study. *Br. J. Ophthalmol.* 2006;90:1014-8.
[44] Cimetta DJ, Cimetta AC. Intraocular pressure changes after clear corneal phacoemulsification in nonglaucomatous pseudoexfoliation syndrome. *Eur. J. Ophthalmol.* 2008;18:77-81.
[45] Sharma TK, Nessim M, Kyprianou I, et al. Vitreous loss during phacoemulsification in glaucoma patients: long-term intraocular pressure control. *J. Cataract Refract. Surg.* 2008;34:831-4.
[46] Rainer G, Menapace R, Schmetterer K, et al.: Effect of dorzolamide and latanoprost on intraocular pressure after small incision cataract surgery. *J. Cataract Refract. Surg.* 1999;25:1624–1629.
[47] Rainer G, Menapace R, Findl O, et al.: Randomised fellow eye comparison of the effectiveness of dorzolamide and apraclonidine on intraocular pressure following phacoemulsification cataract surgery. *Eye.* 2000;14:757–760.

[48] Pohjalainen T, Vesti E, Uusitalo RJ, Laatikaninen L. Intraocular pressure after phacoemulsification and intraocular lens implantation in nonglaucomatous eyes with and without exfoliation. *J. Cataract Refract. Surg.* 2001;27:426-3.

[49] Takmaz T, Can I, Gurdal C, et al. Effect of bimatoprost on intraocular pressure after phacoemulsification in eyes with exfoliation syndrome. *Acta Ophthalmol. Scand.* 2007;85:262-6.

[50] Levkovitch-Verbin H, Habot-Wilner Z, Burla N, et al. Intraocular pressure elevation within the first 24 hours after cataract surgery in patients with glaucoma or exfoliation syndrome. *Ophthalmology.* 2008;115:104-8.

[51] Lin JC, Katz LJ, Spaeth GL, Klancnik JM Jr. Intraocular pressure control after Nd:YAG laser posterior capsulotomy in eyes with glaucoma. *Br. J. Ophthalmol.* 2008;92:337-9.

[52] Shin DH, Kim YY, Sheth N, et al.: The role of adjunctive mitomycin C in secondary glaucoma triple procedure as compared to primary glaucoma triple procedure. *Ophthalmology.* 1998;105:740–745.

[53] Shin DH, Ren J, Juzych MS, et al.: Primary glaucoma triple procedure in patients with primary open-angle glaucoma: the effect of mitomycin C in patients with and without prognostic factors for filtration failure. *Am. J. Ophthalmol.* 1998;125:346–352.

[54] Shin DH, Iskander NG, Ahee JA, et al.: Long-term filtration and visual field outcomes after primary glaucoma triple procedure with and without mitomycin-C. *Ophthalmology.* 2002;109:1607–1611.

[55] Casson RJ, Salmon JF: Combined surgery in the treatment of patients with cataract and primary open-angle glaucoma. *J. Cataract Refract. Surg.* 2001;27:1854–1863.

[56] Chang L, thigarajan M, Moseley M, et al. Intraocular pressure outcome in primary 5FU phacotrabeculectomies compared with 5FU trabeculectomies. *J. Glaucoma.* 2006;15:475-81.

[57] Siriwardena D, Kotecha A, Minassian D, et al. Anterior chamber flare after trabeculectomy and after phacoemulsification. *Br. J. Ophthalmol.* 2000;84:1056–1057.

[58] Jampel HD, Roche N, Stark WJ, Roberts AB. Transforming growth factor-beta in human aqueous humor. *Curr. Eye Res.* 1990;9:963-969.

[59] Tripathi RC, Li J, Chan WF, Tripathi BJ. Aqueous humor in glaucomatous eyes contains an increased level of TGF-beta 2. *Exp. Eye Res.* 1994;59:723-7.

[60] Simone JN, Whitacre MM. Effects of anti-inflammatory drugs following cataract extraction. *Curr. Opin. Ophthalmol.* 2001;12:63-67.

[61] Cordeiro MF, Reichel MB, Gay JA, D'Esposita F, Alexander RA, Khaw PT. Transforming growth factor-beta1, -beta2, and -beta3 in vivo: effects on normal and mitomycin C-modulated conjunctival scarring. *Invest. Ophthalmol. Vis. Sci.* 1999;40:1975-1982.

[62] Cordeiro MF, Bhattacharya SS, Schultz GS, Khaw PT. TGF-beta1, -beta2, and -beta3 in vitro: biphasic effects on Tenon's fibroblast contraction, proliferation, and migration. *Invest. Ophthalmol. Vis. Sci.* 2000;41:756-763.

[63] Rossetti L, Bucci L, Miglior S, et al.: Temporal corneal phacoemulsification combined with separate-incision superior trabeculectomy vs standard phacotrabeculectomy. A comparative study. *Acta Ophthalmol. Scand.* 1997;Suppl:39.

[64] Wyse T, Meyer M, Ruderman JM, et al.: Combined trabeculectomy and phacoemulsification: a one-site vs a two-site approach. *Am. J. Ophthalmol.* 1998;125:334–339.

[65] Borggrefe J, Lieb W, Grehn F: A prospective randomized comparison of two techniques of combined cataract-glaucoma surgery. *Graefes Arch. Clin. Exp. Ophthalmol.* 1999;237:887–892.

[66] el Sayyad F, Helal M, el Maghraby A, et al.: One-site versus 2-site phacotrabeculectomy: a randomized study. *J. Cataract Refract. Surg.* 1999;25:77–82.

[67] Shingleton BJ, Price RS, O'Donoghue MW, Goyal S. Comparison of 1-site versus 2-site phacotrabeculectomy. *J. Cataract Refract. Surg.* 2006;32:799-802

[68] Buys YM, Chipman ML, Zack B, et al. Prospective randomized comparison of one-versus two-site Phacotrabeculectomy two-year results. *Ophthalmology.* 2008;115:1130-1133.

[69] Cotran PR, Roh S, McGwin G. Randomized comparison of 1-Site and 2-Site phacotrabeculectomy with 3-year follow-up. *Ophthalmology.* 2008;115:447-454.

[70] Jampel HD, Friedman DS, Lubomski LH, et al.: Effect of technique on intraocular pressure after combined cataract and glaucoma surgery: an evidence based review. *Ophthalmology.* 2002;109:2215–2224.

[71] Li G, Kasner O. Review of consecutive phacotrabeculectomies supplemented with early needle revision and antimetabolites. *Can. J. Ophthalmol.* 2006;41:457-63.

[72] Tham CC, Li FC, Leung DY et al. Microincision bimanual phacotrabeculectomy in eyes with coexisting glaucoma and cataract. *J. Cataract Refract. Surg.* 2006;32:1917-20.

[73] Dada T, Muralidhar R, Sethi HS. Insertion of a foldable hydrophobic IOL through the trabeculectomy fistula in cases with microincision cataract surgery combined with trabeculectomy. *BMC Ophthalmol.* 2006;6:14.

[74] Rotchford AP, Vernon SA. Phaco-microtrabeculectomy: technique and intraocular pressure control in comparison with microtrabeculectomy. *Clin. Experiment Ophthalmol.* 2007;35:812-7.

[75] Jin GJ, Crandall AS, Jones JJ. Phacotrabeculectomy: assessment of outcomes and surgical improvements. *J. Cataract Refract. Surg.* 2007;33:1201-8.

[76] Lu D, Liu W, Li H, Ji J. The application of human anterior lens capsule autotransplantation in phacotrabeculectomy: a prospective, comparative and randomized clinical study. *Eye.* 2008 Apr 11.

[77] Hong S, Seong GJ, Hong YJ. Long-term intraocular pressure fluctuation and progressive visual field deterioration in patients with glaucoma and low intraocular pressures after a triple procedure. *Arch. Ophthalmol.* 2007;125:1010-3.

[78] Hong S, Kim CY, Seong GJ. Long-term intraocular pressure fluctuation and visual field progression in glaucoma patients with low intraocular pressure after post-trabeculectomy phacoemulsification. *J. Ocul. Pharmacol. Ther.* 2007;23:571-6.

[79] Ambresin A, Shaarawy T, Mermoud A: Deep sclerectomy with collagen implant in one eye compared with trabeculectomy in the other eye of the same patient. *J. Glaucoma.* 2002;11:214–220.

[80] Chiselita D: Non-penetrating deep sclerectomy versus trabeculectomy in primary open-angle glaucoma surgery. *Eye.* 2001;15:197–201.

[81] Carassa RG, Bettin P, Fiori M, et al. Viscocanalostomy vs. trabeculectomy: a 12 month prospective trial. *Invest. Ophthalmol. Vis. Sci.* 2000;41;s744.

[82] Jonescu-Cuypers C, Jacobi P, Konen W, Krieglstein G. Primary viscocanalostomy versus trabeculectomy in white patients with open-angle glaucoma: A randomized clinical trial. *Ophthalmology.* 2001;108:254-258.

[83] Dietlein TS, Luke C, Jacobi PC, et al. Does the dissection depth and thickness of the deep scleral flap affect intraocular pressure after viscocanalostomy? A cilinico-pathologic correlation. *Klin. Monatsbl. Augenheilkd.* 2001;18:168-173.

[84] Gimbel HV, Anderson Penno EE, Ferensowicz M. Combined cataract surgery, intraocular lens implantation, and viscocanalostomy. *J. Cataract Refract. Surg.* 1999;25:1370-1375.

[85] Hassan KM, Awadalla MA. Results of combined phacoemulsification and viscocanalostomy in patients with cataract and pseudoexfoliative glaucoma. *Eur. J. Ophthalmol.* 2008;18:212-9.

[86] Park M, Tanito M, Chihara E. Outcomes of combined phacoemulsification, intraocular lens implantation and viscocanalostomy. *Nippon Ganka Gakkai Kaishi.* 2002;106:173-177.

[87] Shoji T, Tanito M, Takahashi H, et al. Phacoviscocanalostomy versus cataract surgery only in patients with coexisting normal-tension glaucoma: midterm outcomes. *J. Cataract Refract. Surg.* 2007;33:1209-16.

[88] Tanito M, Park M, Nishikawa M, Ohira A, Chihara E. Comparison of surgical outcomes of combined viscocanalostomy and cataract surgery with combined trabeculotomy and cataract surgery. *Am. J. Ophthalmol.* 2002;134:513-520.

[89] Park M, Hayashi K, Takahashi H, et al. Phaco-viscocanalostomy versus phaco-trabeculotomy: a middle-term study. *J. Glaucoma.* 2006;15:456-61.

[90] Wishart MS, Dagres E. Seven-year follow-up of combined cataract extraction and viscocanalostomy. *J. Cataract Refract. Surg.* 2006;3:2043-9.

[91] Yuen NS, Chan OC, Hui SP, Ching RH. Combined phacoemulsification and nonpenetrating deep sclerectomy in the treatment of chronic angle-closure glaucoma with cataract. *Eur. J. Ophthalmol.* 2007;17:208-15.

[92] Chiou AG, Mermoud A, Jewelewicz DA. Post-operative inflammation following deep sclerectomy with collagen implant versus standard trabeculectomy. *Graefes Arch. Clin. Exp. Ophthalmol.* 1998;236:593-596.

[93] D'Eliseo D, Pastena B, Longanesi L, et al. Comparison of deep sclerectomy with implant and combined glaucoma surgery. *Ophthalmologica.* 2003,217:208–211.

[94] Gianoli F, Schnyder CC, Bovey E, et al. Combined surgery for cataract and glaucoma: phacoemulsification and deep sclerectomy compared with phacoemulsificationand trabeculectomy. *J. Cataract Refract. Surg.* 1999;25:340–346.

[95] Wishart PK, Wishart MS, Porooshani H. Viscocanalostomy and deep sclerectomy for the surgical treatment of glaucoma: a long term follow-up. *Acta Ophthalmol. Scand.* 2003;81:343–348.

[96] Luke C, Dietlein TS, Luke M, et al. Prospective trial of phaco-trabeculotomy combined with deep sclerectomy versus phaco-trabeculectomy. *Graefes*. 2008;246:1163-8.
[97] Unlu K, Aksunger A. Descemet membrane detachment after viscocanalostomy. *Am. J. Ophthalmol.* 2000;130:833-834.
[98] Luke C, Dietlein T, Jacobi P, Konen W, Kriegelstein GK. Intracorneal inclusion of high-molecular-weight sodium hyaluronate following detachment of Descemet's membrane during viscocanalostomy. *Cornea.* 2000;19:556-557.
[99] Kim CY, Seong GJ, Koh HJ, Kim EK, Hong YJ. Descemet's membrane detachment associated with inadvertent viscoelastic injection in viscocanalostomy. *Yonsei Med. J.* 2002;43:279-281.
[100] Ocakoglu O, Ustundag C, Devrannoglu K, Yildirim R, Ozkan S. Repair of Descemet's membrane detachment after viscocanalostomy. *J. Cataract Refract. Surg.* 2002;28:1703-1706.
[101] Ravinet E, Tritten JJ, Roy S, Gianoli F, Wolfensberger T, Schnyder C, Mermound A. Descemet membrane detachment after nonpenetrating filtering surgery. *J. Glaucoma* 2002;11:244-252.
[102] Fujimoto H, Mizoguchi T, Kuroda S, Nagata M. Intracorneal hematoma with Descemet membrane detachment after viscocanalostomy. *Am. J. Ophthalmol.* 2004;137:195-196.
[103] Gimbel HV, Meyer D: Small incision trabeculotomy combined with phacoemulsification and intraocular lens implantation. *J. Cataract Refract. Surg.* 1993;19:92–96.
[104] Gimbel HV, Meyer D, DeBroff BM, et al.: Intraocular pressure response to combined phacoemulsification and trabeculotomy ab externo versus phacoemulsification alone in primary open-angle glaucoma. *J. Cataract Refract. Surg.* 1995;21:653–660.
[105] Tanito M, Ohira A, Chihara E: Surgical outcome of combined trabeculotomy and cataract surgery. *J. Glaucoma.* 2001;10:302–308.
[106] Hoffmann E, Schwenn O, Karallus M, et al. Long-term results of cataract surgery combined with trabeculotomy. *Graefes Arch. Clin. Exp. Ophthalmol.* 2002;240:2–6.
[107] Inatani M, Tanihara H, Muto T, et al. Transient intraocular pressure elevation after trabeculotomy and its occurrence with phacoemulsification and intraocular lens implantation. *Jpn. J. Ophthalmol.* 2001;45:288–292.
[108] Kubota T, Touguri I, Onizuka N, et al. Phacoemulsification and intraocular lens implantation combined with trabeculotomy for open-angle glaucoma and coexisting cataract. *Ophthalmologica*. 2003;217:204–207.
[109] Nassiri N, Nassiri N, Sadeghi PYarandi S, et al. Combined phacoemulsification and Ahmed valve glaucoma drainage implant: a retrospective case series. *Eur. J. Ophthalmol.* 2008;18:191-8.
[110] Rivier D, Roy S, Mermound A. Ex-PRESS R-50 miniature glaucoma implant insertion under the conjunctiva combined with cataract extraction. *J. Cataract Refract. Surg.* 2007;33:1946-52.
[111] Maris PJ Jr, Ishida K, Netland PA. Comparison of trabeculectomy with Ex-PRESS miniature glaucoma device implanted under scleral flap. *J. Glaucoma.* 2007;16:14-9.
[112] Stewart RM, Diamond JG, Ashmore ED, Ayyala RS. Complications following ex-press glaucoma shunt implantation. *Am. J. Ophthalmol.* 2005;140:340-1.

[113] Dietlein TS, Jordan JF, Schild A, et al. Combined cataract-glaucoma surgery using the intracanalicular Eyepass glaucoma implant: first clinical results of a prospective pilot study. *J. Cataract Refract. Surg.* 2008;34:247-52.

[114] Simon G. 12-month clinical experience with a Gold Micro-shunt for glaucoma treatment. In the Proceeding of World Ophthalmology Congress 2008, ppA15, Hong Kong, 2008.

[115] Lin SC. Endoscopic and transscleral cyclophotocoagulation for the treatment of refractory glaucoma. *J. Glaucoma.* 2008;17:238-47.

[116] Carter BC, Plager DA, Neely DE, et al. Endoscopic diode laser cyclophotocoagulation in the management of aphakic and pseudophakic glaucoma in children. *JAPPOS.* 2007;11:34-40.

[117] Jurowski P, Gos R. Phacosclerothalamotomy--new surgical procedure in the treatment of coexisted cataract with glaucoma. Essence of technique surgery. *Klin. Oczna.* 2007;109:276-9.

[118] Shingleton B, Tetz M, Korber N. Circumferential viscodilation and tensioning of Schlemm canal (canaloplasty) with temporal clear corneal phacoemulsification cataract surgery for open-angle glaucoma and visually significant cataract: one-year results. *J. Cataract Refract. Surg.* 2008;34:433-40.

[119] Tanito M, Ohira A, Chihara E. Factors leading to reduced intraocular pressure after combined trabeculotomy and cataract surgery. *J. Glaucoma.* 2002;11:3–9.

In: Eye Research Developments
Editor: Alan N. Westerhouse

ISBN: 978-1-60741-177-2

Chapter II

Current Trends in Glaucoma: What about Neuroprotection?

Sergio Pinar [1] and Elena Vecino [*2]
[1] Cruces Hospital, Bilbao.
[2]Universidad del País Vasco, Vizcaya, SPAIN

Abstract

Glaucoma is an optic neuropathy, considered as the second leading cause of blindness worldwide. Glaucoma is characterized by selective death of retinal ganglion cells (RGC) and a progressive loss of vision.

Elevated intraocular pressure (IOP) is one of the most important risk factors for developing glaucoma, so we mainly focus on lowering IOP to arrest the progression of glaucoma. However, many patients continue to demonstrate a clinically downhill course despite the control of initially raised IOP. In fact, some patients develop what is called Normal Tension Glaucoma, not associated to an increased IOP. This emphasizes that several pressure-independent mechanisms are responsible for the development and progression of glaucomatous neuropathy and that high intraocular pressure (IOP) and vascular insufficiency in the optic nerve head are only risk factors for the development of glaucoma, and are not the only target for the treatment of glaucoma. The reason is that the process of RGC death is thought to be biphasic, and the primary injury is followed by a slower secondary degeneration related to a noxious environment surrounding the apoptotic cells. This environment is characterized by changes in the extra-cellular ionic concentrations, increased amounts of free radicals, neurotrophins depletion and increased glutamate induced excitotoxicity due to high extra-cellular glutamate levels, which binds to N-methyl-D-aspartate (NMDA) receptors leading to an abnormally high intracellular $Ca2+$ concentration.

Neuroprotection is a process that attempts to preserve the remaining cells that are still vulnerable to damage, and the main aim of neuroprotective therapy is to employ pharmacologic or other means to attenuate the hostility of the environment surrounding the degenerating cells, or to supply the cells with the tools to deal with this aggression, providing resilience to the insult.

* Corresponding Author: Elena Vecino, Departamento de Biología Celular e Histología, Grupo de Oftalmo-Biología Experimental (GOBE), Facultad de Medicina, Universidad del País Vasco, 48940 Leioa, Vizcaya, SPAIN, e.mail: elena.vecino@ehu.es

Several agents have been reported neuroprotective in glaucoma, both in clinical assays, such as Ca2+ channel blockers, and in experimental studies, such as betaxolol, brimonidine, NMDA antagonists, Nitric Oxide Synthase inhibitors, neurotrophins and ginkgo biloba extract.

Most neuroprotective agents for glaucoma have probed beneficial effects over RGC, not showing effects over IOP. However, when analyzing classically used medications for glaucoma, it becomes difficult to understand if its effect over the progression of glaucoma is due to neuroprotective pathways or by means of lowering IOP.

The ideal anti-glaucoma drug would be one that when applied topically, reduces IOP, but also probes to reach the retina in appropriate amounts, and activates specific receptors in the retina to attenuate retinal ganglion cell death.

1. Introduction

1.1. Glaucoma

Glaucoma is an optic neuropathy that affects nearly 60 million people, being expected to reach 79,6 million by year 2020 [Quigley et al., 2006]. Nowadays it is considered the second leading cause of blindness worldwide. Glaucoma is associated with selective death of retinal ganglion cells (RGC) [García-Valenzuela et al., 2005; Quigley, 1995; Mittag et al., 2000; Cordeiro et al., 2004; Libby et al., 2005; Urcola et al., 2006; Hernández et al., 2008] and structural changes in the optic nerve head (fig. 1). This loss of RGC and previous axonal dysfunction are thought to be the cause of visual field changes in those affected by glaucoma [Buckingham et al., 2008].

The cause of glaucoma is not yet well known. Elevated intraocular pressure (IOP) has been established as the main risk factor for developing glaucoma. However, glaucoma is more than just an elevated IOP; it is considered as a multifactorial disease. IOP is regulated by aqueous humour dynamics in the front of the eye, and the neuropathological changes in glaucoma occur in the posterior portion of the eye. It is known that ocular hypertension is due to impairment in the removal of aqueous humour via the trabecular meshwork of multiple causes. Trabecular meshwork inducible glucocorticoid response (TIGR) gene at fault has been identified in juvenile glaucoma, being responsible for 13% of all cases of primary open-angle glaucoma [Stone et al., 1997].

Electroretinography in glaucoma eyes can also show deterioration. ERG demonstrates an attenuation of both a-waves and b-waves after the induction of ocular hypertension using cauterization of episcleral vein experimental glaucoma model in animals [Bayer et al., 2001; Mittag et al., 2000], and also a deterioration of inner retinal function, measured by an attenuation of positive and negative scotopic threshold response (STR) [Li et al., 2006].

Primary open-glaucoma (POAG) is considered to be the most common subtype of glaucoma, and its pathogenesis remains a fascinating area for new research studies. It is almost certain that POAG develops in a multifactorial manner, and some of the risk factors may determine the appearance of the damaged glaucomatous optic nerve head [Broadway et al., 1999] (Figure 1).

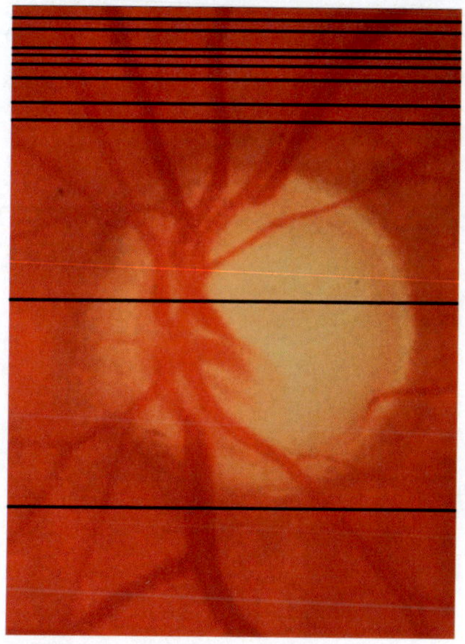

Figure 1.

1.2. Risk Factors

POAG is dependent on the presence of varying risk factors and the presence of a greater combination of these risk factors that makes it easier to develop glaucoma [Broadway et al., 1999].

Numerous potential secondary risk factors for the development of glaucoma have been studied. First of all, high ocular tension (above the normal population level, 21 mmHg) is established as the primary risk factor [Hart et al., 1979; Leibowitz et al., 1980; Armaly et al., 1980; Drance et al., 1981; Sommer, 1989; Quigley et al., 1994]. However, the existence of patients with normal-tension glaucoma (NTG) has suggested that secondary factors play an important role in the development of glaucomatous optic neuropathy in these patients whose IOPs lie within the normal statistical range [Broadway et al., 1999].

Cardiovascular disease has also been implicated as potential risk factors [Carter et al. , 1990; Demailly et al., 1984; Drance et al., 1978; Freyler et al., 1988; Goldberg et al. , 1981; Schulzer et al., 1990; Spaeth et al., 1975]. Other specific cardiovascular risk factors have also been proposed, such as systemic hypertension [Tielsch et al., 1995; Wilson et al., 1987], hypotension, diabetes [Graham et al., 1995; Gramer et al., 1985; Hayreh et al., 1994; Tielsch et al., 1995], increased blood viscosity or platelet aggregation [Hoyng et al., 1992; Klaver et al., 1985; Trope et al., 1987], vasospasm [Drance et al., 1988; Flammer et al., 1987; Gasser and Flammer, 1987; Gasser and Flammer, 1991; Gasser et al., 1990] and migraine [Corbett et al., 1985; Phelps and Corbett, 1985]. Increasing age, family history of glaucoma and black race are also identified risk factors for developing glaucoma [Drance et al., 1978; Hart et al., 1979; Hollows and Graham., 1996; Quigley et al., 1994; Shin et al., 1977; Sommer et al., 1991].

Myopia has also been identified as a risk factor for developing glaucoma [Daubs and Crick, 1981]. Probably, thin eye wall and large globe increases the influence of intraocular pressure over the optic disk.

RISK FACTORS ASSOCIATED WITH INCREASED PREVALENCE OF GLAUCOMA DAMAGE

Glaucomatous damage in the fellow eye
High intraocular pressure
Age
Race
Thin cornea
Pseudoexfoliation
Myopia > 4 dioptres
Vascular risk factors:
Local
 Disc haemorrhage
 Peripapillar atrophy
Systemic
 Cerebral disease
 Cardiovascular disease
 Vasospasm: Cold hands and feet, Raynaud's phenomena, migraine
 Systemic hypotension with nocturnal pressure drops
 Low perfusion pressure
 Hypercholesterolemia/ hyperlipidemia
 Diabetes Mellitus
Family history in first degree relatives

1.3. Intraocular Pressure

Although glaucoma is considered a multivariate and complex genetic disease, the most important risk factor, so far, is elevated intraocular pressure (IOP). Approximately 10,000 RGCs are lost per year, and by age 80, an individual with normal IOP will preserve approximately 70% of their RGCs. However, elevated IOP can accelerate RGC loss [Brubaker, 1996]. It is reasonable to think that increased IOP applies some critical stress to the ganglion cells and their axons [Nickels, 2007].

That's why a frequent and repetitive examination of IOP has great value when following patients diagnosed with glaucoma. However, single IOP measurements do not necessarily provide adequate information about pressure, as the normal diurnal variation in IOP can be on the order of 6 mm Hg, and even larger in eyes with glaucoma, reaching 30 mm Hg [Kitazawa and Horie, 1975; Newell and Krill, 1964]. Furthermore, the fact that measurement of IOP alone is of limited value is reinforced by the existence of patients with NTG, where we can find evidence of optic nerve damage, and IOP measurements within the normal statistical range. This concept emphasizes the important role played by other pressure-independent risk factors in the development and progression of glaucomatous neuropathy. In addition, progression of glaucomatous damage continues in many patients (up to one-sixth of patients with glaucoma) despite attenuation of the initial injury (control of initially raised IOP) [Brubaker, 1996; Lisegang, 1996].

Another important clinical observation in glaucoma that would help to understand the important role of neuroprotection is the fact that patients with severe pre-existing damage are more likely to deteriorate than those previously diagnosed and treated, in spite of reaching the same or even lower IOPs [Yoles and Schwartz, 1998].

1.4. Pathogenesis

The exact mechanism of how glaucoma develops, and the way RGC degenerate is still not well-known, although there is increasing evidence for a biphasic theory.

1.4.1. Initial Injury

It is still unclear what stimulates the axons of retinal ganglion cells to begin to degenerate. Some authors believe that the initial site of damage in glaucoma is the lamina cribosa [Quigley and Addicks, 1980; Quigley et al., 1981; Quigley and Addicks, 1981]. A combined effect of vascular risk factors susceptibility and the triggering effect of increased intraocular pressure would lead to an initial damage of the axons at the level of lamina cribosa. However, another possibility will be that the direct damage of the pressure applied to the retinal ganglion cell bodies at the level of the retina will induce changes in the molecular structure of these cells and thus induce the apoptosis of the RGCs.

The classical **"mechanical damage model"** predicts that the compression of the axons because of increased intraocular pressure leads to their degeneration. This theory will explain that elevated IOP could induce the optic disk cupping causing optic nerve axonal compression at the lamina cribosa, and blockage of axoplasmic retrograde flow of the RGC axons. However, another hypothesis will indirectly explain the physical damage to the axons through the glial cells present in the optic nerve head and lamina cribosa that will have modified their homeostasis at this level and thus influence the RGC axons [Ransom and Behar, 2003]. These glial cells support neurons, regulate extracellular K+ levels, remove glutamate and GABA neurotransmitters (specially in synapses), renew precursor in the synthesis of glutamate, regulate extracellular pH levels and osmolarity and supply to the neuron the energy needed by the provision of lactate and glucose from glycogen stores [Ransom et al., 2003]. This primary insult may alter the gene expression of glial cells and their behaviour. In addition, both retrograde and anterograde axonal transport is blocked at the lamina cribosa in glaucomatous eyes [Minckler et al., 1977; Radius and Anderson, 1981; Dandona et al., 1991]. Some studies have identified astrocytes as the key cell type involved in the altered remodelling of the extracellular matrix (ECM) in the optic nerve head, including collagen I, IV, transforming growth factor ß2 (TGF-ß2) and matrix metalloproteine (MMP)-1 in experimental animal models of glaucomatous damage [Hernandez, 2000]. In another study, Guo et al. demonstrated that RGC apoptosis in glaucoma correlates strongly with elevated IOP, showing a link with MMP-9, and laminin degradation, suggesting that this abnormal ECM remodelling in glaucomatous retinas may increase RGC death [Guo et al., 2005].

On the other hand, the **"vascular damage model"** can also be placed in the initial insult to the optic nerve head. Although the density of capillaries is similar in normal eyes and those affected by glaucoma [Quigley et al., 1984], increased IOP may lead to reduced blood flow in the capillaries of the optic nerve head, probably because of a faulty autorregulation of blood flow in the optic disk [Grunwald et al., 1984]. Astrocytes may also induce vasoconstriction of regional small capillaries by the release of vasoactive peptides during stress, associated to increased intracellular Ca2+ [Mulligan and MacVicar, 2004]. This isquemic condition and the deplection of energy stores can affect axonal Na+/K+ ATPase, that would increase intracellular Na+, leading to an overload of intracellular Ca2+ due to a greater Na+/Ca2+ exchanger activity [Osborne and Schwartz, 1994; Stys et al., 2004].

Both mechanical and vascular initial damage could estimulate axonal degeneration due to the lack of energy supply, neurotrophin withdrawal because of axoplasmic transport block, or the local involvement of the glial cells residing in the optic nerve head and lamina cribosa. This initial damage could trigger a cell self-destruction program, of which there are mainly 2 basic patterns [Beirowski et al., 2005]. The first one could be that those axons that suffered severe damage undergo what is called Wallerian degeneration, with a rapid breakdown of microfilaments and microtubules and swelling of the mitochondria [Whitmore et al., 2005; Raff et al., 2002]. The second one, which is supposed to be the most common pattern in glaucoma, would be a less severe insult to the axon resulting in a slower degeneration [Schlamp et al., 2006]. Whatever the axon degeneration pattern is, RGC's death occurs through a final common pathway (apoptosis) [García-Valenzuela et al., 1995], and it has been speculated that the primary cause of its activation is neurotrophin deprivation [Nickels, 2007]. Apoptosis of RGCs in glaucoma follows the "intrinsic" pathway, generating reactive oxygen species, a loss of ATP production and releasing cytochrome C [Green and Reed, 1998].

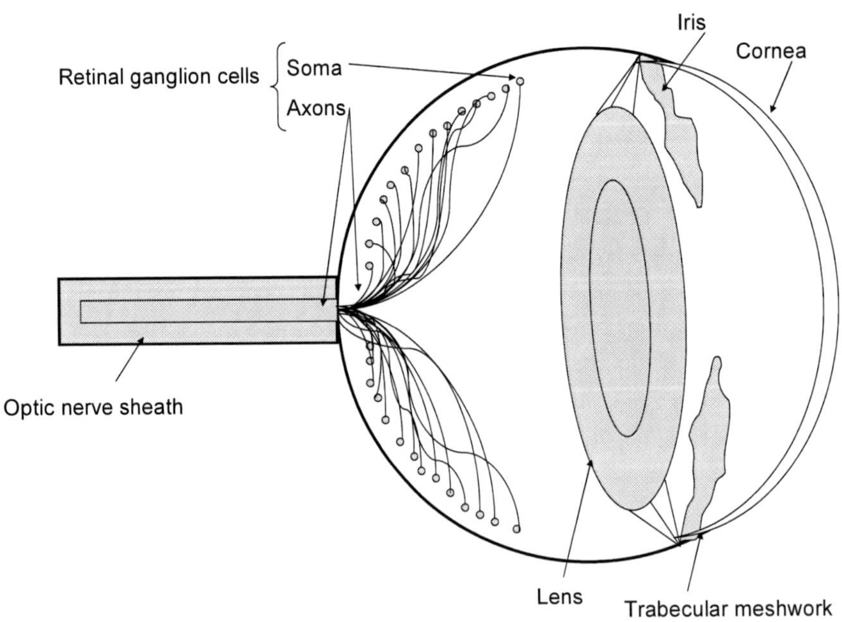

Figure 2.

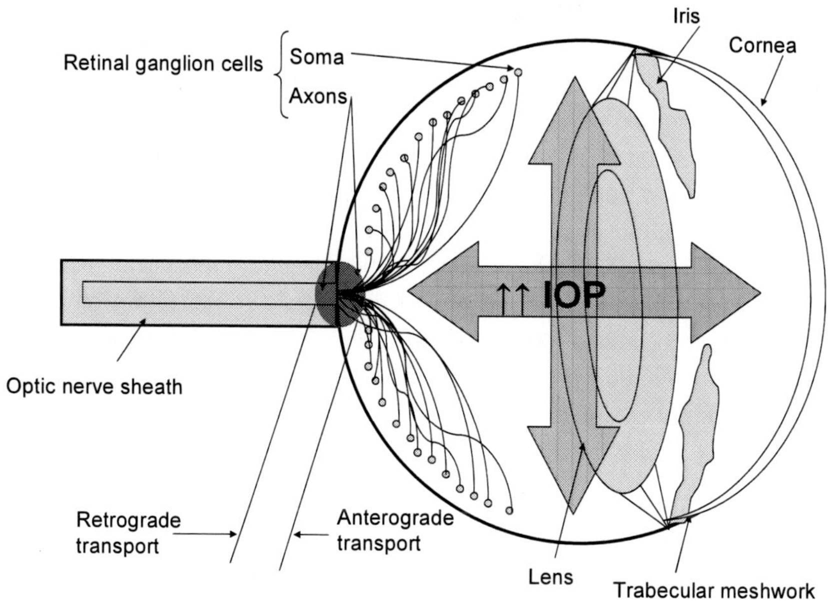

Figure 3.

1.4.2. Secondary Degeneration

After an initial insult, which distorts the normal function of axons and astroglia in the optic nerve head and lamina cribosa, several changes occur, leading to the death of the injured neurons and the neighbouring intact neurons through secondary degeneration.

A). Neurotrophin Deprivation

Both retrograde and anterograde transport is blocked in glaucomatous eyes [Minckler et al., 1977; Radius and Anderson, 1981; Dandona et al., 1991], causing an alteration of axoplasmic transport of soluble growth factors called neurotrophins from target neurons in the superior colliculus and lateral geniculate nucleus in the brain [McKinnon, 1997]. RGCs, as all other neurons in CNS, require support of neurotrophins, as these small peptides regulate cellular metabolism by the activation of neuronal target-cell receptors. RGCs seem to be especially dependent upon brain-derived neurotrophic factor, neurotrophin-4, ciliary nerve trophic factor, and glial-cell derived neurotrophic factor [Mansour-Robaey et al., 1994; Sawai et al., 1996; Klocker et al., 1997; Ji et al., 2004]. Neurotrophins interact with specific receptors, including tyrosine kinase receptors (TrkA, TrkB, and TrkC), primarily activated by nerve growth factor (NGF), brain-derived neurotrophic factor (BDNF), both neurotrophin 4,5 (NT-4/5) and neurotrophin 3 (NT-3), respectively. After activation, neurotrophin/receptor complexes are retrogradely sent to the cell body [Di Stefano et al., 1992; Ehlers et al., 1995; von Bartheld et al., 1996; von Bartheld et al., 1996; Ricci et al., 1977). Immunohistochemical findings provide evidence for experimental glaucoma that induces abnormal TrkB axonal distribution, focal accumulations of TrkB and BDNF, increased label for TrkB in Ganglion Cell Layer (GCL), and increased TrkB label in glia (Pease et al., 2000). However, other results from our lab indicated that it may be other reason than the retrograde transport of BDNF to explain the RGC survival in glaucoma. Thus, the presence of TrkB and BDNF in the complete population of the RGCs has been demonstrated [Vecino et al. 1998, 2002]. Moreover, the capacity of RGCs to survive inculture in absence of external BDNF has also been demonstrated [García et al. 2002, 2003] indicating that the deprivation of extrinsic BDNF due to the interruption of retrograde transport is not the only reason for RGCs to die in glaucoma. This is important because movement of BDNF is mediated by the TrkB receptor, and BDNF is an important trophic factor for RGCs, that inhibits apoptosis, supports survival of retinal explants and cultures and increases the rate of axonal elongation but not only when is present in the axonal terminals [Johnson et al., 1986; Thanos et al., 1989; Mansour-Robaey et al., 1994; Cohen-Cory and Fraser, 1995; Frade et al., 1997]. Neurotrophin deprivation triggers intrinsic apoptosis and activation of c-Jun N-terminal kinases, that stimulates expression of BH-3-containing proteins, that facilitate the actions of a proapoptotic protein that causes mitochondrial dysfunction (BAX) (Nickells, 2004; Putcha et al., 2003].

B)"Activation" Response of Glial Cells

After the primary injury to the optic nerve head, glia surrounding damaged axons alter their gene expression profile, characterized by the expression of two intermediate filament proteins: glial fibrillary acidic protein (GFAP) and vimentin.

This "activated" microglia can directly cause damage to axons and neighbouring cells as it has been suggested to synthesize and release nitric oxide [Neufeld et al., 1999; Liu and Neufeld, 2000]. Nitric oxide neurotoxicity occurs through a reaction with superoxide anion, forming peroxynitrite and free radical species. Peroxinitrite S-nitrosilates both proteins and nucleic acids in neighbouring cells and axons [Farkas and Grosskreutz, 2001].

C) Astrocyte Induced Vasoconstriction

Activated glia may induce vasoconstriction of regional small capillaries in the optic nerve head. During time of stress (under conditions of increased intracellular Ca^{2+}), astrocytic end-feet, that surround small capillaries would release vasoactive peptides [Mulligan and MacVicar, 2004]. This secondary vasoconstriction associated to the initial vascular primary injury caused by mechanical compression of the optic nerve head and lamina cribosa may lead to reduced blood flow in the capillaries of the optic nerve head.

D) Activation of the Caspase Enzyme Family

RGC injury in ONT and experimental glaucoma involve activation of caspases 3 and 8, as well as the mitogen-activated protein kinase pathway (specially p38 mitogen-activated protein kinase and c-jun, facilitating mitochondrial dysfunction and destruction of RGCs [Kikuchi et al., 2000; Isenmann and Bahr., 1997; Levkovitch-Verbin et al., 2005].

E) Glutamate Induced Excitotoxicity

Glutamate is an excitatory neurotransmitter in the CNS, present in neurons in high concentrations, An excess of glutamate in the retina could damage the neurons hyperstimulating the ionotropic N-methyl-D-aspartate (NMDA) receptors, and thus generating a toxic influx of extracellular $Ca2+$. Abnormally high $Ca2+$ concentration leads to inappropriate activation of nucleases, proteases and lipases, that directly leads to the generation of free radicals and activation of the nitric oxide pathway [Naskar and Dreyer,

2001]. The final consecuence is DNA nitrosylation, fragmentation and activation of the apoptosis. Glaucoma has classically been associated to increased levels of glutamate in the vitreous [Dreyer et al., 1996; Dreyer and Lipton, 1993], and RGCs contain a high concentration of NMDA receptors, resulting very sensitive to elevated concentrations of glutamate. Moreover, Müller glial cells that normally take up glutamate fail to do so in glaucoma [Napper et al., 1999]. In addition, there is evidence that the glutamate-glutamine cycle is altered in glaucomatous eyes [Martin et al., 2002].

F) ATP Releases

There is evidence that acute glaucoma leads to an elevation in extracellular ATP levels that damages RGCs. The rise in vitreal ATP in hypertensive eyes is a physiologic response, and pannexines, stable hemichannels in the membrane, could contribute [Dahl and Locovei, 2006; Spray et al., 2006]. Pannexines gate open in response to increased pressure and release ATP from the inner retina [Bao et al., 2004]. When ATP stimulates P2X7 receptor on RGCs intracellular calcium is elevated and RCGs in vitro die [Zhang et al., 2006; Zhang et al., 2006; Zhang et al., 2005]. In adittion, ATPase apyrase and P2X7 receptor antagonists reduce RGC damage in experimental models of glaucoma [Resta et al., 2007].

G) Implication of TNF-a

Tumor necrosis factor-alpha (TNF-α) is a proinflammatory cytokine implicated in the immune response. TNF-α is produced by macrophages, lymphoid cells, endothelial cells, fibroblastas and also by glial cells, and, growing evidence supports that it may lead to neuronal cell death [Downen et al., 1999]. TNF-α is increased in the retina and optic nerve head in glaucomatous eyes. TNF-α is secreted by stressed glial cells and it can induce RGC death through TNF receptor-1-mediated caspase cascade, mitochondrial dysfunction, and oxidative damage (accumulation of reactive oxygen species (ROS)) [Tezel and Wax, 2000; Tezel and Yang, 2004]. In adittion, immunohistochemical analysis of human eyes revealed an increased immunolabeling for TNF-α and TNF-R1 in the optic nerve head [Yan et al., 2000] and retina [Tezel et al., 2001] of glaucomatous eyes relative to controls, showing a predominant localization in RGCs and their axons, which are the sensitive targets for cytotoxic effects of TNF-α. Findings have also demonstrated an upregulation in gene expression for TNF-α and TNF-R1 in ocular hypertensive eyes [Ahmed et al., 2004]. Other findings provide evidence that TNF death receptor signaling is involved in the secondary degeneration of RGCs associated with JNK signaling [Tezel et al., 2004]. TNF-α in glaucoma may also be associated with another neurodestructive role by its ability to induce a highly potent secondary oxidant, nitric oxide [Goureau et al., 1997].

TNF-α also activates matrix metalloproteinases [Gottschall and Yu, 1995], associated with neurotoxicity [Guo et al., 2005]. TNF-α is also a potent stimulator of endothelin-1 (ET-1) synthesis and secretion in optic nerver head astrocytes, a potent vasoactive peptide associated with glaucomatous neurodegeneration [Desai et al., 2004].

TNF-α appears to play an important role in the immune response, ranging effects from inflammation to apoptosis, through Wallerian degeneration [Liefner et al., 2000] (Figure 4).

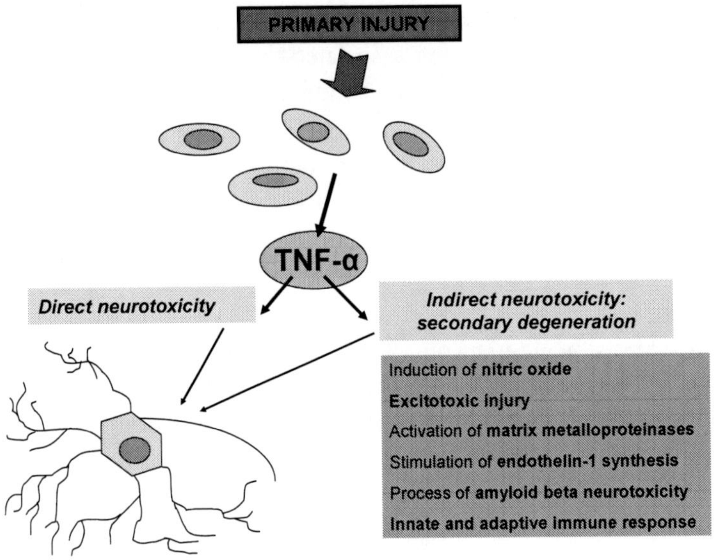

Figure 4.

H) Oxidative Stress and Free Radicals

RGCs have special sensitivity to oxidative stress. Neurons lack an appropriate defences against excitotoxicity and elevated levels of reactive oxygen species (ROS), produced because of the augmented use of O2 and ATP synthesis of these tissues. ROS get accumulated in cells that undergo oxidative stress, and they react with nitric oxide producing free radicals. As a final consecuence, this oxidative chain leads to mitochondrial dysfuncticon, DNA degradation, and cell failure. Free radicals cause extensive damage to the RGCs and their axons [Oku et al., 1997; Levkovitch-Verbin et al., 2000; Tezel, 2006].

I) Increased Accumulation of Self-Proteins

This phenomenon is common for many neurodegenerative diseases. As in Alzheimer's disease, the accumulation of amyloid precursor protein has been reported in glaucoma [McKinnon et al. 2002].

J) Increased Expression of Pro-Apoptotic Genes

During glaucoma there is an unbalance between pro-apoptotic and anti-apoptotic proteins. In fact, there is an increased expression of pro-apoptotic genes, such as bax [Oltvai and Korsmeyer, 1994] and a downregulation of anti-apoptotic genes, such as bcl-xL [Levin et al., 1997].

1.5. Treatment

IOP lowering by means of antiglaucoma drugs, laser or incisional surgery is currently the only therapy approved by regulatory agencies for the treatment of glaucoma. A recent report from the Advanced Glaucoma Intervention Study (AGIS), showed that eyes with 100% of visits and IOP less than 18 mmHg over 6 years had mean changes close to zero during follow-up [The AGIS Investigators, 2000].

However, therapeutically, we need to reduce intraocular pressure, stabilize ocular blood flow, and reduce oxidative stress.

SIX FAMILIES OF ANTIGLAUCOMA AGENTS

ADRENERGIC AGONISTS
Non-selective
Dipivefrin 0,1%
Epinephrine 0,25-2%
Alpha-2 selective
Apraclonidine 0,5-1%
Brimonidine 0,2%
Clonidine 0,125-0,5%
ADRENERGIC ANTAGONISTS
Beta-1 selective
Betaxolol 0,5-0,25%
Non-selective
Befunolol 0,5%
Levobunolol 0,25-0,5%
Metipranolol 0,1-0,3%
Timolol 0,1, 0,25, 0,5%
With ISA (Intrinsic Sympathomimetic Activity)
Carteolol 0,5-2%
Pindolol 2%
CARBONIC ANHYDRASE INHIBITORS
Topical
Brinzolamide 1%
Dorzolamide 2%
Systemic
Acetazolamide
Dichlorphenamide
Methazolamide
PARASYMPATHOMIMETICS (CHOLINERGIC DRUGS)
Direct
Pilocarpine 0,5-4%
Aceclidine 2%
Carbachol 0,75-3%
Acetylcholine 1%
Indirect
Demecarium bromide 0,125, 0,25%
Ecothiophate iodide 0,03-0,25%
Physostigmine
PROSTAGLANDIN DERIVATES AND PROSTAMIDES
Bimatoprost 0,03%
Latanoprost 0,005%
Travoprost 0,004%
Unoprostone 0,12, 0,15%
OSMOTICS
Glycerol 1-1,5 g/kg orally
Manitol 1-1,5 g/kg intravenously

LASER SURGERY

Laser Iridotomy
Trabeculoplasty
Iridoplasty

Cyclophotocoagulation

INCISIONAL SURGERY

Penetrating glaucoma surgery
Trabeculectomy
Trabeculotomy

Non penetrating glaucoma surgery (Deep sclerectomy)

Drainage devices
Molteno
Krupin
Baerveldt
Ahmed
Sbocket

2. Neuroprotection in Glaucoma

2.1. What is Glaucoma Neuroprotection?

Neuroprotection was initially investigated for disorders of the central nervous system such as amyotrophic lateral sclerosis, Alzheimer's disease, Parkinson and head trauma, but only few therapies have been approved (nemantine for Azheimer's dementia).

By definition, glaucoma neuroprotection must be considered independent of IOP lowering, and the target neurons should be in the central visual pathway, including RGCs.

Chronic progressive loss of retinal ganglion cells (RGC) is thought to be biphasic: initiation of damage is caused by a primary injury associated to the main risk factors of glaucoma (elevated IOP, cardiovascular risk factors, age, vasospasm…), and there's a delayed (secondary) degeneration of neurons that either escaped the injury or were only partially damaged. The secondary degeneration may be an outcome of a hostile environment created by damaged neurons. Some factors have been identified as mediators of this secondary neuronal degeneration: high levels of potassium and calcium ions, nitric oxide, amounts of free radicals and excitatory aminoacids such as glutamate and aspartate.

Neuroprotection in glaucoma consists in preventing the death of marginally damaged neurons and the secondary denegaration of those undergoing the hostile environment created by the initial insult. In other words, neuroprotection attempts to provide protection to such retinal ganglion cells that continue to remain at risk [Chew and Ritch, 1997] (Figure 5).

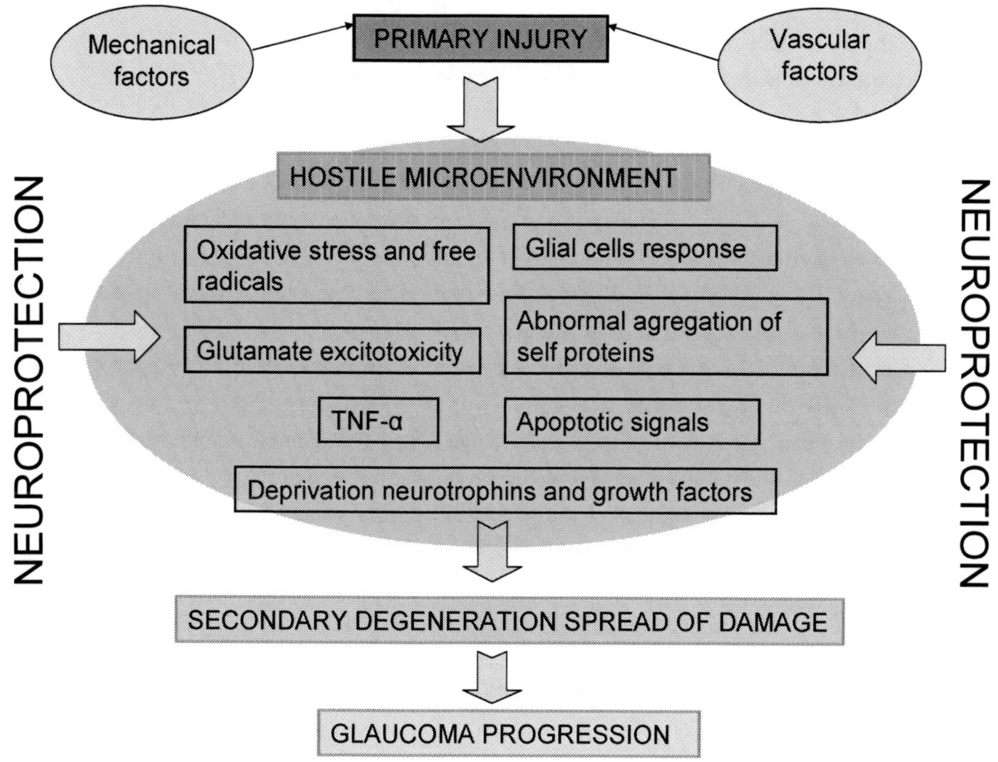

Figure 5.

2.3. Is Neuroprotective Treatment Available for Glaucoma Patients?

A neuroprotective drug is expected to prevent death of RGC in presence of chronic stress by attenuating the hostility of the environment or supplying the cells with the tools to deal with those chances [Kaufman et al., 1999].

The pharmacological profile of neuroprotective drugs should fulfil these four criteria [Wheeler et al., 2001]:

i. To have a specific target (receptors) in the retina
ii. To exhibit neuroprotective activity and have a measurable effect on RGC survival
iii. To reach the retina/vitreous in neuroprotective concentrations after clinical dosing
iv. (First three criteria must be obtained in animal models)
v. Neuroprotective activity must be demonstrated in randomized, controlled, clinical trials in humans.

Glaucoma neuroprotection offers potential as a complementary therapy to IOP-lowering for patients with previous severe damage and for those in whom pressure-lowering agents are ineffective to stop progression.

However, efficacy for neuroprotective agents has not yet been proven in glaucoma, and although there is laboratory evidence for glaucoma neuroprotection by several drugs, evidence from randomized clinical trials is still lacking [Weinreb, 2007].

2.4. Clinical Trials of Neuroprotection in Ophthalmology

To establish neuroprotective drugs for glaucoma, well-designed clinical trials are required, specially randomized clinical trials comparing neuroprotective treatments to a placebo, but there are few of them in ophthalmology.

In order to design clinical trials for neuroprotection, primary outcome measures can be:

- Functional visual acuity (The Ischemic Optic Neuropathy Decompression Trial Research Group, 2000),
- Visual field loss, although it may require several years before meaningful changes appear. Measurements of visual field have become a standard way to assess the functional progression of glaucoma.
- Some new methods for assessing visual function, like:
    - Electrophysiological testing [Berson et al., 1993]
    - Frecuency Doubling Technology (FDT),
    - Short Wave Length Automated Perimetry (SWAP),
    - Contrast sensitivity,
    - The Heidelberg Retinal Tomograph (HRT) (*)
    - The GDx nerve fiber analyzer (*)
    - The optical Coherence Tomograph (OCT) (*).

2.5. Neuroprotective Drugs in Glaucoma

Some agents have been reported as having neuroprotective activity for RGCs in experimental research as well as clinical studies.

2.4.1. Antibiotics

Minocycline

Minocycline hydrochloride is a second-generation tetracycline, commonly used in humans because of its beneficial antimicrobial and anti-inflammatory actions. Minocycline effectively crosses the blood-brain barrier [Aronson, 1980]. This drug also has remarkable neuroprotective qualities in animal models of cerebral ischemia, traumatic brain injury, Huntington disease, and Parkinson disease [Arvin et al., 2002; Du et al., 2001; Tikka and Koistinaho 2001; Yrjanheikki et al. 1999; Yrjanheikki et al., 1998].

Levkovitch-Verbin et al. in 2006 demonstrated that systemic administration of minocycline significantly delays apoptosis of RGCs after severe injury of optic nerve transaction (ONT) [Levkovitch-Verbin et al., 2006]. Its effect is associated with inhibition of inducible nitric oxide synthase [Du et al. 2001], caspase 1 and caspase 3 expression [Chen et al., 2000; Sanchez et al., 2001]. It also inhibits p38 mitogen-activated protein kinase [Yrjanheikki et al., 1999; Yrjanheikki et al., 1998] and cytochrome c release [Zhu et al., 2002]. It also depresses oxygen radical release and matrix metalloproteinase activity [Brundula et al., 2002; Gabler and Creamer. 1991; Power et al. 2003; Ryan et al. 2001; Sadowski and Steinmeyer. 2001; Golub et al. 1991]. It has also been found to be neuroprotective in models of photoreceptor death [Baptiste et al., 2004; Hughes et al., 2004; Zhang et al., 2004].

Doxycycline

Doxycycline is another semisynthetic second-generation tetracycline. It also penetrates the blood-brain barrier, with well-known effects of neuroprotection [Gabler et al., 1992; Smith and Gabler, 1994; Smith and Gabler, 1995]. However, it hasn't shown as much neuroprotective effect as minocycline in most studies.

2.4.2. Antiglaucomatous Agent

Antiglaucoma agents typically used in clinical practice exert neuroprotective effects on RGCs via distinct mechanisms.

a-2 Agonists (Brimonidine)

Brimonidine is a drug used daily in clinical practice. Brimonidine reduces the production of aqueous humor and facilitates its exit via the trabecular meshwork.

Treatment with intraperitoneal brimonidine leads to a total rescue of RGCs in glaucomatous eyes; however, the intraperitoneal application of brimonidine in animals has not been found to reduce IOP [Hernández et al., 2008]. The neuroprotective effect of brimonidine has been studied in several experimental models of optic neuropathy, including optic nerve injury [Yoles et al., 1999; Ruiz et al., 2000], transitory ischemia [Donello et al., 2001; Lafuente et al., 2001], and experimental glaucoma [Ahmed et al. , 2001; Wheeler and Woldemussie, 2001; Wheeler et al., 2003; Hernández et al., 2008].

Brimonidine treatment may exert its neuroprotective effect through inhibition of the apoptotic cascade, reduction of glutamate toxicity, or enhancing the expression of BDNF. Thus, brimonidine could activate an anti-apoptotic pathway in RGCs by inducing the expression of anti-apoptotic genes such as bcl2 and bcl-xl [Lai et al., 1999]. Activation of RGC alpha-2 adrenergic receptors may inhibit pro-apoptotic mitochondrial signaling [Wheeler et al., 2001; Wheeler et al., 2001]. Also, brimonidine-mediated neuroprotection could also be due to the inhibition of glutamate-mediated excitiotoxicity [Vorwerk et al., 1996]. Brimonidine could also exert its beneficial effects via neurotrophins. Thus, intravitreal injection of brimonidine has been shown to upregulate brain-derived neurotrophin factor (BDNF) expression in rat RGCs [Gao et al., 2002].

ß Blockers (Betaxolol, Metipranolol and Timolol)

The ability to confer neuroprotection to retinal neurones is a common feature of three ophthalmic beta adrenoceptor antagonists (betaxolol, metipranolol and timolol).

Beta(1)-selective adrenoceptor antagonist, betaxolol, is able to protect retinal neurones in vitro and ganglion cells in vivo from the detrimental effects of either ischemia reperfusion or from excitotoxicity, after topical application. The neuroprotective effect of betaxolol is thought not to be elicited through an interaction with beta-adrenoceptors, but by its ability to reduce influx of sodium and calcium through voltage-sensitive calcium and sodium channels. Betaxolol has also been shown to increase blood flow velocity in the optic nerve head tissue [Tamaki et al., 1999]. Improvements have been made in measuring ocular blood flow velocity, but measurement difficulties still persist [Harris et al., 1999].

It has also been shown that the non-selective beta-adrenoreceptor antagonists, metipranolol and timolol when topically applied behave like betaxolol. They all attenuate the detrimental effect of ischemia-reperfusion. Protection of the retina was determined by evaluating changes in the electroretinogram and by assessing the loss of mRNA for Thy-1, which is expressed in retinal ganglion cells. In addition, studies conducted on neurones in mixed retinal cultures demonstrated that betaxolol>metipranolol>timolol were all able to partially counteract anoxia-induced cell loss and viability reduction and also to attenuate ligand-induced stimulation of calcium and sodium entry into neuronal preparations. The influence of timolol was, however, not significant [Wood et al., 2003].

Muscarinic Receptor Agonist (Pilocarpine)

Some studies demonstrated that pretreatment of pilocarpine could prevent glutamate-induced neuron death through M1 muscarinic receptor, as its effect was blocked by the non-selective antagonist atropine and the M1-selective muscarinic receptor antagonist pirenzepine. The antiapoptotic effect of pilocarpine was associated with maintaining calcium homeostasis, recovering mitochondrial membrane potential, and regulating the expression of Bcl-2 and Caspase-3 [Zhou et al. 2008].

2.4.3. Ca 2+ Channel Blockers

In an interesting article, fifty-six patients with either open-angle or low-tension glaucoma, concurrently taking calcium channel blockers were compared to similar groups not taking such medications for a mean follow-up period of 3.4 years. In patients with low-tension glaucoma, there was a significant difference in the progression of visual field defects, with only two of 18 eyes (11%) of patients taking calcium channel blockers, compared to ten of 18 eyes (56%) of controls showing new visual field defects. Similarly, low-tension glaucoma patients taking calcium channel blocker therapy demonstrated no evidence of progressive optic nerve damage, compared to eight of 18 control eyes (44%). However, such differences didn't appear in patients with open-angle glaucoma, suggesting that calcium channel blockers may be useful in the management of low-tension glaucoma [Netland et al., 1993]. However, excessive blood-pressure lowering properties might also decrease perfusion in the optic nerve, worsening glaucomatous damage [Caprioli, 1997].

Nifedipine

In a clinical study, it was demonstrated that in a significant number of patients with NTG who took nifedipine, visual field got improved after 6 months follow-up [Kittazawa et al., 1989].

Flunarizine

Flunarizine is a selective calcium entry blocker with calmodulin binding properties and histamine H1 blocking activity. It is effective in the prophylaxis of migraine, occlusive peripheral vascular disease, vertigo of central and peripheral origin, and as an adjuvant in the therapy of epilepsy. It may help to reduce the severity and duration of attacks of paralysis associated with the more serious form of alternating hemiplegia. Flunarizine has been demonstrated to enhance RGC survival after optic nerve transection in mice [Eschweiler and Bahr, 1993].

2.4.4. Antioxidants

Both an activation of glial cells and an oxidative stress in the axons play an important role in the secondary degeneration. Various natural compounds possess potential antioxidative value. Reduction of oxidative stress at the level of mitochondria can be achieved by gingko biloba. Polyphenolic compounds, such as tea, red wine, dark chocolate, or coffee have antioxidative properties. Coffee contains 3-methyl-1,2-cyclopentanedione (MCP), capable of scavenging peroxynitirite. Red wine-polyphenols (e.g., resveratrol), exert vasoprotective effects by inhibiting the synthesis of endothelin-1. Dark chocolate decreases blood pressure and improves endothelium-dependant vasorelaxation. Omega-3-fatty acids and magnesium can also improve blood flow regulation Anthocyanosides (bilberries) owe their antioxidant effects to their particular chemical structure. Other antioxidants include ubiquinone and melatonin, and heat shock proteins can be induced naturally by the use of sauna baths [Mozaffarieh et al., 2008; Mozaffarieh and Flammer, 2007].

Natural compounds with antioxidative value

Polyphenolic Flavonoids
Tea
Coffee
Wine
Dark Chocolate
Ginkgo Bilboa
Anthocyanosides
Vaccinium Myrtillus (Bilberry)
Vitamins
Alpha Lipoic Acid (ALA)
Thiamin (Vitamin B1)
Cobalamin (Vitamin B12)
Miscellaneous
Ubiquinone (Coenzyme Q10)
Melatonin

2.4.5. Cannabinoids

Since the early 1970s it was reported that smoking marijuana cigarettes could lower IOP by up to 45% (Hepler and Frank. 1971). Later works showed that delta-9-tetrahydrocannabinol (Δ9-THC) lowered IOP intravenously [Purnell and Gregg, 1975], orally [Merritt et al., 1980] or by inhalation [Merritt et al., 1980]. Other results suggested that topical application of a synthetic cannabinoid receptor agonist (WIN55212-2), lowers IOP in human glaucoma, and that the IOP-lowering effects of WIN55212-2 are, probably, mediated through CB1 cannabinoid receptors [Porcella et al., 2001].

Nowadays, there is important progress in the role of cannabinoids in affording neuroprotection in traumatic, ischemic, inflammatory and neurotoxic damage in neurons [Van der Stelt and Di Marzo, 2005; de Lago and Fernández-Ruíz, 2007; Mechoulam and Shohami, 2007].

Rat retina has a functional endocannabinoid system and high IOP-induced ischemia-reperfusion reduces the endogenous anandamide (AEA) via enhanced expression of fatty acid amide hydrolase (FAAH), implicating this phenomenon in retinal cell loss caused by high IOP. It has been shown that FAAH inhibition or the administration of a stable analogue of AEA reduces cell loss in the RGC layer caused by ischemia-reperfucion. This effect seems to occur via activation of CB1 and TRPV1 receptors, suggesting a neuroprotective effect through engagement of these receptors [Nucci et al., 2007].

Other studies have shown that CB1 agonists (THC and cannabidiol) protect RGCs from glutamate-induced excitotoxicity [El Remessy et al., 2003; Opere et al., 2006], and ischemia secondary to an experimental model of glaucoma in rat [Crandall et al., 2007].

HU-211 is a nonpsychotropic cannabinoid that behaves as a noncompetitive NMDA antagonist [Feigenbaum et al., 1989], and systemic administration provides neuroprotection for RGCs after nerve axotomy [Yoles et al., 1996].

2.4.6. NMDA Antagonists, P38 MAPK, and Caspase Inhibitors

Glutamate mediates synaptic transmission essential for normal function of the nervous system. Hence, complete blockade of NMDA receptor activity causes unacceptable side effects. Open-channel blocker of the NMDA receptors, memantine, blocks only excessive NMDA receptor activity while leaving normal function relatively intact.

This NMDA antagonist is neuroprotectant in several ways: preventing excessive calcium influx by inhibition of over-stimulation of the NMDA receptor, and inhibiting OPA1 release from mitochondria by blockage of NMDA receptor. OPA1 effect is accompanied by increased Bcl-2 expression, decreased Bax expression and apoptosis blockade [Ju et al., 2008].

Memantine effectively blocks the excitotoxic response of retinal ganglion cells both in culture and in vivo [Vorwerk et al., 1996]. Memantine reduced ganglion cell loss when is systemically aplayed in a rat model of retinal ischemia [Lagreze et al., 1998]. Although memantine has demonstrated exciting results for neuroprotection in laboratories, the phase III clinical trial of Memantine failed to prove such activity [Ge, 2008].

NMDA receptors and downstream signaling pathways, triggered by p38 mitogen activated protein kinase (MAPK) and caspases, are also potential targets of intervention for glaucoma, and improved memantine derivatives, p38 MAPK, and caspase inhibitors seem plausible therapeutics to prevent RGC death [Seki and Lipton, 2008]

2.4.7. Nitric Oxide Synthase (NOS-2) Inhibitors

Nitric-oxide synthase (NOS-2) is elevated in the optic nerve heads from human glaucomatous eyes and from rat eyes with chronic, moderately elevated IOP.

Aminoguanidine

Aminoguanidine is a relatively specific inhibitor of NOS-2. It has been shown that aminoguanidine protects RGCs in a rat model of glaucoma; after unilateral induction of monolateral ocular hipertension, some animals were treated for 6 months. At 6 months, untreated animals had pallor and cupping of the optic disks in the eyes with elevated IOP, but aminoguanidine-treated animals with similar elevations of IOP appeared normal. After quantification, eyes with elevated IOP in the untreated group lost 36% of their retinal ganglion cells, and eyes with similarly elevated IOP in the aminoguanidine-treated group lost less than 10% of their retinal ganglion cells. Pharmacological neuroprotection by inhibition of NOS-2 may prove useful for the treatment of patients with glaucoma [Neufeld et al., 1999].

2.4.8. Gingko Biloba Extract (GBE)

This freely available nutritional supplement exerts protective effects against free radical damage and lipid peroxidation, preserves mitochondrial metabolism and ATP production and also behaves as a scavenger of superoxide radicals and nitric oxide [Janssens et al., 1995].

Ginkgo biloba extract (GBE) on glaucoma patients improves ocular blood flow. A Phase I cross-over trial of GBE with placebo control in 11 healthy volunteers was performed. Color Doppler imaging was used to measure ocular blood flow before and after treatment. Ginkgo biloba extract did not alter arterial blood pressure, heart rate, or IOP; but significantly increased diastolic velocity in the ophthalmic artery in the ophthalmic artery [Chung et al., 1999].

2.4.9. 17beta-Estradiol

17beta-estradiol (E2) is a steroid hormone, which has been shown to increase the viability, survival, and differentiation of primary neuronal cultures from different brain areas including amygdala, hypothalamus, and neocortex.

17 beta-estradiol (E2), has shown cytoprotective activities in animal models of stroke, myocardial infarct and neurodegenerative diseases.

Systemic administration of E2 significantly reduces RGC loss induced by acute increase of IOP in rat. In addition, pretreatment with E2, 30 min before ischemia, minimizes the elevation of glutamate observed during the reperfusion period. These effects seem to be in part mediated by the activation of the estrogen receptor, since a pre-treatment with ICI 182-780, a specific estrogen receptor antagonist, partially counteracts the neuroprotection afforded by the estrogen [Russo et al., 2008].

Later studies suggested the possible involvement of estrogen receptor/Akt/CREB/ thioredoxin-1, and estrogen receptor/MAPK/NF-kappaB, in estrogen-mediated retinal ganglion cell protection [Zhou et al., 2007].

However, three synthetic estrogen analogues (ZYC-1, ZYC-3, ZYC-10) showed efficacy of neuroprotection against glutamate-induced RGC cell death. These compounds seem to affect neuroprotection via pathways independent of the classical estrogen receptors, as inclusion of an estrogen receptor antagonist (ICI 182,780) did not reverse their neuroprotective properties against glutamate insult. These results support the hypothesis that estrogen analogues may be useful in neuroprotection of retinal ganglion cells in ocular pathologies such as glaucoma [Kumar et al., 2005]. This receptor –independent effect may be explained by the fact that estrogens and novel analogs prevent cell death in large measure by maintaining functionally intact mitochondria [Simpkins et al., 2005].

2.4.10. Erythropoietin

Erythropoietin is a glycoprotein hormone that controls erythropoiesis. It is produced by the liver and kidney. It is the precursor or erythrocites in the bone marrow, and it also has other known biological functions. For example, erythropoietin plays an important role in the brain's response to neuronal injury [Siren et al., 2001]. EPO is also involved in the wound healing process [Haroon et al., 2003].

In the DBA/2J mouse model of glaucoma EPO promoted RGC survival without affecting IOP. These results suggest that EPO may be a potential therapeutic neuroprotectant in glaucoma [Zhong et al., 2007].

3. What's next? New Neuroprotective Treatment Targets in Glaucoma

Elucidation of specific signalling pathways is crucial to finding new treatment targets. Targeted proteomic approaches are expected to indentify signalling molecules in glaucomatous neurodegeneration.

3.1. Neurotrophins

Neurotrophin administration in glaucoma is being evaluated; however the main problem may be in delivering these substances so that they could reach the retina.

BDNF, ciliary neurotrophin factor and basic fibroblastic growth factor have been shown to protect human RGC from death in culture and in vivo [Rabacchi et al., 1994]. Glial cell line–derived neurotrophic factor also showed neuroprotection of RGCs in mice and it's still under study [Ward et al., 2007].

3.2. Immunomodulatory Compounds

T lymphocytes also provide a certain neuroprotection by freeing neurotrophins or growth factors for microglia and monocytes, according to a specific and active process involving antigen-presenting cells. Activated. Such activated microglia and macrophages can take up glutamate, debris, and produce growth factors. But those T cells are controlled by regulatory T cells, part of the physiological immune network. Glaucoma appears to be characterized by an increase in both TNF-alpha of the glia in the optic-nerve head and its type 1 receptor in the ganglion cells of the retina, which makes them particularly easy to stimulate by TNF-alpha.

Glial cells, both activated during glaucoma and by TNF-alpha, and secreting TNF -alpha, could serve as antigen-presenting cells and thus constitute a new way to neuroprotection [Baudouin and Liang, 2006].

3.3. Glatiramer Acetate(Ga) (Copolymer A® Copraxone®)

It is a synthetic 4-amino-acid copolymer, currently used for multiple sclerosis. In a rat model of experimental chronic glaucoma, vaccination slowed down the progression of glaucoma, by making milieu of the nerve and retina less hostile to RGC survival [Schwartz et al., 2007]. Prevention of ganglion cells loss was also observed by prior immunization of animals using a synthetic polymer close to myelin (COP1), capable of stimulating a specific lymphocyte reaction of neuronal impairment without inducing uveitis [Baudouin and Liang, 2006].

3.4. Anti-TNF-a STRATEGIES

There is growing evidence that TNF-α-mediated neurotoxicity plays a key role in the neurodegenerative injury in glaucoma. Targeting TNF-α signaling for RGC rescue should block the caspase cascade and improve the ability of these neurons to survive. However, ability of anti- TNF-α strategis against axonal injury also needs to be clarified.

3.5. Gene Therapy

Several gene families have been identified to play roles in RGCs apoptosis or survival. Caspases stimulate apoptosis and carry out disassembly of the cells [Hetts, 1998]. Tumor suppression protein, p53 can upregulate the expression of the pro-apoptotic gene bax and down-regulate the expression of the anti-apoptotic gene bcl-2 [Nickells, 1999].

On the other hand, Bcl-2 and related proteins are important inhibitors of apoptosis. They inhibit intermediate proteins that activate caspases [Adams and Cory, 1998].

Transgenic mice allowed expression of the apoptosis-inhibiting gene Bcl-2 in rat neurons, with a 50% increase in retinal ganglion cell number. A gene can be delivered to the damaged tissue via viruses, artificial liposomes, and direct transfer, and even induce the cell to express some genes by its own regulatory pathways.

Recently, rat RGCs were able to be transfected by recombinant adeno-associated virus – BDNF (rAAV-BDNF) in vitro. The transfected cells could express BDNF gene at the level of both mRNA and protein. Apoptosis rate was lower in the transfected cells. This study indicated that rAAV-BDNF transfection can be used for the potential gene therapy in glaucomaneuroprotection [Li et al., 2008].

3.6. siRNA

Since its discovery in plants in the early 1990s, RNA interferente (RNAi) has begun to emerge as a promising technology to apply to therapeutics. This phenomenon consists of a specific and selective inhibition of gene expression in an efficient manner. RNAi is mediated by small interfering RNA (siRNA), consisting of 19-23 nucleotide double-stranded RNA, that promote specific nucleolytic cleavage of mRNA targets through an RNA-induced silencing complex. In this way, siRNAs offers a powerful tool that can be used to determine functional significance of newly identified molecules as treatment targets. This technology can also serve along with other genomic or pharmacologic treatments to provide neuroprotection in glaucoma.

Besides, siRNA can be locally and topically administrated for glaucoma in controlled doses, avoiding treating the whole body.

3.7. Stem Cells

Numerous stem cell sources exist, with embryonic and fetal stem cells liable to be superseded by adult-derived cells. Stem cell transplantation is currently being explored as a therapy for many neurodegenerative diseases including glaucoma. Cellular therapies have the potential to provide chronic neuroprotection after a single treatment, and possible neuroprotective mechanisms offered by stem cell transplantation include the supply of neurotrophic factors and the modulation of matrix metalloproteinases and other components of the CNS environment to facilitate endogenous repair [Bull et al., 2008].

References

[1] Adams, JM; Cory, S. The Bcl-2 functions in an antioxidant pathway to prevent apoptosis. *Science*, 1998; 281: 1322-1326.

[2] Ahmed, F; Brown, KM; Stephan, DA; Morrison, JC; Johnson, EC; Tomarev, SI. Microarray analysis of changes in mRNA levels in the rat retina after experimental elevation of intraocular pressure. *Invest Ophthalmol Vis Sci*, 2004; 45: 1247-1258.

[3] Ahmed, F; Hegazi, K; Chaundhray, P; Sharma, SC. Neuroprotective effect of α2 agonist (brimonidine) on adult rat retinal ganglion cells after increased intraocular pressure. *Brain Res*, 2001; 913: 133-139.

[4] Armaly, MF; Krueger, DE; Maunder, L; Becker, B ; Hetherington, JJr; Kolker, AE; Levene, RZ; Maumenee, AE; Pollack, IP; Shaffer, RN. Biostatistical analysis of the collaborative glaucoma study. I. Summary report of the risk factors for glaucomatous visual-field defects. *Arch Ophthalmol,* 1980; 98: 2163-2171.

[5] Aronson, AL. Pharmacotherapeutics of the newer tetracyclines. *J Am Vet Med Assoc,* 1980; 176: 1061-1068

[6] Arvin, KL; Han, BH; Du, Y; Lin, SZ; Paul, SM; Holtzman, DM. Minocycline markedly protects the neonatal brain against hypoxic-ischemic injury. *Ann Neurol*, 2002; 52: 54-61.

[7] Bao, L; Locovei, S; Dahl, G. Pannexin membrane channels are mechanosensitive conduits for ATP. *FEBS Lett* 2004, 572: 65–68.

[8] Baptiste, DC; Hartwick, AT; Jollimore, CA; Baldridge, WH; Seigel, GM; Kelly, ME. An investigation of the neuroprotective effects of tetracycline derivatives in experimental models of retinal cell death. *Mol Pharmacol,* 2004; 66: 1113-1122.

[9] Baudouin, C; Liang, H. Vaccine for glaucoma, myth or reality? *J Fr Ophtalmol,* 2006; 29 (2):9-12

[10] Bayer, AU; Danias, J; Brodie, S; Maag, KP; Chen, B; Shen, F; Podos, SM; Mittag TW. Electrorretinographic abnormalities in a rat glaucoma model with chronic elevated intraocular pressure. *Exp Eye Res,* 2001; 72: 667-77.

[11] Beirowski, B; Adalbert, R; Wagner, D; Grumme, DS; Addicks, K; Ribchester, RR; Coleman, MP. The progressive nature of Wallerian degeneration in wild-type and slow Wallerian degeneration (WldS) nerves. *BMC Neurosci,* 2005; 6: 1-27.

[12] Berson, EC; Rosner, B; Sandberg, MA; Hayes, KC; Nicholson, BW; Weisel-Di Franco, C; Willett W. A randomized trial of vitamin A and vitamin E supplementation for retinitis pigmentosa. *Arch Ophthalmol 1*993; 111(6): 761-772.

[13] Broadway, DC; Nicolela, MT; Drance, SM. Optic disk appearance in primary open-angle glaucoma. *Surv Ophthalmol,* 1999; 43 (1): 223-243.

[14] Brubaker, RF. Delayed functional loss in glaucoma. *Am J Ophthalmol*, 1996. 121: 473-483.

[15] Brundula, V; Rewcastle, NB; Metz, LM; Bernard, CC; Yong, VW. Targeting leukocyte MMPs and transmigration: minocycline as a potential therapy for multiple sclerosis. *Brain*, 2002; 125: 1297-1308.

[16] Bull, ND; Johnson, TV; Martin, KR. Stem cells for neuroprotection in glaucoma. *Prog Brain Res,* 2008; 173: 511-519.

[17] Caprioli, J. Neuroprotection of the optic nerve in glaucoma. *Acta Ophthalmol Scand,* 1997; 75: 364-367.

[18] Carter, CJ; Brooks, DE; Doyle, DL; Drance, SM. Investigations into a vascular etiology of low-tension glaucoma. *Ophthalmology*, 1990; 97: 49-55.

[19] Chen, M; Ona, VO; Li, M ; Ferrante, RJ; Fink, KB; Zhu, S; Bian, J; Guo, L; Farrell, LA; Hersch, SM; Hobbs, W; Vonsattel, JP; Cha, JH; Friedlander, RM. Minocycline inhibits caspase-1 and caspase-3 expression and delays mortality in a transgenic mouse model of Huntington disease. *Nat Med,* 2000; 6: 797-801.

[20] Chew, SJ; Ritch, R. Neuroprotection: the next break through in glaucoma? Proceedings of the third Annual Optic Nerve Rescue and Restoration Think Tank. *J Glaucoma,* 1997; 6: 263-266.

[21] Chung, HS; Harris, A; Kristinsson, JK; Ciulla, TA; Kagemann, C; Ritch, R. Ginkgo biloba extract increases ocular blood flow velocity. *J Ocul Pharmacol Ther,* 1999; 15(3):233-240.

[22] Cohen-Cory, S; Fraser, SE. Effects of brain-derived neurotrophic factor on optic axon branching and remodelling in vivo. *Nature*, 1995; 378: 192-196.

[23] Corbett, JJ; Phelps, CD; Eslinger, P; Montague, PR. The neurologic evaluation of patients with low-tension glaucoma. *Invest Ophthalmol Vis Sci*, 1985; 26: 1101-1104.

[24] Cordeiro, MF; Guo, L; Luong, V; Harding, G; Wang, W; Jones, HE; Moss, SE; Sillito, AM; Fitzke, FW. Real-time imaging of single nerve cell apoptosis in retinal neurodegeneration. *Proc Natl Acad Sci USA*, 2004; 101: 13352–13356.

[25] Crandall, J; Matragoon, S; Khalifa, YM; Borlongan, C; Tsai, NT; Caldwell, RB; Liou, GI. Neuroprotective and intraocular pressure-lowering effects of Delta9-tetrahydrocannabinol in a rat model of glaucoma. *Ophthalmic Res,* 2007; 39: 69-75.

[26] Dahl, G; Locovei, S. Pannexin: To gap or not to gap, is that a question? *IUBMB Life,* 2006; 58: 409–419.

[27] Dandona, L; Hendrickson, A; Quigley, HA. Selective effects of experimental glaucoma on axonal transport by retinal ganglion cells to the dorsal lateral geniculate nucleus. *Invest Ophthalmol Vis Sci*, 1991; 32: 484–491.

[28] Daubs, JG; Crick, RP. Effect of refractive error on the risk of ocular hypertension and open angle glaucoma. *Trans Ophthalmol Soc* UK, 1981; 101: 121-126.

[29] Demailly, P; Cambien, P; Plouin, PD; Bason, P; Chevallier, B. Do patients with low-tension glaucoma have particular cardiovascular characterisitics? *Ophthalmologica* 1984; 188: 65-75.

[30] Desai, D; He, S; Yorio, T; Krishnamoorthy, RR; Prassana, G. Hypoxia augments TNF-alpha-mediated endothelin-1 release and cell proliferation in human optic nerve head astrocytes. *Biochem Biophys Res Commun*, 2004; 318: 642-648.

[31] Di Stefano, PS; Friedman, B; Radziejewski, C; Alexander, C; Boland, P; Shick, CM; Lindsay, RM; Wiegand, SJ; Schulzer, M; Britton, RJ. The neurotrophins BDNF, NT-3 and NGF display distinct patterns of retrograde axonal transport in peripheral and central neurons. *Neuron*, 1992; 8: 983-993.

[32] Donello, JE; Padillo, EU; Webster, ML; Wheeler, LA; Gil, DW. Alpha (2)-adrenoceptor agonists inhibit vitreal glutamate and aspartate accumulation and preserve retinal function after transient ischemia. *J Pharmacol Exp Ther*, 2001; 1: 216-223.

[33] Downen, M; Amaral, TD; Hua, LL; Zhao, ML; Lee, SC. Neuronal death in cytokine-activated primary human brain cell culture: role of tumor necrosis factor-alpha. *Glia*, 1999; 28: 114-127.

[34] Drance, SM; Douglas, GD; Wijsman, K. et al. Response of blood flow to warm and cold in normal and low-tension glaucoma patients. *Am J Ophthalmol,* 1988; 105: 35-39.

[35] Drance, SM; Schulzer, M; Douglas, GR; Sweeney, VP. Use of discriminant analysis. II. Identification of persons with glaucomatous visual field defects. *Arch Ophthalmol,* 1978; 96: 1571-1573.

[36] Drance, SM; Schulzer, M; Douglas, GR; Sweeney, VP. Use of discriminant analysis. II. Identification of persons with glaucomatous visual field defects. *Arch Ophthalmol,* 1978; 96: 1571-1573.

[37] Drance, SM; Schulzer, M; Thomas, B; Douglas, GR. Multivariate analysis in glaucoma: use of discriminant analysis in predicting glaucomatous visual field damage. *Arch Ophthalmol*, 1981; 99: 1019-1022.

[38] Dreyer, EB; Lipton, SA. *A proposed role of excitatory amino acids in glaucoma visual loss. IOVS*, 1993; 34: 1504.

[39] Dreyer, EB; Zurakowski, D; Schumer, RA; Podos, SM; Lipton, SA. Elevated glutamate levels in the vitreous body of humans and monkeys with glaucoma. *Arch Ophthalmol,* 1996; 114: 299-305.

[40] Du, Y; Ma, Z; Lin, S; Dodel, RC; Gao, F; Bales, KR; Triarhou, LC, Chernet, E; Perry, KW ; Nelson, DL; Luecke, S; Phebus, LA; Bymaster, FP; Paul, SM. Minocycline prevents nigrostriatal dopaminergic neurodegeneration in the MPTP model of Parkinson's disease. *Proc Natl Acad Sci U S A*, 2001; 98:14669-14674.

[41] Ehlers, MD; Kaplan, DR; Price, DL; Koliatsos, VE. NGF-stimulated retrograde transport of TrkA in the mammalian nervous system. *J Cell Biol*, 1995; 130: 149-156.

[42] El Remessy, AB; Khalil, IE; Matragoon, S; Abou-Mohamed, G; Tsai, NJ; Roon, P; Caldwell, RB; Caldwell, RW; Green, K; Liou, GI. Neuroprotective effect of delta(9)-tetrahydrocannabinol and cannabidiol in N-mehyl-D-aspartate-induced retinal neurotoxicity: involvement of peroxynitrite. *Am J Pathol,* 2003; 163: 1997-2008.

[43] Eschweiler, GW; Bahr, M. Flunarizine enhances rat retinal ganglion cells survival after axotomy. *J Neurol Sci,* 1993; 116: 34-40.

[44] Farkas, RH; Grosskreutz, CL. Apoptosis, neuroprotection and retinal ganglion cell death: An overview. *Int Ophthalmol Clin,* 2001; 41:111-130.

[45] Feigenbaum, JJ; Bergmann, F; Richmond, SA; Mechoulam, R; Nadler, V; Kloog, Y; Sokolovsky, M. Nonpsychotropic cannabinoid acts as a functional N-methyl-D-aspartate receptor blocker. *Proc Natl Acad Sci USA*, 1989; 86: 9584-9587.

[46] Flammer, J; Guthauser, U; Mahler, M. Do ocular vasospasms help cause low-tension glaucoma? *Doc Ophthalmol Proc Ser*, 1987; 49: 397-399.

[47] Frade, JM; Bovolenta, P; Martinez-Morales, JR; Arribas, A; Barbas, JA; Rodriguez-Tebar, A. Control of early cell death by BDNF in the chick retina. *Development*, 1997; 124: 3313-3320.

[48] Freyler, H; Menapace, R: Ist die Erblindung an Glauckom vermeidbar? *Spektrum Augenheilkd* 2; 121, 1988;

[49] Gabler WL, Smith J, Tsukuda N. comparison of doxycycline and a chemically modified tetracycline inhibiton of leukocyte functions. *Res Commun Chem Pathol Pharmacol.* 1992; 78: 151-160;

[50] Gabler, WL; Creamer, HR. Suppression of human neutrophil functions by tetracyclines. *J Periodontal Res*, 1991; 26: 52-58.

[51] Gao, H; Qiao, X; Cantor, LB; WuDun, D. Up-regulation of brain-derived neurotrophic factor expression by brimonidine in rat retinal ganglion cells. *Arch Ophthalmol*, 2002; 797-803.

[52] García, M; Forster, V; Hicks, D; Vecino, E. Effects of Müller glia on cell survival and neuritogenesis in adult porcine retina in vitro. *Invest Ophthal Vis Sci*, 2002; 43: 3735-3743.

[53] García, M; Forster, V; Hicks, D; Vecino, E. *In vivo* expression of neurotrophins and neurotrophin receptors is conserved in adult porcine retina *in vitro*. *Invest Ophthal Vis Sci,* 2003; 44: 4532-4541.

[54] Garcia-Valenzuela, E; Shareef, S; Walsh, J; Sharma, SC. Programmed cell death of retinal ganglion cells during experimental glaucoma. *Exp Eye Res*, 1995; 61: 33–44.

[55] Gasser, P; Flammer, J. Blood-cell velocity in the nailfold capillaries of patients with normal-tension and high-tension glaucoma. *Am J Ophthalmol*, 1991; 111: 585-588.

[56] Gasser, P; Flammer, J. Influence of vasospasm on visual function. *Doc Ophthalmol,* 1987; 66: 3-18.

[57] Gasser, P; Flammer, J; Guthauser, U; Mahler, F. Do vasospasms provoke ocular diseases? *Angiology*, 1990; 41: 213-220.

[58] Ge, J. *Glaucoma neuroprotection. How far is it from a dream to reality*. Zhonghua Yan Ke Za Zhi, 2008; 44(5): 385-387 (abstract).

[59] Goldberg, I; Hollows, FC; Kass, MA; Becker, B: Systemic factors in patients with low-tension glaucoma. *Br J Ophthalmol*, 1981; 65: 56.

[60] Golub, LM;, Ramamurthy, NS; McNamara, TF; Greenwald, RA; Rifkin, BR. Tetracyclines inhibit connective tissue breakdown: new therapeutic implications for an old family of drugs. *Crit Rev Oral Biol Med,* 1991; 2: 297-321.

[61] Gottschall, PE; Yu, X. Cytokines regulate gelatinase A and B (matrix metalloproteinase 2 and 9) activity in cultured rat astrocytes. *J Neurochem.* 1995; 64: 1513-1520.

[62] Goureau, O; Amiot, F; Dautry, F and Courtois, Y. Control of nitric oxide production by endogenous TNF-α in mouse retinal pigemented epithelial and Muller glial cells. *Biochem Biophys Res Commun*, 1997; 240: 132-135.

[63] Graham, SL; Drance, SM; Wijsman, K, Douglas, GR; Mikelberg, FS. Ambulatory blood pressure monitoring in glaucoma. T*he nocturnal dip. Ophthalmology,* 1995; 102: 61-69.

[64] Gramer E, Leydhecker W. Glaukom ohne Hochdruck. *Klin Monatsbl Augenheilkd* 1985; 262-267.

[65] Green, DR; Reed, JC. Mitochondria and apoptosis. Science, 1998; 281: 1309–1312.

[66] Grunwald, JE; Riva, CE; Stone, RA; Keates, EU; Petrig, BL. Retinal autoregualtion in open-angle glaucoma. *Ophthalmology*, 1984; 91: 1690-1694.

[67] Guo, L; Moss, SE; Alexander, RA; Ali, RR; Fitzke, FW; Cordeiro, MF. Retinal ganglion cell apoptosis in glaucoma is related to intraocular pressure and IOP-induced effects on extracellular matrix. *Invest Ophthalmol Vis Sci*, 2005; 46: 175-182.

[68] Haroon, ZA; Amin, K; Jiang, X; Arcasoy, MO. "A novel role for erythropoietin during fibrin-induced wound-healing response". *Am J Pathol,* 2003; 163: 993–1000.

[69] Harris, A; Chung, HS; Ciulla, TA; Kagemann, L. Progress in measurement of ocular blood flow and relevance to our understanding of glaucoma and age-related macular degeneration. *Prog Retin Eye Res*, 1999; 18: 669-687.

[70] Hart, WJr; Jablonski, M; Kass, MA; Becker, B. Multivariate analysis of the risk of glaucomatous field loss. *Arch Opthalmol,* 1979; 97: 1455-1458.

[71] Hayreh, SS; Zimmerman, MB; Podhajsky, P; Alward, WL. Nocturnal arterial hypotension and its role in optic nerve head and ocular ischemic disorders. *Am J Ophthalmol,* 1994; 117: 603-624.

[72] Hepler, RS; Frank, IR. Marihuana smoking and intraocular pressure. *JAMA*, 1971. 217: 1392.

[73] Hernandez, M. The optic nerve head in glaucoma: Role of astrocytes in tissue remodelling. *Prog Retin Eye Res.* 2000; 19: 297-321.

[74] Hernández, M; Urcola, JH; Vecino, E. Retinal ganglion cell neuroprotection in a rat model of glaucoma following brimonidine, latanoprost or combined treatments. *Exp Eye Res*, 2008; 86: 798-806.

[75] Hetts, SW. To die or not to die: an overview of apoptosis and its role in disease. *JAMA*, 1998; 279: 300-307.

[76] Hollows, FC; Graham, PA. Intra-ocular pressure, glaucoma and glaucoma suspects in a defined population. *Br J Ophthalmol,* 1996; 50: 570-586.

[77] Hoyng, PFJ; de Jong, H; Oosting, H ; Stilma, J. Platelet aggregation, disc haemorrhage and progressive loss of visual fields in glaucoma. *Int Ophthalmol,* 1992; 15: 65-73.

[78] Hughes, EH; Schlichtenbrede, FC; Murphy, CC; Broderick, C; van Rooijenn, N; Ali RR; Dick, AD. Minocycline delays photoreceptor death in the rods mouse through a microglia-independent mechanism. *Exp Eye Res*, 2004; 78: 1077-1084.

[79] Isenmann, S; Bahr, M. Expression of c-Jun protein in degenerating retinal ganglion cells after optic nerve lesion in the rat. *Exp Neurol,* 1997; 147: 28-36.

[80] Janssens, D; Michiels, C; Delaive, E; Eliaers, F; Drieu, K; Remacle, J. Protection of hypoxia induced ATP decrease in endothelial cells by Ginkgo biloba extract and bilobalide. *Biochem Pharmacol,* 1995; 50: 991-999.

[81] Ji, JZ; Elyaman, W; Yip, HK; Lee, VW; Yick, LW; Hugon, J; So, KF. CNTF promotes survival of retinal ganglion cells after induction of ocular hypertension in rats: the possible involvement of STAT3 pathway. *Eur J Neurosci*, 2004; 19:265–272.

[82] Johnson, JE; Barde, YA; Schwab, M; Thoenen, H. Brain-derived neurotrophic factor (BDNF) supports the survival of cultured rat retinal ganglion cells. *J Neurosci,* 1986; 6: 3031-3038.

[83] Ju, WK; Kim, KY; Angert, M; Duong-Polk, KX; Lindsey, JD; Ellisman, MH; Weinreb, RN. Memantine blocks mitochondrial OPA1 and cytochrome c release, and subsequent apoptotic cell death in glaucomatous retina. *Invest Ophthalmol Vis Sci,* 2008. 20. [Epub ahead of print]

[84] Kaufman, PL; Gabelt, BT; Cynader, M. Introductory comments on neuroprotection. *Surv Ophthalmol,* 1999; 43: 89-90.

[85] Kikuchi, M; Tenneti, L; Lipton, SA. Role of p38 mitogen-activated protein kinase in axotomy-induced apoptosis of rat retinal ganglion cells. *J Neurosci*, 2000; 20: 5037-5044.

[86] Kitazawa, Y; Horie, T. Diurnal variation of intraocular pressure in primary open-angle glaucoma. *Am J Ophthalmol,* 1975; 79: 557-566.

[87] Kittazawa, Y; Shirai, H; Go, FJ. The effect of Ca2+ antagonist on visual field in low-tension glaucoma. *Graefes Arch Clin Exp Ophthalmol,* 1989; 227: 408-412.

[88] Klaver, JHJ; Greve, EL; Golsinga, H; Geijssen, HC, Heuvelmans, JH. Blood and plasma viscosity measurements in patients with glaucoma. *Br J Ophthalmol,* 1985; 69: 765-770.

[89] Klocker, N; Braunling, F; Isenmann, S; Bahr, M. In vivo neurotrophic effects of GDNF on axotomized retina ganglion cells. *NeuroReport,* 1997; 8: 3439–3442.

[90] Kumar, DM; Perez, E; Cai, ZY; Aoun, P; Brun-Zinkernagel, AM; Covey, DF; Simpkins, JW; Agarwal, N. Role of nonfeminizing estrogen analogues in

neuroprotection of rat retinal ganglion cells. *Free Radic Biol Med,* 2005; 15; 39(12): 1676.

[91] Lafuente, MP; Villegas-Pérez, MP; Sobrado-Calvo, P; García Aviles, A; Miralles de Imperial, J; Vidal-Sanz M. Neuroprotective effects of alpha (2)-selective adrenergic agonists against ischemia-induced retinal ganglion cell death. *Invest Ophthalmol Vis Sci,* 2001. 42: 2074-2084.

[92] Lagreze, WA; Knorle, R; Back, M; Feuerstein, TJ. Memantine is neuroprotective in a rat model of pressure-induced retinal ischemia. *Invest Ophthalmol Vis Sci*, 1998; 39: 1063-1066.

[93] Lai, RK; Chun, TY; Hasson, DW; Wheeler, LA. Activation of cell survival signalling pathway in the retina by selective alpha-2 adrenoceptor agonist brimonidine. *Invest Ophthalmol Cis Sci,* 1999; 10: 220-226.

[94] Leibowitz, HM; Krueger, DE ; Maunder LR ; Milton, RC ; Kini, MM ; Kahn, HA; Nickerson, RJ; Pool, J; Colton, TL; Ganley, JP; Loewenstein, JI, Dawber, TR. The Framingham Eye Study monograph: an ophthalmological and epidemiological study of cataract, glaucoma, diabetic retinopathy, macular degeneration, and visual acuity in a general population of 2631 adults, 1973-1975. *Surv Ophthalmol,* 1980; 24: 335-610.

[95] Levin, LA; Schlamp, CL; Spieldoch, RL; Geszvain, KM; Nickells RW. Identification of the bcl-2 family of genes in the rat retina. *Invest Ophthalmol Vis Sci,* 1997; 38: 2545-2553.

[96] Levkovitch-Verbin, H; Harris-Cerruti, C; Groner, Y; Wheeler, LA; Schwartz, M; Yoles, E. RGC death in mice after optic nerve crush injury: oxidative stress and neuroprotection. *Invest Ophthalmol Vis Sci,* 2000; 41: 4169-4174.

[97] Levkovitch-Verbin, H; Kalev-Landoy, M; Habot-Wilner, Z; Melamed, S. Minocycline delays death of retinal ganglion cells in experimental glaucoma and after optic nerve transaction. *Arch Ophthalmol,* 2006; 15: 520-526.

[98] Levkovitch-Verbin, H; Quigley, HA; Martin, KR; Harizman, N; Valenta, DF; Pease, ME; Melamed, S. The transcription factor c-jun is activated in retinal ganglion cells in experimental rat glaucoma. *Exp Eye Res,* 2005; 80: 663-670.

[99] Li, HY; Zhao, JL; Zhang, H. *Transfection of brain-derived neurotrophic factor gene by recombinant adeno-associated virus vector in retinal ganglion cells in vitro*. Zhonghua Yan Ke Za Zhi, 2008; 44(4): 354-60(abstract).

[100] Li, RS; Tay, DK; Chan, HH; So, KF. Changes of retinal functions following the induction of ocular hypertension in rats using argon laser photocoagulation. *Clin Exp Ophthalmol*, 2006; 34: 575-583.

[101] Libby, RT; Li, Y; Savinova, OV; Barter, J; Smith, RS; Nickells, RW; John, SW. Susceptibility to neurodegeneration in a glaucoma is modified by Bax gene dosage. *PLoS Genet,* 2005; 1: 17–26.

[102] Liefner, M; Siebert, H; Sachse, T; Michel, U; Kollias, G; Bruck, W. The role of TNF-alpha during Wallerian degeneration. *J Neuroimmunol,* 2000; 108: 147-152.

[103] Lisegang, TJ. Glaucoma. Changing concepts and future directions. *Mayo Clin Proc,* 1996; 7: 689-694.

[104] Liu, B; Neufeld, AH. Expression of nitric oxide synthase-2 (NOS-2) in reactive astrocytes of the human glaucomatous optic nerve head. *Glia*, 2000; 30: 178–186.

[105] Mansour-Robaey, S; Clarke, DB; Wang, YC; Bray, GM; Aguayo, AJ. Effects of ocular injury and administration of brain-derived neurotrophic factor on survival and regrowth of axotomized retinal ganglion cells. *Proc Natl Acad Sci USA*, 1994; 91: 1632-1636.
[106] Martin, KR; Levkovitch-Verbin, H; Valenta, D; Baumrind, L; Pease, ME; Quigley, HA. Retinal glutamate transporter changes in experimental glaucoma and after optic nerve transection in the rat. *Invest Ophthalmol Vis Sci,* 2002; 43: 2236-2243.
[107] McKinnon, SJ. Glaucoma, apoptosis and neuroprotection. *Curr Opin Ophthalmol,* 1997; 8: 28-37.
[108] McKinnon, SJ; Lehman, DM; Kerrigan-Baumrind, LA; Merges, CA; Pease, ME; Kerrigan, DF; Ransom, NL; Tahzib, NG; Reitsamer, HA; Levkovitch-Verbin, H; Quigley, DJ. and Zack, DJ. Caspase activation and amyloid precursor protein cleavage in rat ocular hypertension. *Invest Ophthalmol,* 2002; 43: 1077-1087.
[109] Merritt, JC; Crawford, WJ; Alexander, PC; Anduze, AL; Gelbart, SS. Effect of marijuana on intraocular and blood pressure in glaucoma. *Ophthalmology*, 1980; 87: 222-228.
[110] Merritt, JC; McKinnon, S; Armstrong, JR; Hatem, G; Reid, LA. Oral Delta(9)-tetrahydrocannabinol, in heterogenous glaucoma. *Ann Ophthalmol,* 1980; 12: 947-950.
[111] Minckler, DS; Bunt, AH; Johanson, GW. Orthograde and retrograde axoplasmic transport during acute ocular hyptertension in the monkey. *Invest Ophthalmol Vis Sci,* 1977; 16: 426–441.
[112] Mittag, TW; Danias, J; Pohorenec, G; Yuan, HM; Burakgazi, E; Chalmers-Redman, R; Podos, SM; Tatton, WG. Retinal damage after 3 to 4 months of elevated intraocular pressure in a rat glaucoma model. *Invest Ophthalmol Vis Sci*, 2000; 41: 3451–3459.
[113] Mozaffarieh, M; Flammer, J. A novel perspective on natural therapeutic approaches in glaucoma therapy. *Expert Opin Emerg Drugs*, 2007; 12(2): 195-198.
[114] Mozaffarieh, M; Grieshaber, MC; Orgül, S; Flammer, J. The potential value of natural antioxidative treatment in glaucoma. *Surv Ophthalmol,* 2008; 53(5): 479-505.
[115] Mulligan, SJ; MacVicar, BA. Calcium transients in astrocyte endfeet cause cerebrovascular constrictions. *Nature*, 2004; 431: 195–199.
[116] Napper, GA; Pianta, MJ; Kalloniatis, M. Reduced glutamate uptake by retinal glial cells under ischemic/hypoxic conditions. *Vis Neurosci,* 1999; 16: 149-158.
[117] Naskar, R; Dreyer, EB. New horizons in neuroprotection. *Surv Ophthalmol,* 2001; 45(3): 250-256.
[118] Netland, PA; Chaturvedi, N; Dreyer, EB. Calcium channel blockers in the management of low tension and open angle glaucoma. *Am J Ophthalmol,* 1993; 115: 608-613.
[119] Neufeld, AH; Sawada, A; Becker, B. Inhibition of nitric oxide synthase-2 by aminoguanidine provides neuroprotection of retinal ganglion cells in a rat model of chronic glaucoma. *Proc Nat Acad Sci USA,* 1999; 96: 9944-9948.
[120] Newell, FW; Krill, AE. Diurnal tonography in normal and glaucomatous eyes. *Trans Am Ophthalmol Soc*, 1964; 62: 349-358.
[121] Nickells, RW. Apoptosis of retinal ganglion cells in glaucoma: an update of the molecular pathways involved in cell death. *Surv Ophthalmol*, 1999; 43: 151-161.
[122] Nickells, RW. From ocular hypertension to ganglion cell death: a theorical sequence of events leading to glaucoma. *Can J Ophthalmol,* 2007; 42: 278-287.

[123] Nickells, RW. The molecular biology of retinal ganglion cell death: caveats and controversies. *Brain Res Bull,* 2004; 62: 439–446.

[124] Nucci, C; Gasperi, V; Tartaglione, R; Cerulli, A; Terrinoni, A; Bari, M; De Simone, C; Finazzi Agró, A; Morrone, LA; Corasaniti, MT; Bagetta, G. and Maccarrone, M. Involvement of the endocannabinoid system in retinal damage after high intraocular pressure-induced ischemia in rats. *Invest Ophthalmol Vis Sci,* 2007; 48: 2997-3004.

[125] Oku, H; Yamaguchi, H; Sugiyama, T; Kojima, S; Ota, M; Azuma, I. Retinal toxicity of nitric oxide released by administration of nitric oxide donor in the albino rabbit. *Invest Ophthalmol Vis Sci,* 1997; 38: 2540-2544.

[126] Oltvai ZN; Korsmeyer SJ. Checkpoints of duelling dimmers foil death wishes. *Cell,* 1994; 79: 189-192.

[127] Opere, CA; Zheng, WD; Zhao, M; Lee, JS; Kulkarni, KH; Ohia, SE. Inhibition of potassium- and ischemia-evoked [3H] D-aspartate release from isolated bovine retina by cannabinoids. *Curr Eye Res*, 2006; 31: 645-653.

[128] Osborne, BA; Schwartz, LM. Essential genes that regulate apoptosis. *Trends Cell Biol,* 1994; 4: 394–399.

[129] Pease, ME; McKinnon, SJ; Quigley, HA; Kerrigan-Baumrind, LA. and Zack, DJ. Obstructed axonal transport of BDNF and its receptor TrkB in experimental glaucoma. *Invest Ophthalmol Vis Sci*, 2000; 41: 764-774.

[130] Phelps, CD; Corbett, JJ. Migraine and low-tension glaucoma. A case-control study. Invest Ophthalmol Vis Sci, 1985; 26; 1105-1108.

[131] Porcella, A; Maxia, C; Gessa, GL; Pani, L. The synthetic cannabinoid WIN55212-2 decreases the intraocular pressure in human glaucoma resistant to conventional therapies. *Eur J Neurosci,* 2001 (13): 490-412.

[132] Power, C; Henry, S; Del Bigio, MR; Larsen, PH; Corbett, D; Imai, Y; Yong, VW; Peeling, J. Intracerebral hemorrhage induces macrophage activation and matrix metalloproteinases. *Ann Neurol*, 2003; 53: 731-742.

[133] Purnell, WD; Gregg JM. Delta(9)-tetrahydrocannabinol, euphoria and intraocular pressure in man. *Ann Ophthalmol,* 1975; 7: 921-923.

[134] Putcha, GV; Le, S; Frank, S; Besirli, CG; Clark, K; Chu, B; Alix, S; Youle, RJ; LaMarche, A; Maroney, AC; Johnson, EMJr. JNK mediated BIM phosphorylation potentiates BAX-dependent apoptosis. *Neuron*, 2003; 38: 899–914.

[135] Quigley HA, Addicks EM. Regional differences in the structure of the lamina cribrosa and their relation to glaucomatous optic nerve damage. *Arch Ophthalmol,* 1981; 99: 137-144.

[136] Quigley, HA. Ganglion cell death in glaucoma: pathology recapitulates ontogeny. *Aust N Z J Ophthalmol*, 1995; 23: 85–91.

[137] Quigley, HA; Addicks, EM. Chronic experimental glaucoma in primates. II. Effect of extended intraocular pressure elevation on optic nerve head and axonal transport. *Invest Ophthalmol Vis Sci*, 1980; 19: 137–152.

[138] Quigley, HA; Addicks, EM; Green, WR; Maumenee, AE. Optic nerve damage in human glaucoma: II. The site of injury and susceptibility to damage. *Arch Ophthalmol,* 1981; 99: 635–649.

[139] Quigley, HA; Engerm, C; Katz, J; Sommer, A; Scottm, R; Gilbertm, D. Risk factors for the development of glaucomatous visual field loss in ocular hypertension. *Arch Ophthalmolol,* 1994; 112; 644-649,

[140] Quigley, HA; Hohman, RM; Addicks, EM; Green, WR. Blood vessels of the glaucomatous optic disk in experimental primate and human eyes. *Invest Ophthalmol Vis Sci,* 1984; 25: 918-931.

[141] Quigley, HS; Broman, AT. The number of people with glaucoma worldwide in 2010 and 2020. *Br J Ophthalmol,* 2006; 90(3): 253-254.

[142] Rabacchi, SA; Ensini, M; Bonfanti, I; Grarina, A; Maffei, L. Nerve growth factor reduces apoptosis of axotomized retinal ganglion cells in the neonatal rat. *Neuroscience*, 1994; 63: 969-973.

[143] Radius, RL; Anderson, DR. Rapid axonal transport in primate optic nerve. *Arch Ophthalmol*, 1981; 99: 650–654.

[144] Raff, MC; Whitmore, AV; Finn, JT. Axonal self-destruction and neurodegeneration. *Science*, 2002; 296: 868–871.

[145] Ransom, B; Behar, T; Nedergaard, M. New roles for astrocytes (stars at last). *TRENDS Neurosci*, 2003; 26: 520–522.

[146] Resta, V; Novelli, E; Vozzi, G; Scarpa, C; Caleo, M; Ahluwalia, A; Solini, A; Santini, E; Parisi, V; Di Virgilio, F; Galli-Resta, L. Acute retinal ganglion cell injury caused by intraocular pressure spikes is mediated by endogenous extracellular ATP. *Eur J Neurosci*, 2007; 25: 2741–2754.

[147] Riccio, A; Pierchala, BA; Ciarallo, CL; Ginty, DD. An NGF-TrkA-mediated retrograde signal to transcription factor CREB in sympathetic neurons. *Science*, 1977; 277: 1037.

[148] Ruiz, G; Wheeler, L; WoldeMussie, E; Wheeler, LA. Time course of pre or post treatment by brimonidine on neuroprotection in rat optic nerve injury model. *Invest Ophthalmol Vis Sci,* 2000; 41: 830.

[149] Russo, R; Cavaliere, F; Watanabe, C; Nucci, C; Bagetta, G; Corasaniti, MT; Sakurada, S; Morrone, LA. 17Beta-estradiol prevents retinal ganglion cell loss induced by acute rise of intraocular pressure in rat. *Prog Brain Res,* 2008; 173: 583-590.

[150] Ryan, ME; Usman, A; Ramamurthy, NS; Golub, LM; Greenwald, RA. Excessive matrix metalloproteinase activity in diabetes: inhibition by tetracycline analogues with zinc reactivity. *Curr Med Chem*, 2001; 8: 305-316.

[151] Sadowski, T; Steinmeyer, J. Effects of tetracyclines on the production of matrix metalloproteinases and plasminogen activators as well as of their natural inhibitors, tissue inhibitor of metalloproteinases-1 and plasminogen activator inhibitor-1. *Inflamm Res,* 2001; 50: 175-182.

[152] Sanchez Mejia, RO; Ona, VO; Li, M; Friedlander, RM. Minocycline reduces traumatic brain injury-mediated caspase-1 activation, tissue damage, and neurological dysfunction. *Neurosurgery*, 2001; 48: 1393-1401.

[153] Sawai, H; Clarke, DB; Kittlerova, P; Bray, GM; Aguayo, AJ. Brain-derived neurotrophic factor and neurotrophin-4/5 stimulate growth of axonal branches from regenerating retinal ganglion cells. *J Neurosci*, 1996; 16: 3887–3894.

[154] Schlamp, CL; Li, Y; Dietz, JA; Janssen, KT; Nickells, RW. Progressive ganglion cell loss and optic nerve degeneration in DBA/2J mice is variable and asymmetric. *BMC Neurosci,* 2006; 7: 66.

[155] Schulzer, M; Drance, SM; Carter, CJ; Brooks, DE; Douglas, GR; Lau, W. Biostatistical evidence for two distinct chronic open angle glaucoma populations. *Br J Ophthtalmol,* 1990: 74: 196-200.

[156] Schwartz, M. Modulating the immune system: a vaccine for glaucoma? *Can J Ophthalmol*, 2007; 42: 439-441.

[157] Seki, M, Lipton, SA. Targeting excitotoxic/free radical signaling pathways for therapeutic intervention in glaucoma. *Prog Brain Res,* 2008; 173: 495-510.

[158] Shin, DH; Becker, B; Kolker, AE. Family history in primary open-angle glaucoma. *Arch Ophthalmol,* 1977; 95: 598-600.

[159] Simpkins, JW; Wang, J; Wang, X; Perez, E; Prokai, L; Dykens, JA. Mitochondria play a central role in estrogen-induced neuroprotection. *Curr Drug Targets CNS Neurol Disord*, 2005; 4(1): 69-83.

[160] Sirén, AL; Fratelli, M; Brines, M; Goemans, C; Casagrande, S; Lewczuk, P; Keenan, S; Gleiter, C; Pasquali, C; Capobianco, A; Mennini, T; Heumann, R; Cerami, A; Ehrenreich, H; Ghezzi, P. "Erythropoietin prevents neuronal apoptosis after cerebral ischemia and metabolic stress". *Proc Natl Acad Sci USA,* 2001; 98: 4044–4049.

[161] Smith, JR; Gabler, WL. Protective effects of doxycycline in mesenteric ischemia and reperfusion. *Res Commun Mol Pathol Pharmacol*, 1995; 88: 303-315.

[162] Smith, JR; Gabler, WL. Effects of doxycycline in two rat models of ischemia/reperfucion injury. *Proc West Pharmacol So*, 1994; 37: 3-4.

[163] Sommer, A ; Tielsch, JM ; Katz, J. et al. Relationship between intraocular pressure and primary open angle glaucoma among white and black Americans. The Baltimore Eye Survey. *Arch Ophthalmol*, 1991; 109: 1090-1095.

[164] Sommer, A. Intraocular pressure and glaucoma. *Am J Ophthalmol,* 1989; 107: 186-188.

[165] Hart, WMJr; Yablonski, M; Kass, MA; Becker, B. Multivariate analysis of the risk of glaucomatous visual field loss. *Arch Ophthalmol,* 1979; 97: 1455-1458.

[166] Spaeth, GL. Fluorescein angiography: its contributions towards understanding the mechanisms of visual loss in glaucoma. *Trns Am Ophthalmol Soc,* 1975; 73: 491-553.

[167] Spray, DC; Ye, ZC; Ransom, BR. Functional connexion "hemichannels": a critical appraisal. *Glia*, 2006; 54: 758–773.

[168] Stone, EM; Fingert, JH; Alward, WLM; Nguyen, TD; Polansky, JR; Sunden, SLF; Nishimura, D; Clark, AF; Nystuen, A; Nichols, BE; Mackey, DA; Ritch, R; Kalenak, JW; Craven, ER; Sheffield, VC. Identification of a gene that causes primary open angle glaucoma. *Science*, 1997; 275: 668-670.

[169] Stys, PK. White matter injury mechanisms. *Curr Mol Med*, 2004; 4: 113–130.

[170] Tamaki, Y; Araie, M; Tomita, K; Nagahara, M. Effect of topical betaxolol on tissue circulation in the human optic nerve head. J Ocul Pharmacol Ther, 1999; 15: 313-321.

[171] Tezel, G. and Wax, MB. Increased production of tumor necrosis factor-alpha by glial cells exposed to simulated ischemia or elevated hydrostatic pressure induces apoptosis in cocultured retinal ganglion cells. *J Neurosc*i, 2000; 20: 8693-8700.

[172] Tezel, G. and Yang, X. Caspse-independent component of retinal ganglion cell death, in vitro. *Invest Ophthalmol Vis Sci*, 2004; 45: 4049-4059.

[173] Tezel, G; Li, LY; Patil, RV. and Wax, MB. Tumor necrosis factor-alpha and its receptor-1 in the retina of normal and glaucomatous eyes. *Invest Ophthalmol Vis Sci,* 2001; 42: 1787-1794.

[174] Tezel, G; Yang, X; Yang, J. and Wax, MB. Role of tumor necrosis factor receptor-1 in the death of retinal ganglion cells following optic nerve crush injury in mice. *Brain Res,* 2004; 996: 202-212.

[175] Tezel, G. Oxidative stress in glaucomatous neurodegeneration: mechanisms and consequences. *Prog Retin Eye Res,* 2006; 25: 490-513.

[176] Thanos S, Bahr M, Barde YA, Vanselow J. Survival and axonal elongation of adult rat retinal ganglion cells: in vitro effects of lesioned sciatic nerve and brain-derived neurotrophic factor (BDNF). *Eur J Neurosci*, 1989; 1: 19-26.

[177] The AGIS Investigators. The Advanced Glaucoma Intervention Study (AGIS): 7. The relationship between control of intraocular pressure and visual field deterioration. *Am J Ophthalmol*, 2000; 130(4): 429-440.

[178] The Ischemic Optic Neuropathy Desompression Trial Research Group. Optic nerve descompression surgery for nonarteritic anterior ischemic optic neuropathy (NAION) is not effective and may be harmful. The Ischemic Optic Neuropathy Descompression Trial Research Group. *JAMA*, 2000; 273(8): 625-632.

[179] Tielsch, JM; Katz, J; Sommer, A; Quigley, HA; Javitt, JC. Hypertension, perfusion pressure and primary open-angle glaucoma. A population-based assessment. *Arch Ophthalmol,* 1995; 113: 216-221.

[180] Tikka, TM; Koistinaho, JE. Minocycline provides neuroprotection against N-methyl-D-aspartate neurotoxicity by inhibiting microglia. *J Immunol,* 2001; 166: 7527-7533.

[181] Trope, GE; Salinas, SA; Glynn, M. Blood viscosity in primary open-angle glaucoma. *Can J Ophthalmol,* 1987; 22: 202-204.

[182] Urcola, JH; Hernández, M; Vecino, E. Three experimental glaucoma models in rats: Comparison of the effects of intraocular pressure elevation on retinal ganglion cell size and death. *Exp Eye Res,* 2006; 83: 429-437.

[183] Van der Stelt, M; Di Marzo, V. Cannabinoid receptors and their role in neuroprotection. *Neuromolecular Med,* 2005; 7: 37-50.

[184] Vecino, E; Caminos, E; Ugarte, M; Martín-Zanca, D; Osborne, N. Immunohistochemical distribution of neurotrophins and their receptors in the rat retina and the effects of ischemia and reperfusion. *Gen. Pharmacol Vas*, 1998; 30: 305-314.

[185] Vecino, E; García, D; Martinez-Millán, L; Sharma, SCS; Carrascal, E. Rat retina ganglion cells co-express brain derived neurotrophic factor (BDNF) and its receptor TrkB. *Vision Res.* (2002) 42:151-157.

[186] de Lago, E; Fernández-Ruíz, J. Cannabinoids and neuroprotection in motor-related disorders. *CNS Neurol Disord Drug Targets*, 2007; 6: 337-387.

[187] Mechoulam, R; Shohami, E. Endocannabinoids and traumatic brain injury. *Mol Neurobiol,* 2007; 36: 68-77.

[188] von Bartheld, CS; Byers, MR; Williams, R; Bothwell, M. Anterograde transport and axo-dendritic transfer of neurotrophins in the developing visual system. *Nature*, 1996; 379: 830-833.

[189] von Bartheld, CS; Williams, R; Lefcort, F; Clary, DO; Reichardt, LF; Bothwell, M. Retrograde transport of neurotrophins from the eye to the brain in chick embryos: roles of the p75NTR and Trkb receptors. *J Neurosci,* 1996; 16: 2995-3008.

[190] Vorwerk, CK; Lipton, SA; Zurakowski, D; Hyman, BT; Sabel, BA; Dreyer, EB. Chronic low-dose glutamate is toxic to retinal ganglion cells. Toxicity blocked by mementine. *Invest Ophthalmol Vis Sci,* 1996; 37: 1618-1624.

[191] Ward MS; Khoobehi, A; Lavik, EB; Langer, R; Young, MJ. Neuroprotection of retinal ganglion cells in DBA/2J mice with GDNF-loaded biodegradable microspheres. *J Pharm Sci*, 2007; 96: 558-568.

[192] Weinreb, RN. Glaucoma neuroprotection: What is it? Why is it needed? *Can J Ophthalmol*, 2007; 42: 396-398.

[193] Wheeler, LA; Gil, DW; WoldeMussie, E. Role of alpha-2 adrenergic receptors in neuroprotection and glaucoma. Surv Ophthalmol, 2001; 45(3): 290-296.

[194] Wheeler, LA; WoldeMussie, E; Lai, R. Role of alpha-2 agonist in neuroprotection. *Surv Ophthalmol,* 2003; 48: 47-51.

[195] Wheeler, LA; Woldemussie, E. Alpha-2 adrenergic receptor agonists are neuroprotective in experimental models of glaucoma. *Eur J Ophthalmol*, 2001; 11: 30-35.

[196] Wheeler, LA; Tatton, NA; Elstner, M. Alpha-2 adrenergic receptor activation by brimonidine reduces neuronal apoptosis through Akt (protein Kinase B) dependent new synthesis of BCL-2. *Invest Ophthalmol Vis Sci,* 2001; 42: 411.

[197] Whitmore, AV; Libby, RT; John, SWM. Glaucoma: thinking in new ways: a role for autonomous axonal self-destruction and compartmentalised processes? *Prog Retin Eye Res*, 2005; 24: 639–662.

[198] Wilson, MR; Hertzmark, E; Walker, AM; Childs-Shaw, K; Epstein, DL. A case-control study of risk factors in open angle glaucoma. *Arch Ophthalmol,* 1987; 105: 1066-1071.

[199] Wood, JP; Schmidt, KG; Melena, J; Chidlow, G; Allmeier, H; Osborne, NN. The beta adrenoceptor antagonists metipranolol and timolol are retinal neuroprotectants: comparison with betaxolol. *Exp Eye Res*, 2003; 76(4): 505-516.

[200] Yan, X; Tezel, G; Wax, MB; Edward DP. Matrix metalloproteinases and tumor necrosis factor alpha in glaucomatous optic nerve head. *Arch Ophthalmol*, 2000. 118: 666-673.

[201] Yoles, E; Belkin, M; Schwartz, M. HU-211, a nonpsychotropic cannabinoid, produces short- and long-term neuroprotection after optic nerve axotomy. *J Neurotrauma*, 1996; 13: 49-57.

[202] Yoles, E; Schwartz, M. Potential neuroprotective therapy for glaucomatous optic neuropathy. *Surv Opththalmol,* 1998; 42367-42372.

[203] Yoles, E; Wheeler, LA; Schwartz, M. Alpha2-adrenoreceptor agonists are neuroprotective in a rat model of optic nerve degeneration.*Invest Ophthalmol Vis Sci,* 1999; 40: 65-73.

[204] Yrjanheikki, J; Keinanen, R; Pellikka, M; Hokfelt, T; Koistinaho, J. Tetracyclines inhibit microglial activation and are neuroprotective in global brain ischemia. *Proc Natl Acad Sci U S A*, 1998; 95: 15769-15774.

[205] Yrjanheikki, J; Tikka, T; Keinanen, R; Goldsteins, G; Chan, PH; Koistinaho, JA. A tetracycline derivative, micocycline, reduces inflammation and protects against focal cerebral ischemia with a wide therapeutic window. *Proc Natl Acad Sci USA*, 1999; 96: 13496-13500.

[206] Zangwill, LM; Bowd, C; Berry CC; Williams, J; Blumenthal, EZ; Sánchez-Galeana, CA; Vasile, C; Weinreb, RN. Discriminating between normal and glaucomataous eyes using the Heidelberg retina tomography, GDx Nerve Fiber Analyzer, and Optical Coherence Tomograph. *Arch Ophthalmol*, 2001; 119(7): 985-993.

[207] Zhang, C; Lei, B; Lam, TT; Yang, F ; Sinha, D; Tso, MO. Neuroprotection of photoreceptors by minocycline in light-induced retinal degeneration. *Invest Ophthalmol Vis Sci,* 2004; 45: 2753-2759.

[208] Zhang, X; Reigada, D; Zhang, M; Laties, AM; Mitchell, CH. Increased ocular pressure increases vitreal levels of ATP. *Association for Research in Vision and Ophthalmology* (ARVO), 2006; Abstract 426.

[209] Zhang, X; Zhang, M; Laties, AM; Mitchell, CH. Stimulation of P2X7 receptors elevates Ca2_ and kills retinal ganglion cells. *Invest Ophthmol Vis Sci,* 2005; 46: 2183–2191.

[210] Zhang, X; Zhang, M; Laties, AM; Mitchell, CH. Balance of purines may determine life or death as A3 adenosine receptors prevent loss of retinal ganglion cells following P2X7 receptor stimulation. *J Neurochem,* 2006; 98: 566-575.

[211] Zhong, L; Bradley, J; Schubert, W; Ahmed, E; Adamis, AP; Shima, DT; Robinson, GS; Ng, YS. Erythropoietin promotes survival of retinal ganglion cells in DBA/2J glaucoma mice. *Invest Ophthalmol Vis Sci*, 2007; 48(3): 1212-1218.

[212] Zhou, W; Zhu, X; Zhu, L; Cui, YY; Wang, H; Qi, H; Ren, QS; Chen, HZ. Neuroprotection of muscarinic receptor agonist pilocarpine against glutamate-induced apoptosis in retinal neurons. *Cell Mol Neurobiol.* 2008; 28(2): 263-275.

[213] Zhou, X; Li, F; Ge, J; Sarkisian, SRJr, Tomita H; Zaharia, A; Chodosh, J; Cao, W. Retinal ganglion cell protection by 17-beta-estradiol in a mouse model of inherited glaucoma. *Dev Neurobiol,* 2007; 67(5): 603-616.

[214] Zhu, S; Stavrovskaya, IG; Drozda, M; Kim, BY; Ona, V; Li, M; Sarang, S; Liu, AS; Hartley, DM; Wu, DC; Gullans, S; Ferrante, RJ; Przedborski, S; Kristal, BS; Friedlander, RM. Minocycline inhibits cytochrome c release and delays progression of amyotrophic lateral sclerosis in mice. *Nature*, 2002; 417: 74-78.

In: Eye Research Developments
Editor: Alan N. Westerhouse

ISBN: 978-1-60741-177-2

Chapter III

Helicobacter Pylori Infection as a Risk Factor for Glaucoma: Geographical Similarities and Diversities

Christos Zavos, Jannis Kountouras**, Georgia Deretzi, Nikolaos Grigoriadis, Dimitrios Tzilves, Panagiotis Katsinelos, Dimitrios Gisakis, Olga Giouleme, Nikolaos Zavos, Ioannis Pilpilidis, Elena Tsiaousi, Dimitrios Tsantilas and Alexandros Karagiannidis

Department of Gastroenterology, Second Medical Clinic,
Aristotle University of Thessaloniki, Ippokration Hospital, Thessaloniki, Greece

Abstract

Decades of epidemiologic research into glaucoma have elucidated several risk factors related in some way to the disease. Moreover, limited data indicate that marked geographical variations have been demonstrated regarding mainly the pseudo-exfoliation glaucoma (XFG). Currently, the best-known causative risk factor is raised intraocular pressure. Among other risk factors, age, ischemia, increased homocysteine levels, changes in endothelium-dependent vascular regulation, impaired blood-brain barrier and ocular blood flow and cytokines have been implicated in the mechanisms underlying glaucoma. Although degenerative diseases, including glaucoma, have an increasingly high impact on aged population, their association with Helicobacter pylori (H. pylori) infection has not been thoroughly researched. This issue has only recently been addressed by Kountouras et al. who documented: a high prevalence of H. pylori infection in Greek patients with primary open-angle glaucoma (POAG) and XFG, a beneficial effect of eradication of H. pylori on glaucoma progression, suggesting a possible causal link between the bacterium and POAG and an increased H. pylori-specific IgG antibody concentration in the aqueous humor of patients with glaucoma the titer of which correlated with the degree of vertical cupping, possibly indicating the severity of glaucomatous damage. A positive association between H. pylori infection serology and glaucoma was also reported by three studies from Turkey, China, and India. An elevation in aqueous humor anti-H. pylori IgG antibodies in XFG was further reported by an Iranian study. Conversely, two other studies from Canada and Israel found no

* Please address correspondence to: Jannis Kountouras, MD, PhD; Professor of Medicine; Gastroenterologist; 8 Fanariou St, Byzantio; 551 33, Thessaloniki, Macedonia, Greece; Tel: +30-2310-892238, Fax: +30-2310-992794; E-mail: jannis@med.auth.gr

association between H. pylori infection and POAG. Apart from a brief description of the potential underlying pathogenetic mechanisms, the data of these studies are herein analyzed according to their geographical similarities and diversities, and the methodological flaws and weaknesses are highlighted, emphasizing the need for larger, randomized, multicenter studies.

A. *Helicobacter Pylori* and Glaucoma Association: Shaping the Hypothesis

Currently glaucoma is recognized as an optic neuropathy and defined as "ocular" Alzheimer disease (AD); it is a chronic neurodegeneration of the optic nerve, the second cause, after cataract, of world blindness and of major public health importance [1-3]. Selective death of retinal ganglion cells (RGC) is the hallmark of glaucoma, also associated with structural changes in the optic nerve head; RGCs' death after axonal injury can be induced by a variety of different stimuli [4]. The process of RGC death is thought to be biphasic: a primary injury responsible for initiation of damage followed by a slower secondary degeneration related to noxious environment surrounding the degenerating cells. Decades of epidemiologic research into glaucoma have elucidated several risk factors related in some way to the disease. The most important risk factor for glaucoma is increased intraocular pressure. However, other factors may also damage the neural tissue in glaucomatous optic neuropathy. The most prominent of these is vascular dysregulation [4]. According to recent evidence, this disease may be associated with changes in endothelium-dependent vascular regulation [4-11]. In addition, impaired ocular blood flow due to blood hyperviscosity (increased platelet aggregation on atheromatous plaques in the elderly) [12-19] and cytokines may also be involved in the pathogenesis of this disease [20-22]. A working knowledge of the environmental risk factors for the induction and progression of the disease is essential to our clinical practices and helps those patients at greater risk of disease progression and blindness; a major priority is to achieve a better understanding of the risk factors, likely to involve gene-environment interactions.

Evidence for the possibility of an infectious agent comes from reports in younger patients with pseudo-exfoliative glaucoma (XFG) after intraocular surgery or trauma with iris surgery in infancy and childhood or after penetrating keratoplasty from elderly donors [23]. Moreover, in a Norwegian eye-screening study, the prevalence of XFG in both members of married couples is significantly higher than expected [23], thereby suggesting a common environmental (probably infectious) agent, which may be of etiological significance for the XFG development [24]. In this respect, Koch's postulates regarding a causal association with a disease seem to apply in glaucoma [25], but, until recently, no one had associated any microorganisms with glaucoma. Specifically, although degenerative diseases, including glaucoma or AD, have an increasingly high impact on aged population, their association with *Helicobacter pylori* (*H. pylori*) infection has not been thoroughly researched.

The latter issue has only recently been addressed by Kountouras et al. [26] who first shaped the hypothesis that a theoretical relationship between glaucoma and *H. pylori* infection exists: a. both are diseases of older adults in the developed world [27-29]; b. chronic *H. pylori* infection has been associated with extradigestive disorders, such as functional vascular disorders caused by vascular dysregulation due to the release of vasoactive and pro-inflammatoty substances [30-38]; and c. *H. pylori* infection is associated with arteriosclerosis-induced increased platelet activation and aggregation [39, 40]. *H. pylori* may also contribute to atherosclerosis through an auto-immune process against endothelial cells or an increased concentration of blood homocysteine due to decreased levels of folic acid and cobalamin, and/or hypertension, all of which have been found to be risk factors for glaucoma and other neurodegenerative disorders such as AD [3, 41], mainly by impairing blood-brain barrier (BBB), a common denominator associated with glaucoma and various degrees of dementia including AD [3, 42, 43].

B. Pathogenetic Mechanisms via which *H. Pylori* May Be Linked to Glaucoma

H. pylori infection may influence the pathophysiology of glaucoma by promoting platelet and platelet-leukocyte aggregation, releasing proinflammatory and vasoactive substances, such as cytokines [interleukin (IL)-1, IL-6, IL-8, IL-10, IL-12, tumor necrosis factor (TNF)-α, interferon-γ], eicosanoids (leukotrienes, prostaglandins) and acute phase proteins (fibrinogen, C-reactive protein), involved in a number of vascular disorders (migraine, systemic hypertension, Raunaud's phenomenon, cardiovascular disease and possibly glaucoma) [44, 45], stimulating mononuclear cells to induce a tissue factor-like procoagulant activity that converts fibrinogen into fibrin, causing the development of cross mimicry between endothelial and *H. pylori* antigens, producing oxidative stress and circulating lipid peroxides, and influencing the apoptotic process; these parameters may also exert their own effects in the induction and/or progression of glaucomatous neuropathy [44, 45] and other neurodegenerative disorders [AD, Guillain-Barré syndrome (GBS), Parkinson's disease] associated with both *H. pylori* infection and glaucoma [45, 46]. In particular, increased endothelin (ET)-1 (a potent constrictor of arterioles and venules), nitric oxide (NO) and inducible nitric oxide synthase (iNOS) levels are associated with *H. pylori* infection [45, 46]. In glaucoma, weaker BBB renders circulating molecules, such as ET-1, capable to directly access smooth vascular muscle cells and pericytes both in the prelaminar part of the optic nerve head and in adjacent retinal tissue. This potentially results in vasoconstriction as noticed in the peri-papillary retinal vessel in glaucoma patients, thereby provoking retinal vein occlusion. The direct access of these molecules also influences the barrier function. If ET-1 reduces endothelial tight junctions and moreover matrix metalloproteinase-9 degrades the basement membrane, not only macromolecules but even red blood cells may cross the BBB and lead to what is clinically observed as optic disk hemorrhages. Therefore, the diffusion of ET-1 and metalloproteinases to the surrounding of the optic nerve head results in a local vasoconstriction in glaucoma, increases the risk for venous occlusion and weakens the BBB, which in extreme situations leads to splinter hemorrhages [42, 43]. Apart from ET-1-induced vasoconstriction of the anterior optic nerve vessels, NO modulation of vascular tone in the ophthalmic artery may also produce glaucomatous damage. NO, a rapidly diffusing gas, is a potent neurotoxin that may facilitate the apoptotic death of retinal ganglion cells in glaucomatous optic neuropathy [45, 46]. Support for the consideration of NO neurotoxicity in glaucoma is provided by experimental evidence demonstrating that retinal ganglion cell apoptosis is attenuated by neutralizing antibodies against TNF-α or by selective inhibitors of iNOS, thereby suggesting that the inhibitions of TNF-α or the inducible isoform NOS2 may provide novel therapeutic targets for neuroprotection in the treatment of glaucomatous optic neuropathy.

Importantly, geographical variations in *H. pylori* infection have been reported [47]; there are differences in the clinical presentation in various geographical regions resulting from variations in the genetic make-up of *H. pylori*. Comparable limited data indicate that marked geographical variations also have been demonstrated regarding mainly the XFG. Therefore, relative glaucoma studies from different parts of the world are needed to elucidate the aforementioned potential involvement of *H. pylori* infection in glaucomatous neuropathy more thoroughly.

C. Greek Data

In 2001, by using histology, representing the practical gold standard for *H. pylori* infection diagnosis, Kountouras and colleagues documented for the first time a high prevalence of *H. pylori* infection in Greek patients with primary open-angle glaucoma (POAG) and XFG, establishing a relationship between *H. pylori* infection and glaucoma [26]. The initial study showed a histological prevalence of *H. pylori* infection in 87.5% of the POAG patients (28 of 32), in 88.9% of the XFG patients (8 of 9) and in 46.7% of the anemic controls (14 of 30) (*P*[POAG vs. controls]=0.0006 and *P*[XFG vs. controls]=0.02). The authors concluded that these results may indicate either a common factor that causes susceptibilities to both glaucoma and *H. pylori* infection or that *H. pylori* may be a causal factor for developing glaucoma. Establishing firm proof of the association of *H. pylori* and glaucoma as well as the benefit of *H. pylori* eradication in the clinical course of glaucoma is vital because this may have a major impact on the treatment of glaucoma. Nevertheless, before antibiotic therapy of *H. pylori* infection becomes an established step in the management of POAG, sufficient evidence should be provided that glaucoma parameters are positively influenced by the eradication of *H. pylori* infection.

In a subsequent study published in 2002 [48], the same investigators reported a beneficial effect of *H. pylori* eradication on glaucoma progression. Specifically, the authors evaluated the effect of *H. pylori* eradication on 2 well-established clinical parameters in glaucoma: intraocular pressure and visual field indices. The study reported that *H. pylori*-positive patients in whom *H. pylori* was successfully eradicated showed a statistically significant reduction in intraocular pressure at both 1 and 2 years post-treatment. A similar improvement occurred in visual field data (mean short-term fluctuation and corrected loss variance) at 1 and 2 years' follow-up. These results in *H. pylori*-positive POAG patients are of interest because it is unusual for these parameters to improve over time. It should be noted that these changes occurred while patients were maintained on the same glaucoma regimen. On the other hand, *H. pylori*-positive POAG patients, in whom the bacterium was not eradicated, showed a slight deterioration in visual field indices mean values after 2 years of follow-up. These data suggest a possible causal link between the *H. pylori* infection and glaucoma. It was thus important to further investigate the role of *H. pylori* in POAG and XFG initiation, progression, or susceptibility, by documenting its qualitative and quantitative presence in the aqueous humor of these patients.

In a third study published in 2003 at the *Graefe's Archive for Clinical and Experimental Ophthalmology* [49], Kountouras et al. investigated the presence of *H. pylori*-specific IgG antibodies in the aqueous humor of patients with POAG and XFG, and compared their levels with those in age-matched normal cataract controls to determine whether *H. pylori* plays a role in these two common glaucomas. Specifically, aqueous humor was aspirated at the beginning of glaucoma surgery from 26 eyes of 26 patients with POAG, 27 eyes of 27 patients with XFG, and at the beginning of phacoemulsification cataract surgery from 31 eyes of 31 age-matched normotensive cataract patients. Serum samples were obtained the day before surgery from all patients. Anti-*H. pylori* IgG concentration in the aqueous humor and serum was measured by an enzyme-linked immunosorbent assay (ELISA). The mean concentration of anti-*H. pylori* IgG antibodies in the aqueous humor of patients with POAG was significantly higher than that observed in the aqueous humor of age-matched control patients (14.27±3.86 U/mL vs. 4.67±1.07 U/mL; P=0.006). Likewise, the mean concentration of anti-*H. pylori* IgG in the aqueous humor of patients with XFG (14.25±3.39 U/mL) was also significantly greater than that of the age-matched control patients (P=0.003). Moreover, the concentration of this antibody correlated with the degree of vertical cupping, possibly indicating the severity of glaucomatous damage [49].

Interestingly, molecular mimicry of host structures by the saccharide portion of lipopolysaccharides of the gastrointestinal pathogens *Campylobacter jejuni* (*C. jejuni*) and *H. pylori* is thought to be connected with the development of autoimmune sequelae observed in neuropathies. *C. jejuni*, a principal cause of gastroenteritis, and *H. pylori* are crucial antecedent infections in GBS, an inflammatory neuropathy [50]. Chemical analyses of the core oligosaccharides of neuropathy-associated *C. jejuni* strains have revealed structural homology with human gangliosides. Serum antibodies against gangliosides are found in one third of patients with GBS but are generally absent in enteritis cases. Collective data suggest that the antibodies are induced by an antecedent infection with *C. jejuni*, and subsequently react with nerve tissue causing damage [49]. In addition, several IgG antibodies against *H. pylori* proteins are found in the cerebrospinal fluid (CSF) in 57% of patients with GBS. No cross reactivity against *C. jejuni* is observed and these antibodies may also be involved in the immune responses of patients with GBS [51]. Similarly, 46% of patients with GBS have specific IgG antibodies to VacA of *H. pylori* in the CSF, and the sequence homology found between VacA and human Na^+/K^+-ATPase A subunit suggests that antibodies to VacA involve ion channels in abaxonal Schwann cell plasmalemma resulting in demyelination in some patients with in the CSF [52]. In view of all above-mentioned data, Kountouras et al. collectively suggested that the titer of anti-*H. pylori* IgG in the aqueous humor of glaucoma patients might indirectly offer evidence of the damage of glaucomatous optic neuropathy possibly induced by this organism via molecular mimicry autoimmune sequelae.

The authors admitted some limitations in their study, i.e., the relatively small number of patients, and that the aqueous humor antibody titers were not normalized to another protein to serve as control, such as IgG or albumin. The latter was due to the fact that the aqueous humor samples obtained were not sufficient to perform measurement of the total IgG titer.

Finally, Kountouras et al. also obtained comparable data for AD which is associated with and shares similar risk factors and pathogenetic mechanisms with glaucoma [3, 53-57]. Indeed, an association between *H. pylori* infection and AD/mild cognitive impairment patients in a Greek cohort has been found, *H. pylori* eradication may positively influence AD manifestations, and *H. pylori*-specific IgG antibody levels are significantly increased in the CSF of AD patients; its concentration in CSF might reflect the AD severity, thereby supporting a role for this common infection in the pathobiology of the disease [54-57]. An association between *H. pylori* infection and other glaucoma-related neurodegenerative disorders including multiple sclerosis (MS) and GBS in Greek cohorts have also been observed [58, 59].

D. Turkish Data

Kountouras et al.'s results from Greece, analyzed previously, were initially presented orally at the 6th Congress of the European Glaucoma Society in London in 2000 [60]. At the same Congress, Ozturk et al. from neighboring Turkey presented as an abstract similar results to theirs, which also showed a possible relationship between glaucoma and *H. pylori* infection by using serology [61].

E. Canadian Data

Two years after Kountouras's first full-text publication in *Ophthalmology* [26], a paper from Canada published in the same journal attempted to investigate the association between *H. pylori* and glaucoma, by using serology [62]. Specifically, Galloway et al. further investigated the prevalence of exposure to *H. pylori* infection in patients with different subtypes of glaucoma compared with normal control participants by using a prospective case-control methodology. Their study included 38 patients with POAG, 19 with normal pressure glaucoma, 16 with XFG, and 24 with ocular hypertension, whereas 94 age-matched participants without glaucoma served as a control population. The investigators analyzed the serum of the participants for the presence of *H. pylori*-specific IgG antibodies by ELISA. The results of this study were unable to provide additional confirmation of a link between *H. pylori* and glaucoma. Specifically, a total of 26.0% of POAG patients demonstrated serologic evidence of *H. pylori* infection, whereas *H. pylori* antibodies were detected in 20.2% of control participants.

The potential weaknesses of this study are criticized in a letter to the Editor published by Kountouras et al. in a successive issue of this Journal [63]. The ELISA method used to detect *H. pylori* infection has suboptimal sensitivity and specificity (85% and 79%, respectively). The diagnostic gold standard, used in the Greek studies, remains the histologic detection of *H. pylori*. The alternative urea breath test is widely used as the noninvasive alternative diagnostic test of choice, with a sensitivity and specificity of about 95%, particularly in elderly patients, who refuse to undergo the endoscopic/histologic procedure. Therefore, the

Canadian study, by introducing the less reliable serologic method, may not support definite conclusions.

Furthermore, a higher *H. pylori* prevalence in the Canadian control group had to be expected, because, in Canada, *H. pylori* prevalence seems to be around 50% at 60 to 70 years [64], similar to that observed in our Greece. Moreover, in some aboriginal Canadian communities *H. pylori* prevalence is as high as 95%. The very low *H. pylori* prevalence (20.2%) in the Canadian control group may perhaps be attributed to the fact that the authors have not excluded patients treated with antibiotics for past infections or for medication use that may interfere with *H. pylori* serology. Galloway et al. admit this fact indirectly by stating that had they used the urea breath test they might have excluded many patients with past treated infections. Moreover, it is known that socioeconomic status and education play a role in *H. pylori* prevalence. The subjects in the Canadian study seem to be at the higher educational level associated with lower *H. pylori* prevalence than the low educational level participants [65, 66], thereby altering the Canadian study's estimations.

F. Iranian Data

An Iranian study published in the *Iranian Journal of Immunology* in 2006 by Razeghinejad et al. aimed at investigating the level of anti *H. pylori* IgG in the aqueous humor of POAG, XFG and cataract patients as control participants for any role of *H. pylori* infection in glaucomatous neuropathy [67]. The study employed 41 cases of glaucoma (21 with XFG and 20 with POAG), comparable to the Greek study, and 39 cases of cataract patients as controls. Aqueous humor was aspirated at the beginning of glaucoma or phacoemulsification cataract surgery in glaucoma and cataract patients, respectively. Anti-*H. pylori* IgG concentration was measured by ELISA. The authors found that the aqueous levels of anti-*H. pylori* IgG in POAG (0.44±0.64 U/mL) had no significant difference with cataract (0.24±0.52 U/mL) and XFG glaucoma group (0.63±0.71 U/mL) (P=0.18 and 0.44, respectively). However, the concentration of this antibody was higher in the aqueous humor of XFG glaucoma patients compared to the control group (p=0.03). The study concluded that a relationship between *H. pylori* infection and POAG was not supported, and that the elevated concentration of anti-*H. pylori* IgG in XFG glaucoma compared to cataract patients may be due to the breakdown of blood-aqueous-barrier. However, the latter finding does not exclude a possible role of these antibodies in XFG glaucoma pathophysiology, because this was not the case for POAG Iranian patients.

In a subsequent letter to the Editor published by Kountouras et al. the limitations of this study were highlighted [68]. Specifically, in the original Iranian study there was no discussion of: (a) the relatively small sample size, (b) the limited power of the study, (c) the possibility that the control group represents a selected group resulting in bias, and (d) the absence of normalization of aqueous antibody titers to another serum protein to serve as control, such as IgG or albumin.

G. Chinese Data

A case-control study by Hong et al. published in the *Asian Journal of Ophthalmology* in 2007 aimed to investigate the prevalence of *H. pylori* infection in Chinese patients with different stages of POAG compared with healthy control individuals [69]. The study enrolled 24 patients with glaucoma (the vast majority of whom had POAG) and equal number of healthy control participants without glaucoma from the same Ophthalmology department. All subjects were tested for *H. pylori* infection using the mentioned ^{13}C-urea breath test, broadly used as the non-invasive diagnostic test of choice. The results showed a significantly higher prevalence of *H. pylori* infection in glaucoma patients compared with controls (54.2% vs. 20.8%; p=0.017). The authors found no association between *H. pylori* infection and glaucoma stage, as estimated by mean visual defect and cup-disc ratio in 13 and 11 patients, *H. pylori* positive and negative, respectively. The authors suggested that the reason for that was that the mean visual field defect and cup-disc ratio of patients with glaucoma showed no significant differences between patients who were *H. pylori* positive or negative.

Commenting on the difference in the Chinese and Greek data concerning the association between *H. pylori* infection and glaucoma stage, Kountouras et al. published a letter in the same Journal in 2009 claiming that their findings suggest that only mean vertical cupping correlated significantly with the titer of anti-*H. pylori*-specific IgG in the aqueous humor, thereby reflecting the severity of glaucomatous damage [70]. Therefore, the data presented by Hong et al. are not comparable to the Greek ones. Moreover, Kountouras et al. noted that measurements in such a small number of patients means that their study is underpowered and of limited value, and thus further recruitment should be encouraged. Furthermore, it would be of particular interest if the Chinese investigators could report any differences or similarities with Kountouras et al.'s data with respect to mean intraocular pressure, short term fluctuation, or corrected loss of variance between *H. pylori* positive and negative patients. Finally, it is important to note that, because *H. pylori* prevalence is significantly lower in gastro-esophageal reflux disease (GERD) patients from East Asia, including China, than in those from Western countries, possibly indicating a protective role against GERD, comparable data did not explain its association with glaucoma development in the Chinese population [70].

H. Israeli Data

In April 2008 a series from Israel was presented in the *Journal of Glaucoma* [71]. Kurtz et al. evaluated the association of *H. pylori* infection and CagA seropositivity and the occurrence of glaucoma in an Israeli cohort of 51 consecutive glaucoma patients versus 36 cataract control subjects. The authors stressed that cagA gene is one of several genes of a pathogenicity island (PAI) called the cag-PAI, and studies emphasizing on the functional importance of this island have reported higher levels of IL-8 production and higher grades of gastric inflammation and atrophy among *H. pylori* strains possessing cag-PAI than cagA-negative strains. Serum samples obtained from all participants were analyzed for *H. pylori* and CagA seropositivity using a commercial immunoblot analysis kit, consisting of Western blot membrane strips prepared by using a surface antigen-enriched preparation of *H. pylori*. The bacterium was detected in 31 of 51 (60.8%) glaucoma patients, compared with 22 of 36 (61.1%) cataract (control) patients (*P*=NS), and 26 of 51 glaucoma patients (51%) and 19 of 6 cataract patients (52.8%) were infected by CagA-positive *H. pylori* strains (P=NS). *H. pylori* infection and CagA-positive strain rates were similar in all glaucoma subgroups and were not statistically different from those of cataract control subjects.

In their discussion, Kurtz et al. attempted to dispel the discrepancy between their results and Greek findings by mentioning epidemiologic studies that demonstrated that both countries share similar patterns in *H. pylori* infection occurrence rates. Addressing this rationale, Kountouras et al. published a Letter to the Editor in the same Journal pointing out that the prevalence of *H. pylori* infection is decreasing due to wide use of eradication practices [72]. Over a 10-year period, Apostolopoulos et al. [73], who conducted one of the epidemiologic studies mentioned by Dr Kurtz, found a significant decrease in *H. pylori* infection in Greece. Likewise, in Tel Aviv, by using the mentioned ^{13}C-urea breath test, broadly used as the non-invasive diagnostic test of choice, having a significantly higher diagnostic accuracy than serology particularly in older subjects [74], Niv Y et al. also found a rather lower prevalence of *H. pylori* infection in 33% of the elderly people studied [75]. Surprisingly, Dr Kurtz reported a much higher prevalence of *H. pylori* infection in his age- and ethnicity-matched controls (61.1%). The reason for this remarkable difference in the prevalence of *H. pylori* infection in the control groups between the studies of Dr Kurtz and Dr Niv may be explained by the very small number of subjects (n=36) included in the first study (n=36 vs. n=2128, respectively).

More importantly, the same group of investigators observed, again in Tel Aviv, by using ^{14}C-urea breath test, a seasonal variation in the prevalence of *H. pylori* infection [76]. Specifically, they found a significant decrease in *H. pylori* prevalence during the summer (July-September) compared with winter (December-January) (42.3% vs. 60.9%, $p<0.007$, results from 371 *H. pylori*-positive participants). According to the results in the study by Dr Kurtz, all their participants might have been recruited during the winter since they found such a high prevalence of *H. pylori* infection. On the other hand, had their subjects been recruited mainly in the summer (42.3%), a statistical difference in *H. pylori* prevalence between their glaucoma patient and controls might have been observed. In any case, the most significant limitation in this study is the very low number of patients enrolled.

From another viewpoint, *H. pylori* positivity in Israel is also associated with ethnic variations [Sephardic (Asian and African origins) versus Ashkenazi (European and American origins)] [77], which should have been taken into consideration in order to determine the prevalence of *H. pylori* infection in both glaucoma patients and control subjects.

In addition, Kountouras et al. used mainly female controls with iron deficiency anemia (IDA) in their studies including glaucoma (*H. pylori* incidence: 53.3%) and MS (*H. pylori* incidence: 44%). In this respect, relative Israeli studies in pre-menopausal female subjects with IDA, comparable to Kountouras's MS female controls, reported an *H. pylori* incidence of only 16% among participants [78].

In view of the above-mentioned data, the explanation offered by Dr Kurtz for the discrepancy between his and Greek studies stemming from different *H. pylori* infection occurrence rates between Greece and Israel was certainly not dispelled by some epidemiologic studies that demonstrated that both countries share similar patterns, since different patterns do exist.

With regard to the potential argument that Kountouras et al. also used a small number of patients, in their studies *H. pylori* infection was mainly determined by histologic detection of the bacteria in mucosal biopsy specimens, considered to be the mentioned actual gold standard for the diagnosis of this infection. It is important to note that the serological test has limitations because it does not discriminate between current and old infections. Such a distinction is essential because current *H. pylori* infection induces humoral and cellular immune (predominant *H. pylori*-specific Th1 response with a Th1-type cytokine production leading to gastric epithelial cell apoptotic damage) responses that, owing to the sharing of homologous epitopes (molecular mimicry), cross-react with components of nerves, thereby affecting or perpetuating neural tissue damage including glaucomatous optic neuropathy. Moreover, eradication of *H. pylori* infection seems to delay glaucoma progression, particularly at early disease stages. Although Kountouras et al. admit it was too difficult to obtain consent of their glaucoma patients to be submitted to an upper gastrointestinal endoscopy, they managed to recruit a number of 41 by using this gold diagnostic standard, and thus they consider this number as rather reliable for their conclusions.

Moreover, Kountouras et al. indicated that differences might exist particularly in the prevalence of XFG glaucoma between Greek and other populations, with a high incidence in Greece and Scandinavia.

Finally, apart from CagA of *H. pylori* possibly being involved in some neurodegenerative disorders [79], the well-established VacA of *H. pylori* also appears to be involved in peripheral and central nervous system neuropathies including GBS and the prion encephalopathies [59, 80]. In this respect, the patients with anti-r-VacA IgG show appreciable demyelination of the peripheral nerves [52, 81]. Therefore, future VacA-relative studies in glaucoma patients may cast light on *H. pylori* VacA cytotoxin involvement in glaucomatous pathophysiology.

I. Indian Data

Underscoring the fact that the prevalence of *H. pylori* infection may vary in the general population and may be dependent upon cultural, socioeconomic, and geographic differences, a well-designed study from an Indian group of investigators led by Deshpande et al. was published in the *Journal of Glaucoma* in December 2008 [82]. The authors performed a prospective case-control analysis aiming to investigate the prevalence of exposure to *H. pylori* in subjects with POAG and exfoliation glaucoma in a South Indian population. The investigators enrolled 150 participants (50 with POAG, 50 with XFG, and 50 age-matched controls undergoing cataract surgery for senile cataract). Inclusion and exclusion criteria matched those in the Greek studies. The Indian investigators obtained 60 μL of aqueous humor before creating the sclera flap in glaucoma surgery and before fashioning a corneoscleral tunnel in the phacoemulsification group. In addition, they drew 3 mL venous blood from each subject on the same day of surgery. All samples were analyzed for presence of *H. pylori* by ELISA, and a cut-off value for the aqueous humor was established by the Indian investigators in exactly the same way with the study by Kountouras and associates.

Serum analysis of anti-*H. pylori* IgG antibodies revealed that the POAG group had significantly higher titers than the XFG group (52.26±52.51 vs. 25.22±35.27; P=0.01). Moreover, anti-*H. pylori* IgG antibodies were significantly higher in the serum of POAG versus control subjects (54.05±55.04 vs. 33.83±41.73; P=0.04). Qualitative data showed that the prevalence of *H. pylori* infection in POAG patients was significantly higher than XFG patients and cataract controls (POAG: 70%, XFG: 44%, controls: 66%; *P*[POAG vs. XFG]=0.009, *P*[POAG vs. controls]=0.04, *P*[XFG vs. controls]=0.67). The authors failed to show any statistical differences in the titers of anti-*H. pylori* IgG antibodies in the aqueous humor among the 3 groups. Finally, the mean vertical cupping in POAG and XFG was statistically higher compared with control group (0.82±0.10 vs. 0.48±0.22, *P*=0.02; and 0.79±0.15 vs. 0.48±0.22; *P*=0.08, respectively).

In their discussion, the authors hypothesized that auto-immune injury to the optic nerve from *H. pylori* antibodies is initiated early in life and manifests in the later decades, which could partly explain the increasing POAG prevalence with increasing age, while the *H. pylori* infection progressively declined at the same time [82].

Moreover, commenting on the lack of association between XFG and *H. pylori* infection the authors hypothesized that this could be owing to the different pathogenic mechanisms underlying these glaucoma groups. XFG is a form of open-angle glaucoma secondary to blockade of trabecular meshwork by exfoliation material and the release of pigments or both leading to high intraocular pressure and subsequent glaucomatous optic nerve head damage, and thus it is less likely to be directly related to serum anti-*H. pylori* status of these individuals.

Finally, the authors point 2 limitations in their study, the first being the age difference between glaucoma patients and cataract controls, and the second being the fact that their population was fairly homogenous. In the South Indian population, the infection rate of *H. pylori* is 83.3%, thereby requiring a very large population to be screened to prove the statistical difference in *H. pylori* infection among subjects with glaucoma and general population. Despite this fact, the observed statistical increased incidence in *H. pylori* infection among a small number of such populations with glaucoma compared with cataract controls, make these findings rather reliable for conclusions. In conclusion, the Indian data support a possible role for *H. pylori* infection as a causative mechanism of POAG [82].

J. Italian Metanalysis

In a 2009 issue of the *British Journal of Ophthalmology*, Izzotti et al. [83] published collective data in order to elucidate any ethnic correlation between glaucoma and *H. pylori* infection and if both diseases share common pathogenetic mechanisms, mainly oxidative injury. Consistent associations were found between the mentioned Greek data and POAG and/or XFG data from China (using ^{13}C-urea breath test), Turkey (using serology), and Iran (investigating aqueous humor antibody concentrations). In contrast, in their paper, Izzotti and colleagues report that the two studies from Canada and Israel found no association between seropositivity for *H. pylori* infection and the occurrence of glaucoma.

In an Editorial which accompanied the metanalysis by Izzotti et al., Prof. Kountouras, by adding the more recent data from India indicating the role of *H. pylori*-specific IgG antibodies in causative mechanisms for glaucoma, stressed that geographical and ethnic similarities or differences in *H. pylori* prevalence in glaucoma patients appear to exist [84]. Therefore, further relative large studies should be considered, particularly in populations at greater risk of *H. pylori* infection and glaucoma development and progression [46, 85] before reaching a final conclusion. The last is essential because eradication of *H. pylori* infection might delay the progression of glaucoma and other glaucoma-associated neurodegenerative diseases [50, 59, 86-89], particularly at early disease stages.

Izzotti and colleagues described a comprehensive focus on *H. pylori*-induced oxidative stress involved in the pathogenesis of neurodegenerative diseases, mainly including glaucoma. Importantly, oxidative stress is an essential underlying cause of neuroinflammatory and neurodegenerative diseases including glaucoma and BBB damage connected to them; oxidative stress activates protein tyrosine kinase and matrix metalloproteinases resulting in BBB dysfunction [43, 90].

Specifically, a series of factors have been implicated in inducing BBB disruption, including inflammatory mediators (e.g., cytokines and chemokines induced by *H. pylori* infection) and oxidative stress [91, 92]. *H. pylori* could indirectly affect the brain and other target organs, e.g. the heart, through the release of numerous cytokines such as TNF-α acting at a distance; TNF-α is involved in BBB disruption through a mechanism involving matrix metalloproteinases upregulation [93]. TNF-α and IL-6 (TNF-α is the main trigger for the production of IL-6 by a variety of cells) play important roles in the regulation of the synthesis of other acute phase proteins which are established risk factors for atherosclerosis, such as fibrinogen and factor VIII. These cytokines also have profound effects on lipid metabolism directly at the site of the atherosclerotic lesion, but could influence the atheroma process through blood circulating levels, distant production of cytokines, or through stimulating circulating white blood cells to produce them, thereby contributing to BBB disruption and pathogenesis of heart and brain neurodegenerative diseases [94-96]. In addition, *H. pylori*-induced cytotoxin VacA exhibits chemotactic activities to the bone marrow-derived mast cells (BMDMCs) and induces BMDMCs to produce proinflammatory cytokines including TNF-α [97]; BMDMCs reside adjacent to blood and lymphatic channels, mainly under epithelial surfaces including the BBB and gastrointestinal tract [98]. *H. pylori* stimulates mast cells directly or via gastrin induction and mast cells are actively involved in the pathogenesis of *H. pylori*-associated pathologies [98]. Apart from activated mast cells, vascular endothelial growth factor (VEGF), IL-8, chymase or tryptase (a serine endoprotease released by mast cells) and mast cell growth factor linked to *H. pylori* infection [91, 98], mast cells themselves can be stimulated by corticotropin-releasing hormone, secreted under stress, to release mediators including histamine, IL-8, tryptase and VEGF, which disrupt the BBB [99].

BBB disruption could play an important role in promoting entry of immune cell infiltration and pathogens into the brain resulting in the development of brain pathologies [102]. In this regard, the influx of activated monocytes infected with *Chlamydia pneumoniae* (*C. pneumoniae*) through the BBB could have dire consequences in the brain leading to the development of degenerative diseases, including AD [100] and possibly glaucoma; infectants including *herpes simplex virus 1*, *C. pneumoniae*, and even *Borrelia* species have been found in brain regions demonstrating significant AD pathology.

Apart from BBB disruption, an infection-based animal model demonstrated that following intranasal inoculation of BALB/c mice with *C. pneumoniae*, amyloid plaques/deposits consistent with those observed in the AD brain develop, thereby implicating this infection in the etiology of AD [100]. Specifically, the intranasal route of inoculation was used for the following reasons: the recognized olfactory deficits in AD; the previous PCR findings of *C. pneumoniae* presence in human olfactory bulbs; and the respiratory nature of this pathogen providing direct access to the nasal olfactory neuroepithelium. In this respect, after intranasal inoculation, light microscopy and electron microscopy revealed the presence of *C. pneumoniae* in the olfactory bulbs of animals. Upon labeling for typical pathology in areas of the brain associated with AD pathology (e.g., hippocampus, endorhinal cortex) and in a region less affected in AD (e.g., cerebellum), the most striking finding was the presence of β-amyloid immunoreactive amyloid plaques, thereby suggesting that amyloid plaque formation in the brain is a consequence of infection with *C. pneumoniae* [100]. Comparably, the intranasal *H. pylori* colonization [101] may also represent a route of its subsequent access the eyes, resulting in the development of *H. pylori*-related ocular pathologies, possibly including glaucoma.

Besides, autoimmune injury to the optic nerve may occur directly by autoantibodies or indirectly via a "mimicked" autoimmune response to a sensitizing antigen, which, in turn, damages RGC. Specific antibodies are found in increased levels in glaucoma patients sera, and when these antibodies access the brain due to BBB disruption, they are capable of killing retinal cells, thereby contributing to glaucoma pathologies [49]. Specifically, comparable data could also be considered in the presence of blood-ocular barrier (BOB) dysfunction. In this respect, *H. pylori* antibodies circulating in the bloodstream can enter the aqueous circulation due to BOB disruption possibly contributing to glaucoma development and progression [49].

K. Concluding Remarks

A significant body of evidence on the association between *H. pylori* infection and glaucoma from various geographical areas of the world is being built up. Table 1 summarizes all available data to date. Studies published so far have limitations and are difficult to compare and incorporated in a meta-analysis, mainly owing to the heterogeneity of the ethnic populations, and of the methods for the detection of *H. pylori* infection. Currently available studies are generally small, indicating the difficulty persuading asymptomatic from the upper gastrointestinal tract glaucoma patients to undergo an investigation for *H. pylori* infection.

A number of pathogenetic mechanisms have been proposed, but so far the published studies focus on clinical and epidemiological parameters, mainly involving the prevalence of *H. pylori* infection in different glaucoma cohorts. Certainly all the aforementioned speculations concerning the pathogenesis that links *H. pylori* and POAG merit future in-depth investigation.

Table 1. A synopsis of all the studies available concerning the role of *Helicobacter pylori* infection in glaucoma

Year	First author	Country	Outcome	Method used	Sample used
2000	Kountouras J [60]	Greece	Higher prevalence	Histology/ELISA	Biopsy/Serum
2000	Ozturk F [61]	Turkey	Higher prevalence	ELISA	Serum
2001	Kountouras J [26]	Greece	Higher prevalence	Histology/ELISA	Biopsy/Serum
2002	Kountouras J [48]	Greece	Eradication improved glaucoma	Histology/ELISA /Visual field indices	Biopsy/Serum
2003	Kountouras J [49]	Greece	Higher anti-*H. pylori* IgG titer in aqueous humor	ELISA	Aqueous humor/Serum
2003	Galloway PH [62]	Canada	No difference in prevalence	ELISA	Serum
2006	Razeghinejad MR [67]	Iran	Higher anti-*H. pylori* IgG titer in aqueous humor only in XFG	ELISA	Aqueous humor
2007	Hong Y [69]	China	Higher prevalence	^{13}C-urea breath test	Breath test
2008	Kurtz S [71]	Israel	No difference in CagA-positive strain rates	Immunoblot analysis kit	Serum
2008	Deshpande N [82]	India	Higher prevalence and higher anti-*H. pylori* IgG titer in aqueous humor only in POAG	ELISA	Aqueous humor/Serum
2009	Izzotti A [83]	Italy	Meta-analysis		

References

[1] Johnson GJ, Foster PJ. Can we prevent angle-closure glaucoma? *Eye*, 2005 19, 1119-1124.

[2] McKinnon SJ. Glaucoma: ocular Alzheimer's disease? *Front Biosci,* 2003 8, s1140-s1156.

[3] Kountouras J, Gavalas E, Zavos C, et al. Alzheimer's disease and *Helicobacter pylori* infection: defective immune regulation and apoptosis as proposed common links. *Med. Hypotheses.* 2007 68, 378-388.

[4] Orgul S, Prunte C, Flammer J. Endothelium-derived vasoactive substances relevant to normal-tension glaucoma. *Curr. Opin. Ophthalmol.* 1998 9, 88-94.

[5] Luscher TF, Meyer P, Haefliger IO, Flammer J. Endothelial mediators as regulators of the ophthalmic circulation. In: Drance SM, Anderson DR, eds. *Optic Nerve in Glaucoma.* New York: Kugler Publications, 1995 259-281.

[6] Orgul S. Physiology of optic nerve perfusion. In: Drance SM, ed. Vascular Risk Factors and Neuroprotection in Glaucoma: Update 1996. New York: Kugler Publications, 1997 pp. 1-14.

[7] Sugiyama T, Moriya S, Oku H, Azuma I. Association of endothelin-1 with normal tension glaucoma: clinical and fundamental studies. *Surv. Ophthalmol.* 1995 39(Suppl 1), S49-S56.
[8] Gass A, Flammer J, Linder L, et al. Inverse correlation between endothelin-1-induced peripheral microvascular vasoconstriction and blood pressure in glaucoma patients. *Graefes Arch. Clin. Exp. Ophthalmol.* 1997 235, 634-638.
[9] Noske W, Hensen J, Wiederholt M. Endothelin-like immunoreactivity in aqueous humor of patients with primary open angle glaucoma and cataract. *Graefes Arch. Clin. Exp. Ophthalmol.* 1997 235, 551-552.
[10] Tezel G, Kass MA, Kolker AE, et al. Plasma and aqueous humor endothelin levels in primary open-angle glaucoma. *J. Glaucoma.* 1997 6, 83-89.
[11] Cioffi GA, Sullivan P. The effect of chronic ischemia on the primate optic nerve. *Eur. J. Ophthalmol.* 1999 9(Suppl 1), S34-S36.
[12] Hoyng PF, Greve EL, Frederikse K, et al. Platelet aggregation and glaucoma. *Doc. Ophthamol.* 1985 61, 167-173.
[13] Babizhayev MA, Mucha AI. Modulative effects of cell adhesion peptide (Arg-Gly-Asp-Ser) on the aggregation of stimulated platelets from ophthalmic patients. *Clin. Chim. Acta.* 1991 196, 77-85.
[14] Hoyng PF, de Jong N, Oosting H, Stilma J. Platelet aggregation, disc haemorrhage and progressive loss of visual fields in glaucoma. A seven year follow-up study on glaucoma. *Int. Ophthalmol.* 1992 16, 65-73.
[15] Zakharova GP, Kaliteevskii PF, Kaufman OIA. Comparative pathology of the choroid vessels in glaucoma, hypertension and arteriosclerosis. *Arkh. Patol.* 1976 38, 12-16.
[16] Hayreh SS, Bill A, Sperber GO. Effects of high intraocular pressure on the glucose metabolism in the retina and optic nerve in old atherosclerotic monkeys. *Graefes Arch. Clin. Exp. Ophthalmol.* 1994 232, 745-752.
[17] Kaiser HJ, Stümpfig D, Flammer J. Short-term effect of dipyridamole on blood flow velocities in the extraocular vessels. *Int. Ophthalmol.* 1995-1996 19, 355-358.
[18] Drance SM. Glaucoma: a look beyond intraocular pressure. *Am. J. Ophthalmol.* 1997 123, 817-819.
[19] Hayreh SS. Retinal and optic nerve head ischemic disorders and atherosclerosis: role of serotonin. *Prog. Retin. Eye Res.* 1999 18, 191-221.
[20] Wakefield D, Lloyd A. The role of cytokines in the pathogenesis of inflammatory eye disease. *Cytokine.* 1992 4, 1-5.
[21] Frank WA, Limb GA, Stanford MR, et al. Cytokines in human intraocular inflammation. *Curr. Eye Res.* 1992 11(Suppl 1), 187-191.
[22] Cunliffe IA, Richardson PS, Rees RC, Rennie IG. Effect of TNF, IL-1, and IL-6 on the proliferation of human Tenon's capsule fibroblasts in tissue culture. *Br. J. Ophthalmol.* 1995 79, 590-595.
[23] Ritch R. Perspective on exfoliation syndrome. *J. Glaucoma.* 2001 10(5 Suppl 1), S33-S35.
[24] Ringvold A. Epidemiology of the pseudo-exfoliation syndrome. *Acta Ophthalmol. Scand.* 1999 77, 371-375.
[25] Van Buskirk EM. Aphorisms of the hero. *J. Glaucoma.* 2003 12, 189-192.

[26] Kountouras J, Mylopoulos N, Boura P, et al. Relationship between *Helicobacter pylori* infection and glaucoma. *Ophthalmology.* 2001 108, 599-604.
[27] Hart WM. The epidemiology of primary open-angle glaucoma and ocular hypertension. In: Ritch R, Shields MB, Krupin T, eds. *The Glaucomas.* St. Louis: Mosby, 1989 pp. 790-791.
[28] Cave DR. How is *Helicobacter pylori* transmitted? *Gastroenterology.* 1997 113, S9-S14.
[29] Graham DY, Sung JJY. *Helicobacter pylori.* In: Feldman M, Friedman LS, Sleisenger MH, eds. Sleisenger & Fordtran's Gastrointestinal and Liver Disease. 8th ed. Philadelphia: WB Saunders, 2006 pp. 1049-1066.
[30] Mendall MA, Goggin PM, Molineaux N, et al. Relation of *Helicobacter pylori* infection and coronary heart disease. *Br. Heart J.* 1994 71, 437-439.
[31] Kountouras J, Halkides F, Hatzopoulos D, et al. Decrease in plasma fibrinogen after eradication of *Helicobacter pylori* infection in patients with coronary heart disease. *Hell J. Gastroenterol.* 1997 10, 113-117.
[32] McColl KEL. What remaining questions regarding *Helicobacter pylori* and associated diseases should be addressed by future research? View from Europe. *Gastroenterology.* 1997 113, S158-S162.
[33] Gasbarrini A, Franceschi F, Arnuzzi A, et al. Extradigestive manifestations of *Helicobacter pylori* gastric infection. *Gut.* 1999 45(Suppl 1), I9-I12.
[34] Gasbarrini A, Franceschi F, Cammarota G, et al. Vascular and immunological disorders associated with *Helicobacter pylori* infection. *Ital. J. Gastroenterol. Hepatol.* 1998 30, 115-118.
[35] Gasbarrini A, De Luca A, Fiore G, et al. Beneficial effects of *Helicobacter pylori* eradication on migraine. *Hepatogastroenterology.* 1998 21, 765-770.
[36] Bodger K, Wyatt JI, Heatley RV. Gastric mucosal secretion of interleukin-10: relations to histopathology, *Helicobacter pylori* status, and tumour necrosis factor-a secretion. *Gut.* 1997 40, 739-744.
[37] Shimoyama T, Crabtree JE. Bacterial factors and immune pathogenesis in *Helicobacter pylori* infection. *Gut.* 1998 43(Suppl 1), S2-S5.
[38] Akimoto M, Hashimoto H, Shigemoto M, Yokoyama I. Relationship between recurrence of gastric ulcer and the microcirculation. *J. Cardiovasc. Pharmacol.* 1998 31(Suppl1), S507-S508.
[39] Markus HS, Mendall MA. *Helicobacter pylori* infection: a risk factor for ischaemic cerebrovascular disease and carotid atheroma. *J. Neurol. Neurosurg. Psychiatry.* 1998 64, 104-107.
[40] Panes J, Granger DN. Leukocyte-endothelial cell interactions: molecular mechanisms and implications in gastrointestinal disease. *Gastroenterology.* 1998 114, 1066-1090.
[41] Clement CI, Goldberg I, Healey PR, Graham SL. Plasma homocysteine, MTHFR gene mutation, and open-angle glaucoma. *J. Glaucoma.* 2009 18, 73-78.
[42] Flammer J, Mozaffarieh M. What is the present pathogenetic concept of glaucomatous optic neuropathy? *Surv. Ophthalmol.* 2007 52(Suppl 2), S162-S173.
[43] Grieshaber MC, Flammer J. Does the blood-brain barrier play a role in glaucoma? *Surv. Ophthalmol.* 2007 52(Suppl 2), S115-S121.

[44] Kountouras J, Zavos C, Chatzopoulos D. Apoptosis: an overview and a proposed link between glaucoma and *Helicobacter pylori* infection. In: Reece SM (ed). *Trends in Glaucoma Research.* 1st Edn, New York: Nova Biomedical Books, 2005 pp. 1-28.

[45] Kountouras J, Zavos C, Chatzopoulos D. Primary open-angle glaucoma: pathophysiology and treatment. *Lancet.* 2004 364, 1311-1312.

[46] Kountouras J, Zavos C, Grigoriadis N, Deretzi G, Katsinelos P, Tzilves D. *Helicobacter pylori* infection as a risk factor for primary open-angle glaucoma. *Clin. Experiment. Ophthalmol.* 2008 36, 196.

[47] Pajares JM. *Helicobacter pylori* infection and gastric cancer in Spain. *Hepatogastroenterology.* 2001 48, 1556-1559.

[48] Kountouras J, Mylopoulos N, Chatzopoulos D, et al. Eradication of *Helicobacter pylori* may be beneficial in the management of chronic open-angle glaucoma. *Arch. Intern. Med.* 2002 162, 1237-1244.

[49] Kountouras J, Mylopoulos N, Konstas AG, et al. Increased levels of *Helicobacter pylori* IgG antibodies in aqueous humor of patients with primary open-angle and exfoliation glaucoma. *Graefes Arch. Clin. Exp. Ophthalmol.* 2003 241, 884-890.

[50] Kountouras J, Deretzi G, Grigoriadis N, et al. Guillain-Barré syndrome. *Lancet. Neurol.* 2008 7, 1080-1081.

[51] Chiba S, Sugiyama T, Matsumoto H, et al. Antibodies against *Helicobacter pylori* were detected in the obtained from patients with Guillain-Barre syndrome. *Ann. Neurol.* 1998 44, 686-688.

[52] Chiba S, Sugiyama T, Yonekura K, et al. An antibody to VacA of *Helicobacter pylori* in cerebrospinal fluid from patients with Guillain-Barre syndrome. *J. Neurol. Neurosurg. Psychiatry.* 2002, 73, 76-78.

[53] Kountouras J, Zavos C, Chatzopoulos D. Induction of apoptosis as a proposed pathophysiological link between glaucoma and *Helicobacter pylori* infection. *Med. Hypotheses.* 2004 62, 378-381.

[54] Kountouras J, Tsolaki M, Gavalas E, et al. Relationship between *Helicobacter pylori* infection and Alzheimer disease. *Neurology.* 2006 66, 938-940.

[55] Kountouras J, Tsolaki M, Boziki M, et al. Association between *Helicobacter pylori* infection and mild cognitive impairment. *Eur. J. Neurol.* 2007 14, 976-982.

[56] Kountouras J, Boziki M, Gavalas E, et al. Eradication of *Helicobacter pylori* may be beneficial in the management of Alzheimer's disease. *J. Neurol.* 2009 (in press)

[57] Kountouras J, Boziki M, Gavalas E, et al. Increased cerebrospinal fluid *Helicobacter pylori* antibody in Alzheimer's disease. *Int. J. Neurosci.* 2009 (in press)

[58] Gavalas E, Kountouras J, Deretzi G, et al. *Helicobacter pylori* and multiple sclerosis. *J. Neuroimmunol.* 2007 188, 187-189.

[59] Kountouras J, Deretzi G, Zavos C, et al. Association between *Helicobacter pylori* infection and acute inflammatory demyelinating polyradiculoneuropathy. *Eur. J. Neurol.* 2005 12, 139-143.

[60] Kountouras JK, Mylopoulos NM, Boura P, et al. Relation between *Helicobacter pylori* infection and glaucoma. In: Program and abstracts of the 6th Congress of the European Glaucoma Society, London, 2000, p. 98.

[61] Ozturk F, Kurt E, Inan UU, et al. Is *Helicobacter pylori* related to glaucoma? In: Program and abstracts of the 6th Congress of the European Glaucoma Society, London, 2000, p. 108.

[62] Galloway PH, Warner SJ, Morshed MG, Mikelberg FS. *Helicobacter pylori* infection and the risk for open-angle glaucoma. *Ophthalmology.* 2003 110, 922-925.

[63] Kountouras J, Zavos C, Chatzopoulos D. *Helicobacter pylori* and glaucoma. *Ophthalmology.* 2003 110, 2433-2434.

[64] McKeown I, Orr P, Macdonald S, et al. *Helicobacter pylori* in the Canadian arctic: seroprevalence and detection in community water samples. *Am. J. Gastroenterol.* 1999 94, 1823-1829.

[65] Russo A, Eboli M, Pizzetti P, et al. Determinants of *Helicobacter pylori* seroprevalence among Italian blood donors. *Eur. J. Gastroenterol. Hepatol.* 1999 11, 867-873.

[66] Stettin D, Waldmann A, Wolters M, et al. [Infection with *Helicobacter pylori*--outcome of a cross-sectional investigation] *Dtsch. Med. Wochenschr.* 2007 132, 2677-1682.

[67] Razeghinejad MR, Kamali-Sarvestani E, Farvardin M, Pourhabibi A. Aqueous levels of anti-*Helicobacter pylori* IgG antibody in patients with primary open angle and pseudoexfoliation glaucoma. *Iran J. Immunol.* 2006 3, 86-90.

[68] Zavos C, Kountouras J. *Helicobacter pylori* antibodies in the aqueous humor of an Iranian glaucoma cohort. *Iran J. Immunol.* 2006 3, 192-193.

[69] Hong Y, Zhang C, Duan L, Wang W. Relationship between *Helicobacter pylori* infection and open angle glaucoma in China. *Asian J. Ophthalmol.* 2007 9, 205-208.

[70] Kountouras J, Zavos C, Katsinelos P, et al. *Helicobacter pylori* infection and open-angle glaucoma association: comparison of Greek and Chinese data. *Asian J. Ophthalmol.* 2009 (in press)

[71] Kurtz S, Regenbogen M, Goldiner I, et al. No association between *Helicobacter pylori* infection or CagA-bearing strains and glaucoma. *J. Glaucoma.* 2008 17, 223-226.

[72] Kountouras J, Zavos C, Katsinelos P, et al. Greek and Israeli patterns of *Helicobacter pylori* infection and their association with glaucoma: similarities or diversities? *J. Glaucoma.* 2008 17, 503-504.

[73] Apostolopoulos P, Vafiadis-Zouboulis I, Tzivras M, et al. *Helicobacter pylori* (H. pylori) infection in Greece: the changing prevalence during a ten-year period and its antigenic profile. *BMC Gastroenterol.* 2002 2, 11.

[74] Pilotto A, Franceschi M, Leandro G, et al. Noninvasive diagnosis of *Helicobacter pylori* infection in older subjects: comparison of the 13C-urea breath test with serology. *J. Gerontol. A Biol. Sci. Med. Sci.* 2000 55, M163-M167.

[75] Niv Y, Niv G, Koren R. 13C-urea breath test for diagnosis of *Helicobacter pylori* infection in the elderly. *Dig. Dis. Sci.* 2004 49, 1840-1844.

[76] Moshkowitz M, Konikoff FM, Arber N, et al. Seasonal variation in the frequency of *Helicobacter pylori* infection: a possible cause of the seasonal occurrence of peptic ulcer disease. *Am. J. Gastroenterol.* 1994 89, 731-733.

[77] Birkenfeld S, Keter D, Dikman R, et al. Prevalence of *Helicobacter pylori* infection in health-care personnel of primary care and gastroenterology clinics. *J. Clin. Gastroenterol.* 2004 38, 19-23.

[78] Carter D, Maor Y, Bar-Meir S, Avidan B. Prevalence and predictive signs for gastrointestinal lesions in premenopausal women with iron deficiency anemia. *Dig. Dis. Sci.* 2008 53, 3138-3144.

[79] Weller C, Oxlade N, Dobbs SM, et al. Role of inflammation in gastrointestinal tract in aetiology and pathogenesis of idiopathic parkinsonism. *FEMS Immunol. Med. Microbiol.* 2005 44, 129-135.

[80] Kourie JI. Prion channel proteins and their role in vacuolation and neurodegenerative diseases. *Eur. Biophys. J.* 2002 31, 409-416.

[81] Chiba S, Sugiyama T, Yonekura K, et al. An antibody to VacA of *Helicobacter pylori* in the CSF of patients with Miller-Fisher syndrome. *Neurology.* 2004 63, 2184-2186.

[82] Deshpande N, Lalitha P, Krishna das SR, et al. *Helicobacter pylori* IgG antibodies in aqueous humor and serum of subjects with primary open angle and pseudo-exfoliation glaucoma in a South Indian population. *J. Glaucoma.* 2008 17, 605-610.

[83] Izzotti A, Saccà SC, Bagnis A, et al. Glaucoma and *Helicobacter pylori* infection. Correlations and controversies. *Br. J. Ophthalmol.* 2009 (in press)

[84] Kountouras J. *Helicobacter pylori*: an intruder conspiring glaucomatous neuropathy. *Br. J. Ophthalmol.* 2009 (in press)

[85] Kountouras J, Zavos C, Grigoriadis N, et al. *Helicobacter pylori* infection as an enviromental familial clustering risk factor for primary open-angle glaucoma. *Clin. Experiment. Ophthalmol.* 2008 36, 296-297.

[86] Tamura H, Kawakami H, Kanamoto T, et al. High frequency of open-angle glaucoma in Japanese patients with Alzheimer's disease. *J. Neurol. Sci.* 2006 246, 79-83.

[87] Kountouras J, Zavos C, Gavalas E, et al. Normal-tension glaucoma and Alzheimer's disease: *Helicobacter pylori* as a possible common underlying risk factor. *Med. Hypotheses.* 2007 68, 228-229.

[88] Kountouras J, Gavalas E, Boziki M, Zavos C. *Helicobacter pylori* may be involved in cognitive impairment and dementia development through induction of atrophic gastritis, vitamin B-12–folate deficiency, and hyperhomocysteinemia sequence. *Am. J. Clin. Nutr.* 2007 86, 805-806.

[89] Kountouras J, Zavos C, Gavalas E, et al. *Helicobacter pylori* may hold a variable role in multiple sclerosis based on ethnicity. *Med. Hypotheses.* 2008 71, 614-5.

[90] Haorah J, Ramirez SH, Schall K, et al. Oxidative stress activates protein tyrosine kinase and matrix metalloproteinases leading to blood-brain barrier dysfunction. *J. Neurochem.* 2007 101, 566-576.

[91] Kountouras J, Zavos C, Chatzopoulos D, Katsinelos P. New aspects of *Helicobacter pylori* infection involvement in gastric oncogenesis. *J. Surg. Res.* 2008 146, 149-158.

[92] Keep RF, Xiang J, Ennis SR, et al. Blood-brain barrier function in intracerebral hemorrhage. *Acta Neurochir. Suppl.* 2008 105, 73-77.

[93] Candelario-Jalil E, Taheri S, Yang Y, et al. Cyclooxygenase inhibition limits blood-brain barrier disruption following intracerebral injection of tumor necrosis factor-alpha in the rat. *J. Pharmacol. Exp. Ther.* 2007 323, 488-498.

[94] Mendall MA, Patel P, Asante M, et al. Relation of serum cytokine concentrations to cardiovascular risk factors and coronary heart disease. *Heart.* 1997 78, 273-277.

[95] Guerreiro RJ, Santana I, Brás JM, et al. Peripheral inflammatory cytokines as biomarkers in Alzheimer's disease and mild cognitive impairment. *Neurodegener Dis.* 2007 4, 406-412.

[96] Tan ZS, Beiser AS, Vasan RS, et al. Inflammatory markers and the risk of Alzheimer disease: the Framingham Study. *Neurology.* 2007 68, 1902-1908.

[97] Supajatura V, Ushio H, Wada A, et al. Cutting edge: VacA, a vacuolating cytotoxin of *Helicobacter pylori,* directly activates mast cells for migration and production of proinflammatory cytokines. *J. Immunol.* 2002 168, 2603-2607.

[98] Kountouras J, Zavos C, Diamantidis MD, et al. A concept of *Helicobacter pylori* and stress-secreted mast cells' potential involvement in brain metastases. *J. Neuroimmunol.* 2009 Feb 4. [Epub ahead of print]

[99] Theoharides TC, Rozniecki JJ, Sahagian G, et al. Impact of stress and mast cells on brain metastases. *J. Neuroimmunol.* 2008 205, 1-7.

[100] Itzhaki RF, Wozniak MA, Appelt DM, Balin BJ. Infiltration of the brain by pathogens causes Alzheimer's disease. *Neurobiol. Aging.* 2004 25, 619-627.

[101] Kim HY, Dhong HJ, Chung SK, et al. Intranasal *Helicobacter pylori* colonization does not correlate with the severity of chronic rhinosinusitis. *Otolaryngol. Head Neck Surg.* 2007 136, 390-395.

In: Eye Research Developments
Editor: Alan N. Westerhouse

ISBN: 978-1-60741-177-2

Chapter IV

Efficacy of Each Glaucoma Drug in Multiple Drug Therapy in Patients with Open-Angle Glaucoma and Ocular Hypertension

Hiroshi Kobayashi** *and Kaori Kobayashi
[1] Department of Ophthalmology, Kokura Memorial Hospital, Kitakyushu,
[2] Department of Ophthalmology, Kurashiki Central Hospital, Kurashiki, Japan

Abstract

Purpose: Multiple drug therapy is used to treat glaucoma when monotherapy is not effective or sufficient. A combination of several drugs, including prostaglandin analogues, β-blockers, cholinergic agonists, adrenergic agonists, α_2-stimulants, α_1-blockers, and carbonic anhydrase inhibitors has been reported to be effective. These studies are carried out at the time when additional drugs were first administered in patients already receiving one drug. Efficacy of each drug in the patients who continue to administer two or more drugs was unknown. In this study, we studied the efficacy of each drug in these patients with its discontinuation.

Patients and Methods: We conducted 2 series of investigation; 1) thirty patients with open angle glaucoma or ocular hypertension who receiving both latanoprost 0.005% and timolol XE 0.5%. Either latanoprost or timolol XE was discontinued and 8 weeks later was resumed. A change in intraocular pressure was studied. 2) Thirty patients with open angle glaucoma or ocular hypertension who administered latanoprost 0.005%, brinzolamide 2% and timolol XE 0.5% were studied. One of timolol XE, brinzolamide and latanoprost was discontinued and 8 weeks later was resumed. A change in intraocular pressure was studied.

Results: In the patients who administered latanoprost and timolol XE, discontinuation of latanoprost or timolol XE provided an IOP increase of 4.2±1.8mmHg (27.1±13.4%) or 1.3±0.7mmHg (8.7±4.7%), respectively. The IOP increase achieved by the discontinuation of latanoprost was significantly greater compared with timolol XE ($P < 0.0001$). There was no significant difference in mean intraocular pressure between before drug discontinuation and at 8 weeks after drug resumption in any group. In the patients administering latanoprost, timolol XE or brinzolamide, a significant increase in

* Address for correspondence: To Hiroshi Kobayashi MD, PhD; Department of Ophthalmology, Kokura Memorial Hospital; 1-1 Kifune-machi, Kokurakita-ku, Kitakyushu 802-8555, Japan; Phone: 093-921-2231; Fax: 093-921-8497; E-mail: kobi@earth.ocn.ne.jp

mean intraocular pressure was found following drug discontinuation (latanoprost: P = 0.0001; timolol XE: P = 0.0224; brinzolamide: P = 0.0030). Mean change in intraocular pressure by discontinuation of the drug was +4.0 ± 1.2 mmHg (25.3 ± 9.7 %) in the latanoprost group, +1.4±0.7 mmHg (9.2±4.9 %) in the timolol XE group, +4.1±1.9 mmHg (26.7±12.7%) in the latanoprost group, and +1.9±1.0 mmHg (+14.7±5.1%) in the brinzolamide group. The change in the latanoprost group was significantly greater compared with those in the timolol XE and brinzolamide groups ($P< 0.0001$; $P < 0.0001$). The IOP change in the brinzolamide group was significantly greater than that in the timolol XE group (P = 0.0244). No significant difference was in mean intraocular pressure between before drug discontinuation and at 8 weeks after drug resumption in any group.

Conclusions: There was a significant increase in intraocular pressure from discontinuation of timolol XE, brinzolamide, and latanoprost. The hypotensive effect of latanoprost in the multiple drug therapy is significantly greater than those of timolol XE and brinzolamide.

Introduction

Multiple drug therapy is used to treat glaucoma when monotherapy is not effective or sufficient. A combination of several drugs, including prostaglandin analogues, β-blockers, cholinergic agonists, adrenergic agonists, α_2-stimulants, α_1-blockers, and carbonic anhydrase inhibitors (CAIs) have been reported to be effective.[1-7] These studies were carried out at the time when additional drugs were first administered in patients already receiving one drug. Several investigators demonstrated that patients with less dosing showed better adherence and higher persistency.[8-13] When a patient with 2 or 3 anti-glaucomatous drugs has an intraocular pressure low enough to approach the target pressure, ophthalmologists are concerned with whether one of the drugs can be discontinued. However, the efficacy of each drug in the patients who continue to administer two or more drugs is not available. In this study, we studied the efficacy of each drug in these patients with its discontinuation.

Patients and Methods

Patients

We conducted two series of investigation. In Study 1, 30 patients with open angle glaucoma and ocular hypertension who had received timolol XE 0.5% (Timoptol XE, Santen, Osaka, Japan) and latanoprost 0.005% (Xalatan, Pfizer, New York, NY) for at least 6 months were enrolled in this study. In Study 2, we studied 30 patients with open angle glaucoma and ocular hypertension who had received timolol XE 0.5%, latanoprost 0.005% and brinzolamide 2% (Eizopt, Alcon, Fort Worth, TX) for at least 6 months. A diagnosis of glaucoma was based on the appearance of the optic nerve head cupping and visual field alteration according to the guideline of Japanese Glaucoma Society.[14] Excluded were patients with angle closure glaucoma or post-traumatic, uveitic, neovascular or dysgenetic glaucoma, as well as patients with a known life-threatening disease. The study protocol and consent forms were approved by the Human Subjects Committee.

In Study 1, the patients were prospectively randomized to discontinue timolol XE or latanoprost, with only one eye of a patient to be randomized. When both eyes were eligible, the right eye became the study eye. Within 24 hours after enrollment, the patients were randomized using an envelope method. In brief, we prepared each 15 envelopes which contained a card which showed either timolol XE group or latanoprost group. Within 24 hours after enrollment, an envelope was picked-up and the inside card showed the way to discontinue timolol XE or latanoprost. Fifteen patients discontinued timolol XE and the remaining 15 patients discontinued latanoprost. Treatment began within a week after these random assignments.

In Study 2, the patients were prospectively randomized to discontinue timolol XE, latanoprost or brinzolamide with only one eye of a patient to be randomized. When both eyes were eligible, the right eye became the study eye. The patients were randomized using an envelop method in the same way as in Study 1. Each ten patients discontinued timolol XE, latanoprost or brinzolamide. Treatment began within a week after these random assignments.

Evaluation of Outcomes

Patients read and signed an Institutional Review Board-approved informed consent form before any procedures were performed in this study. Patients had ocular and systemic histories taken and underwent slit-lamp biomicroscopy, visual acuity testing, a physical examination, and dilated funduscopy. Goldmann applanation tonometry was carried out at the same time (±1:00) at three visits with a 2-week interval and the mean of the three values was calculated to determine the baseline intraocular pressure. Three measurements per visit were recorded in each eye and the mean of these was used in the calculations. The optic nerve was examined with a Goldmann 3-mirror lens and measurements were taken of the size of the disc, the vertical and horizontal cup/disc ratios, the presence of rim notching or splinter hemorrhage, and the presence of peripapillary atrophy. Visual field testing with a Humphrey visual field analyzer (Humphrey-Zeiss, Dublin, CA) and Program 30-2 SITA STANDARD™ testing were carried out before and 16 weeks after discontinuation of drugs.

In study 1, patients who qualified for the study were instructed to discontinue timolol XE or latanoprost for 8 weeks and then resume taking the discontinued drug. In Study 2, patients who qualified for the study were instructed to discontinue timolol XE, latanoprost or brinzolamide for 8 weeks and then resume taking the discontinued drug. We asked the patients questions concerning their compliance with treatment and discontinuation more than once per visit to increase the accuracy of the compliance rate.[15] The patients were reviewed at the interval of 2 weeks for 12 weeks. Intraocular pressure (IOP) was measured at the same time (±1:00) as at baseline and its change was studied. A single observer (HK) took intraocular pressure measurements in all eyes.

Study End

All patients were meant to reach a 16-week follow-up, but the following were considered as endpoints: (1) the need for any further medical or surgical treatment and (2) failure to attend scheduled visits, allowing for a margin of tolerance.

Statistical Analysis

Evaluation of continuous variables was achieved using the Student's *t* test. To evaluate the difference in IOP between follow-up intervals, the paired *t*-test was implemented. All *t*-tests were 2-tailed. Categoric variables were evaluated with chi-square, the Fisher exact test or the Spearman rank correlation, when appropriate. A level of $P < 0.05$ was accepted as statistically significant.

Results

Baseline

Baseline data in Study 1 are summarized in table 1. Thirty patients were enrolled in this study. Mean age was 62.7±11.3 mmHg in the timolol XE group and 67.8±10.0 mmHg in the latanoprost group. No significant difference was found between the two groups in age, gender, best-corrected visual acuity, Humphrey visual field analyzer 30-2 mean deviation and duration of administration of timolol XE and latanoprost.

Table 1. Demographics of patients in Study One

	Timolol XE group	Latanoprost group
Age (years)	62.7±11.3	67.8±10.0
Gender	11:4	7:8
Intraocular pressure before glaucoma medication (mmHg)	22.7±2.6	22.4±1.5
Intraocular pressure before discontinuation of timolol XE or latanoprost (mmHg)	15.9±1.7	15.9±1.5
Best-corrected visual acuity	1.0 (20/20)	1.0 (20/20)
Humphrey visual analyzer 30-2 mean deviation (dB)	-1.82±2.61	-2.78±3.13
Duration of administration of two drugs (month)	8.3±1.1	7.9±0.9

Table 2. Demographics of patients in Study Two

	Timolol group	Latanoprost group	Brinzolamide group
Age (years)	62.7±11.3	61.9±13.6	66.7±6.7
Gender	6 women, 4men	7 women, 3 men	5 women, 5 men
Intraocular pressure before glaucoma medication	22.7±2.6	22.8±1.5	22.4±1.6
Intraocular pressure before discontinuation of drug	15.9±1.5	15.7±1.07	15.7±1.4
Best-corrected visual acuity	1.0 (20/20)	1.0 (20/20)	1.0 (20/20)
Humphrey visual analyzer 30-2 mean deviation (dB)	-2.12±2.83	-2.58±2.93	-3.28±3.04
Duration of administration of three drugs (months)	8.5±1.2	8.2±1.1	7.8±0.8

In Study 2, 30 patients were enrolled in this study (table 2). Mean age was 62.7±11.3 years in the timolol XE group, 61.9±13.6 years in the latanoprost group, and 66.7±6.7 years in the brinzolamide group; patients in the brinzolamide group were older than those in the other groups, but this difference was not statistically significant. All patients had complete follow-up visits and reported to be compliant.

The Change in IOP

In Study 1, in the patients who administered latanoprost and timolol XE, no significant difference was found in mean baseline IOP between the two groups (table 3). The discontinuation of latanoprost or timolol XE provided an IOP increase of 4.3±1.9 mmHg (27.5±13.4%) or 1.6±0.9 mmHg (10.1±5.9%), respectively (figure 1, 2). The IOP increase achieved by the discontinuation of latanoprost was significantly greater compared with timolol XE ($P < 0.0001$). There was no significant difference in mean IOP between before drug discontinuation and at 8 weeks after drug resumption in any group.

Table 3. Intraocular pressure and its change in Study One

	Timolol XE group	Latanoprost group
Intraocular pressure (mmHg)		
Baseline	15.5±1.4	15.9±0.9
2 weeks	17.0±1.5	19.8±1.5
4 weeks	16.9±2.0	20.1±1.6
6 weeks	17.0±2.0	20.2±1.6
8 weeks	17.0±2.0	20.2±1.6
10 weeks	15.2±1.4	16.0±1.3
12 weeks	15.4±1.5	15.8±0.9
14 weeks	15.5±1.3	16.0±1.3
16 weeks	15.3±1.4	15.9±1.2
Intraocular pressure change (mmHg) (%)		
2 weeks	+1.5±0.7 (+10.1±4.5%)	+4.0±1.8 (+25.4±12.5%)
4 weeks	+1.5±1.0 (+9.4±6.6%)	+4.3±1.9 (+27.5±13.4%)
6 weeks	+1.6±0.9 (+10.1±5.4%)	+4.3±1.9 (+27.5±13.4%)
8 weeks	+1.6±0.9 (+10.1±5.9%)	+4.3±1.9 (+27.5±13.4%)
10 weeks	-0.3±0.7 (-1.5±4.5%)	+0.1±0.9 (+0.5±5.5%)
12 weeks	-0.1±0.9 (-0.4±5.8%)	-0.1±0.9 (-0.4±5.5%)
14 weeks	±0.0±0.9 (+0.2±5.8%)	-0.1±0.8 (+0.8±5.0%)
16 weeks	-0.2±0.8 (-1.2±5.1%)	±0.0±0.9 (+0.1±5.8%)

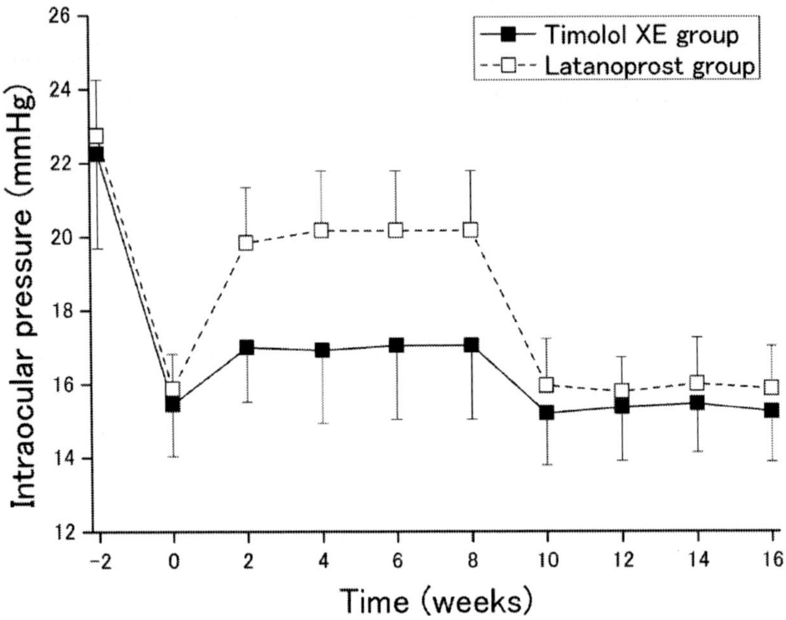

Figure 1. Intraocular pressure. The solid squares and solid line indicate the timolol XE group, and the open squares and broken line indicate the latanoprost group.

In Study 2, in the patients administering latanoprost, timolol XE and brinzolamide, there was no significant difference in mean baseline IOP among the three groups (table 4). A significant increase in mean IOP was found after the drug discontinuation in all groups (latanoprost: P = 0.0001; timolol XE: P = 0.0224; brinzolamide: P = 0.0030) (figure 3). Mean change in IOP by discontinuation of the drugs was +1.5±0.9 mmHg (9.5±8.7 %) in the timolol XE group, +4.1±1.9 mmHg (29.4±13.2%) in the latanoprost group, and +2.1±1.0 mmHg (+14.1±7.2%) in the brinzolamide group (figure 4). The change in the latanoprost group was significantly greater compared with those in the timolol XE and brinzolamide groups (P< 0.0001; P < 0.0001). The IOP change in the brinzolamide group was significantly greater than that in the timolol XE group (P = 0.0244). No significant difference was in mean IOP between before drug discontinuation and at 8 weeks after drug resumption in any group. No adverse events were reported during the discontinuation period in Study 1 and 2.

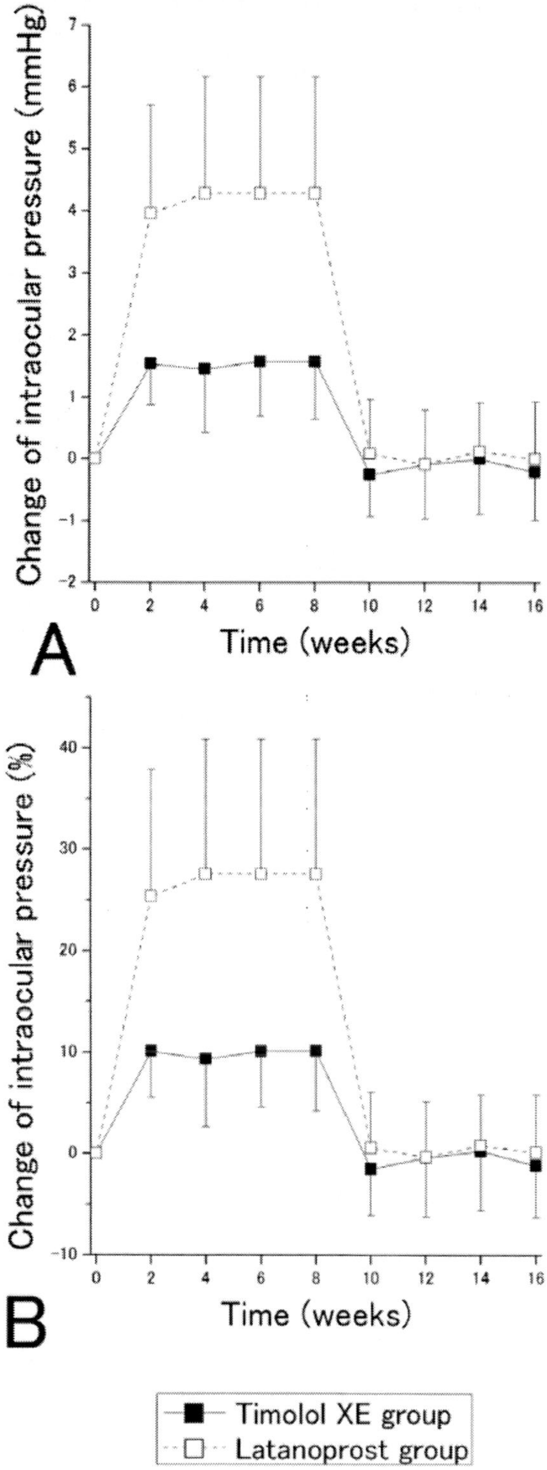

Figure 2. A change of intraocular pressure (mmHg) (A) and (%) (B). The solid squares and solid line indicate the timolol XE group, and the open squares and broken line indicate the latanoprost group.

Table 4. Intraocular pressure and its change in Study Two

	Timolol XE group	Latanoprost group	Brinzolamide group
Intraocular pressure (mmHg)			
Baseline	15.5±1.6	15.9±1.2	15.7±1.7
2 weeks	16.9±1.5	20.0±1.5	17.6±1.0
4 weeks	16.9±2.1	20.2±1.7	17.7±1.3
6 weeks	17.2±1.8	20.2±1.6	17.7±1.3
8 weeks	17.0±2.0	20.4±1.6	17.8±1.4
10 weeks	15.6±1.8	16.2±1.3	15.6±1.3
12 weeks	15.7±1.9	16.1±0.8	15.9±1.7
14 weeks	15.7±1.8	16.2±1.2	15.8±1.6
16 weeks	15.5±1.9	16.0±1.2	15.9±1.7
Intraocular pressure change (mmHg) (%)			
2 weeks	+1.4±0.7 (+9.2±4.9%)	+4.1±1.7 (+26.7±12.7%)	+1.9±1.0 (+13.0±7.6%)
4 weeks	+1.4±1.1 (+9.0±7.2%)	+4.4±1.9 (+28.5±13.9%)	+2.0±0.8 (+13.3±6.5%)
6 weeks	+1.7±1.1 (+10.9±7.3%)	+4.3±1.9 (+28.1±14.0%)	+2.1±0.9 (+13.7±6.7%)
8 weeks	+1.5±1.4 (+9.5±8.7%)	+4.6±1.7 (+29.4±13.2%)	+2.1±1.0 (+14.1±7.2%)
10 weeks	+0.1±0.9 (+0.4±5.5%)	+0.4±0.7 (+2.3±4.7%)	-0.1±0.7 (-0.1±4.5%)
12 weeks	+0.2±1.1 (+1.3±6.8%)	+0.3±0.9 (+2.1±6.2%)	+0.2±0.6 (+1.4±7.2)
14 weeks	+0.1±0.9 (+0.9±5.7%)	+0.4±0.9 (+2.4±6.0%)	+0.1±0.4 (+0.9±2.5%)
16 weeks	±0.0±1.2 (+0.1±7.5%)	+0.1±0.8 (+1.0±4.9%)	+0.2±0.4 (+1.3±2.8%)

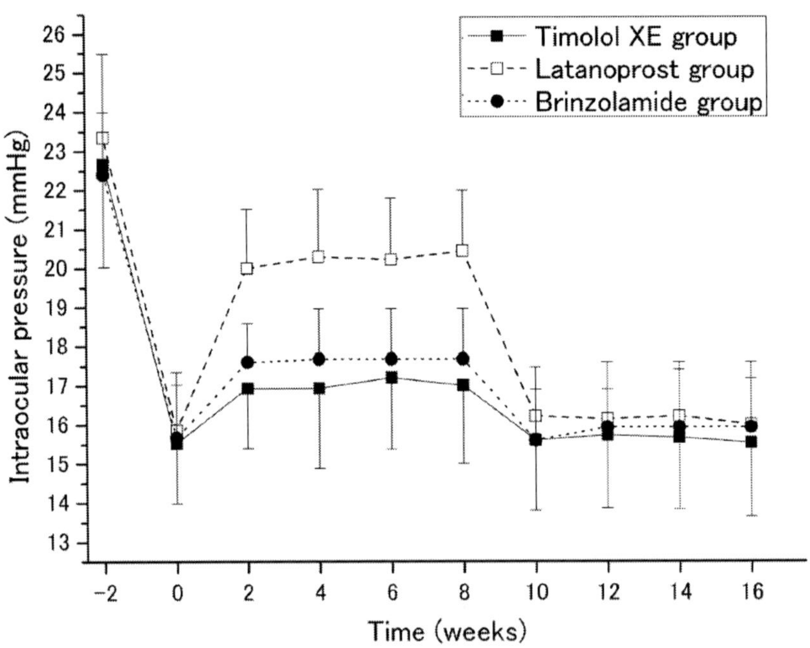

Figure 3. Intraocular pressure. The solid squares and solid line indicate the timolol XE group, the open squares and broken line indicate the latanoprost group, and the open squares and dotted line indicate the brinzolamide group.

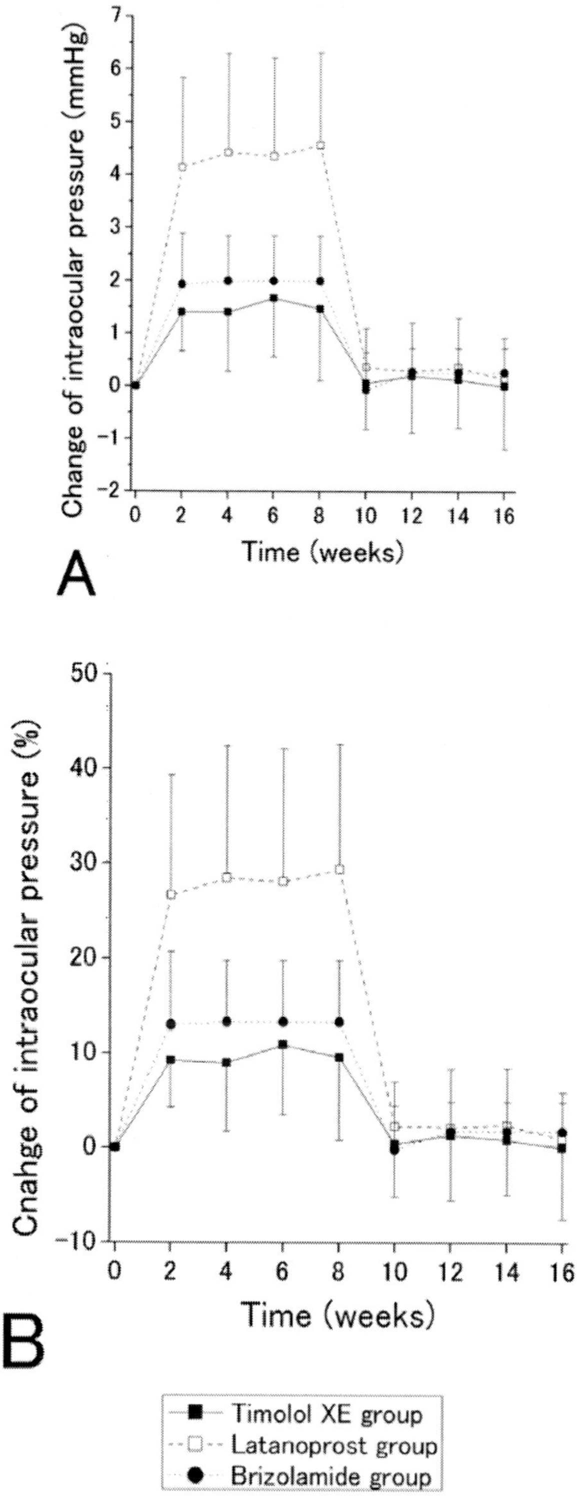

Figure 4. A change of intraocular pressure (mmHg) (A) and (%) (B). The solid squares and solid line indicate the timolol XE group, the open squares and broken line indicate the latanoprost group, and the open squares and dotted line indicate the brinzolamide group.

Discussion

In current study, we demonstrated that the discontinuation of timolol XE 0.5%, latanoprost 0.004% and brinzolamide 1% provided a significant increase in IOP in patients with primary open angle glaucoma or ocular hypertension. The discontinuation of latanoprost produced a significantly greater increase compared with timolol XE and brinzolamide.

In a previous study, although a wide variation existed in washout times among individuals, the mean washout periods of latanoprost, timolol XE and brinzolamide have been reported to be less than 6 weeks and the majority of the patients reached baseline by 8 weeks after the discontinuation of each drug.[16,17] In this study, we assumed that 8 weeks may be sufficient to eliminate the effect of the drugs. Schuman *et al.* demonstrated that the use of systemic β-blocker reduced the IOP lowering efficacy of topical β-blockers.[18] In this study, no patient used systemic β-blockers.

We showed that timolol XE and brinzolamide showed a similar hypotensive effect at the time the drug was first administered in patients already receiving latanoprost.[7] The mean reduction in IOP was 11.5±7.1% by the addition of timolol XE and 12.2±3.8% by the addition of brinzolamide. In this study, the discontinuation of timolol XE increased the IOP significantly less compared with brinzolamide. In spite of the long-term efficacy of timolol therapy, investigators have noted that the IOPs initially well controlled in some patients slowly increased after several months.[19,20] Brubaker also demonstrated fluorophotometrically that the timolol-induced reduction of aqueous flow is less pronounced at 1 year compared with 1 week after beginning treatment.[21] Long-term drift may be related to partial adaptation of the ciliary body to chronic administration of timolol.

Efficacy of anti-glaucomatous drugs as adjunctive therapy has been investigated in various methods. Stewart et al. evaluated the efficacy of currently available ocular hypotensive medicine monotherapy derived from 24-hour studies in a meta-analysis.[22]

1) The Addition of Anti-Glaucomatous Agents to Β-Blockers

All the available evidence shows that β-blockers produce a clinically significant additive ocular hypotensive effect when used in combination with any currently available ocular hypotensive agent. Prostaglandin analogue is additive to β-blocker treatment.[23-27] PGF_2-isopropylester provided a further IOP reduction of 17% compared with timolol alone.[24] Lee et al. demonstrated that the addition of PGF_2-isopropylester produced an additional reduction of 6 to 9 mmHg below the level provided by timolol alone in patients whose IOPs were uncontrollable with timolol.[25] Rulo et al. showed that latanoprost reduced IOP by 13 to 17% compared with timolol.[22] Alm et al. showed that the addition of latanoprost reduced IOP by 28 to 37% over 3 months in patients whose IOP was not controlled under 25 mmHg with timolol.[26]

There were several studies comparing an additional hypotensive effect of various drugs to timolol therapy. Webers et al. demonstrated that the addition of dorzolamide or latanoprost significantly lowers IOP in eyes with timolol in a meta-analysis of randomized clinical trials.[27] Concomitant use of dorzolamide and timolol decreased IOP by 4.1 mmHg at trough and by 4.9 mmHg at peak, and latanoprost and timolol provided a reduction of 6 mmHg. Wang et al, in a monkey study, showed that the addition of brimonidine, dorzolamide and latanoprost to timolol therapy produced a further reduction in IOP of 4.8±0.8 mmHg, 5.6±1.0 mmHg, and 4.3±1.0 mmHg, respectively ($P < 0.01$).[28] Several studies have showed that latanoprost is superior to CAIs and brimonidine as adjunctive therapy to timolol. Stewart et al. demonstrated that the addition of latanoprost provide a further reduction of 6.3±4.1 mmHg, brimonidine 4.2±4.5 mmHg and dorzolamide 3.1±5.1 mmHg at three months.[29] Petounis et al. showed that latanoprost showed a significantly greater reduction compared with brinzolamide and dorzolamide ($P < 0.005$).[30] In another study, a combination of latanoprost and timolol produced a reduction of 7.06 mmHg (32%) from baseline and a combination of dorzolamide and timolol 4.44 mmHg (20%); there was a significant difference between the two groups ($P < 0.001$).[31]

2) The Addition of Anti-Glaucomatous Drugs to Prostaglandin Analogues

I) The Addition of Β-Blockers to Prostaglandin Analogues

β-blockers are additive to latanoprost therapy as well as latanoprost to β-blockers. Adding latanoprost to the eyes treated with timolol provided a reduction of 2.6±1.1 mm Hg (13%), whereas timolol to the eyes receiving latanoprost gave a reduction of 2.6±2.2 mm Hg (14%).[26] Interestingly, in this study, timolol and latanoprost appeared to have a similar IOP-lowering effect in the combined treatment.

II) The Addition of CAIs to Prostaglandin Analogues

Several investigations demonstrated that topical CAIs are additive to latanoprost treatment. In a cross-over study, Kimal Arici et al. demonstrated that the combination of latanoprost and dorzolamide provided a reduction of 10.9 mmHg in patients who received latanoprost first and dorzolamide later, and 10.2 mmHg in patients who received dorzolamide first and latanoprost later.[31] When dorzolamide was added to latanoprost, the additional IOP reduction was 2.8 mm Hg (15%) ($p<0.01$) compared with 5.1 mm Hg (24.1%) ($p<0.01$) when latanoprost was added to dorzolamide. The values obtained in this study were similar to those in our current study, indicating that an IOP-lowering effect may last after a long concomitant therapy of latanoprost and topical CAI.

Shoji et al. reported that brinzolamide, another kind of topical CAI, also has an additional IOP-lowering effect to latanoprost therapy in open-label study.[32] The addition of brinzolamide to latanoprost decreased IOP from 21.1±4.8 mmHg to 15.9±3.1 mmHg at 3 months.[32] In this study, two patients experienced conjunctival hyperemia and three corneal epithelium defect; these complications were mild and self-limiting. Tsukamoto et al. compared ocular discomfort of brinzolamide and dorzolamide in combination therapy with latanoprost and timolol.[33] Substituting brinzolamide for dorzolamide decreased ocular irritation from 63% to 20%.

Nakamoto et al. demonstrated that the combination of latanoprost and brinzolamide demonstrated additive effects in lowering IOP, not only during the day, but also at night.[34] Percent reductions in the diurnal mean IOP and in nocturnal mean IOP were significantly greater in the eyes treated with the combination of latanoprost and brinzolamide (19.8% and 13.4%) than those with latanoprost alone (14.1% and 10.0%) ($P<0.05$).

III) The Addition of Brimonidine to Prostaglandin Analogues

Brimonidine, α_2-stimulant, provides a further reduction of IOP to latanoprost treatment. Erdogan et al. demonstrated that, after a short administration of latanoprost, brimonidine decreased an additional 2.53-3.10 mmHg in IOP compared with placebo [35]. In another study, the addition of brimonidine to latanoprost therapy provided a further of 5.1 mmHg (23%) at peak ($P<.001$) and 2.0 mmHg (9%) at trough ($P=.002$).[36]

IV) The Addition of Cholinergic Agonists to Prostaglandin Analogues

The addition of prostaglandin analogues to topical cholinergic therapy, including pilocarpine, may be problematic, at least theoretically. Cholinergic agent reduces IOP by direct stimulation of ciliary muscle whose contraction opens the trabecular meshwork and improves trabucular outflow.[37] It also reduces the uveoscleral outflow, by reducing the space between muscle fibers. Therefore, cholinergic agents could inhibit the action of prostaglandin analogues, which reduce IOP primarily by increasing aqueous humor .[38] Several studies showed that this is not a problem clinically.[39-42] Firestorm et al. showed that adding latanoprost to pilocarpine provided a further reduction of 2.7 mmHg, whereas adding pilocarpine to latanoprost produced an additional reduction of 1.5 mmHg.[39] Linden and Alm demonstrated that an addition of latanoprost to the potent cholinergic agonist physostigmine provided an additional reduction in normal volunteers.[40] Toris et al. demonstrated that a combination of latanoprost and pilocarpine provided a reduction of 5.2 mmHg in patients who received pilocarpine first and latanoprost later, and 4.9 mmHg in patients who received latanoprost first and pilocarpine later.[41] When pilocarpine was added to latanoprost, the additional IOP reduction was 1.6 mm Hg (11.2%) compared with 2.5 mm Hg (15.4%) when latanoprost was added to dorzolamide. The same author group assessed aqueous humor dynamics to explain the additivity of pilocarpine and latanoprost, and showed that pilocarpine increases outflow facility and does not block or attenuate the uveoscleral outflow effect of latanoprost, resulting in greater IOP reduction when these drugs are used in combination than when either drug is used alone.[42]

V) A Comparison of Efficacy of Anti-Glaucomatous Drugs as Adjunctive Therapy to Prostaglandin Analogues

There were several studies comparing efficacy of various ocular hypotensive agents as an adjunctive therapy of latanoprost. Miura et al. showed that the additional of brinzolamide and timolol to latanoprost significantly decreased IOP by 2.0 mm Hg and 2.7 mm Hg, respectively ($P<0.01$), but there were no significant differences between the two drugs.[43] O'Conner DJ compared IOP-lowering effect of dorzolamide, beta-blocker and brimonidine when added to latanoprost. Dorzolamide lowered an additional 3.9 mm Hg (19.7%), beta-blockers 2.0 mm Hg (12.3%) and brimonidine 2.0 mm Hg (9.3%) for 1 year; Dorzolamide provided a significant greater reduction compared with β-blockers and brinzolamide.[44] In another randomized trial, the efficacy of brimonidine, dorzolamide and latanoprost as an adjunctive therapy was compared, and all three drugs caused a significant reduction in the mean IOP from pretreatment values. Patients with brimonidine experienced a higher incidence of severe side-effects necessitating alteration of therapy.[45]

Travoprost, another type of prostaglandin analogues, is additive to various anti-glaucomatous drugs, including β-blockers, topical CAIs and brimonidine.[46-48] Feldman et al. compared efficacies of adjunctive therapy with brimonidine and adjunctive therapy with brinzolamide in combination with travoprost with diurnal change and showed that brinzolamide provided a significantly greater reduction at the trough.[46] Reis et al. and Holllo et al. demonstrated no significant difference in hypotensive effect between brinzolamide and timolol when administered as an adjuvant to travoprost in the treatment of patients with open-angle glaucoma and ocular hypertension.[47,48] Brinzolamide and timolol produced a significantly greater reduction in IOP compared with brimonidine.[48] The results of our current study were different in the comparison between efficacies of timolol and brinzolamide from these previous studies.

VI) The Addition of A1-Blocker to Prostaglandin Analogues or Β-Blockers

The addition of bunazosin, which is only commercially available α_1-blocer, provided a further reduction of 2.8±2.1 mmHg and 2.8±2.1 mmHg in patients who already administered latanoprost or timolol, respectively.[8]

VII) A Comparison of Efficacy of Various Combinations

Simmons et al. compared the efficacy of brimonidine or latanoprost as an adjunctive agent in patients already administering a β-blocker and dorzolamide or pilocarpine. They found that overall mean IOP reduction at month 1 was 4.60±0.62 mmHg (22.8%) with brimonidine and 3.43±0.62 mm Hg (17.2%) with latanoprost, with no significant differences between groups; however, the two groups before the addition of the drugs had various regimens, which precluded a simple comparison.[5] The same author group compared the efficacy of brimonidine or latanoprost as an adjunctive agent in patients whose IOP was not controlled with timolol; After 1 month of adjunctive therapy, brimonidine and latanoprost provided a comparable IOP reduction; the addition of brimonidine and latanoprost produced a reduction of 4.88 mmHg (22.8%) and 5.01 mmHg (23.5%) , respectively.[49] Netland et al. compared an IOP-lowering effect of the unfixed combination of brimonidine and bimatoprost with timolol and latanoprost. Brimonidine and bimatoprost provided a reduction of 8.5 to 9.0 mmHg and latanoprost and timolol 7.5 to 7.7 mm Hg. More patients achieved low target pressures with brimonidine and bimatoprost (P = 0.024).[50]

Fixed Combination

Treatment of fixed combination has been expected to increase patient compliance as a result of simplifying the dosage regimen.[51-53] Combining two medications in one bottle may reduce the risks associated with washout of the first administered medication and reduce additional benzolkonnium chloride exposure.[54]

There were some fixed combinations; timolol and dorzolamide [27,55-64], timolol and latanoprost [27, 65-72], bimatoprost and timolol [72,73], travoprost and timolol [74-78], brimonidine and timolol [79,80], and pilocarpine and latanoprost [81].

1) Timolol/Dorzolamide Fixed Combination

A fixed combination of dorzolamide/timolol provided an IOP reduction which was not statistically inferior to its concomitant administration. [27,55,58] Webers et al. compared an IOP-lowering effect of adding dorzolamide to timolol therapy in a meta-analysis and demonstrated that the concomitant use and fixed combination of dorzolamide and timolol provided a reduction of 4.1 mmHg at trough and 4.9 mmHg at peak and 3.8 mmHg at trough and 4.9 mmHg at peak, respectively.[27]

Latanoprost and the fixed combination of dorzolamide/timolol showed better adherence and persistency than other anti-glaucomatous drugs.[8-13] They are not only administered once daily but also have better IOP-lowering effects compared with other drugs. Which is superior in hypotensive effect, latanoprost or the fixed combination of dorzolamide/timolol, has been a focus of glaucoma investigations and controversial. Lesk et al. and Konstas et al. showed the superiority of the fixed combination of dorzolamide/timolol to latanoprost [63,82] using switching; In patients with uncontrolled IOP after latanoprost monotherapy, the switch to the fixed combination of dorzolamide/timolol decreased IOP by 5.8±4.9 mm Hg (23.5%). On the contrary, Polo et al. demonstrated the superiority of latanoprost to the fixed combination of dorzolamide/timolol on IOP-lowering.[56,60] Latanoprost provided a reduction of 1.58 mm Hg greater than timolol/dorzolamide at 3 months ($p<0.05$)[56] However, several studies showed the efficacy of IOP reduction of latanoprost is equivalent to the combination of timolol/dorzolamide.[57,59,61] Fetcher et al. concluded in combined analysis of pooled data, that the effect on IOP reduction of latanoprost is similar to combined timolol and dorzolamide; the fixed combination of dorzolamide/timolol and latanoprost provided mean IOP reductions of 12.5 mmHg and 12.6 mmHg, respectively.[61] In most cases, the overall safety profile of latanoprost is better than the fixed combination of timolol/dorzolamide. Sharma and Salmon reported hypotony and choroidal detachment as a complication of the fixed combination of dorzolamide/timolol.[62]

Latanoprost has been reported to be additive to the fixed combination. [57,63,82-84] Sunanna et al. showed that the addition of latanoprost to the combination of timolol and dorzolamide provided a significant IOP reduction of 3.1 mm Hg (16%) from a baseline of 19.3 mm Hg.[83] Lesk et al. showed that the addition of the fixed combination of dorzolamide/timolol to their existing latanoprost therapy provided a further reduction of 6.3±3.6 mmHg (28.1%).in patients with uncontrolled IOP on latanoprost monotherapy.[63] Akman et al. compared the efficacy of latanoprost and brimonidine as an adjunctive therapy to the fixed combination of dorzolamide/timolol; the addition of latanoprost to the fixed combination of dorzolamide/timolol reduced IOP by 4.4 mmHg at peak and 3.5 mmHg at trough at 3 months, and the addition of brimonidine to the fixed combination produced a reduction of 2.9 mmHg at peak and 2.9 mmHg at trough; there was no significant difference in peak/trough reductions.[84]

The efficacy of the fixed combination of dorzolamide/timolol has been compared with other combination of drugs.[64] Shall et al. compared fixed combination of dorzolamide/timolol with concomitant brimonidine and timolol, and showed no significant difference between IOP-lowering effect and the incidence of adverse experience.[64]

2) Latanoprost/Timolol Fixed Combination

The fixed combination of latanoprost and timolol provided a reduction which was greater compared with monotherapy of its components. [66,67] Higginbotham et al. showed that the fixed combination of latanoprost/timolol provided a further reduction in diurnal IOP of 0.9 to 1.2 mmHg and 1.9 to 3.5mmHg compared with latanoprost alone and timolol alone, respectively.[66] Konstas et al. demonstrated in a cross-over study that the fixed combination of latanoprost/timolol provided a better 24-hour IOP control compared with latanoprost alone; mean diurnal IOP curve was 19.2±2.6 mmHg for those who received latanoprost therapy alone and 16.7±2.1 mm Hg for those who received the fixed combination therapy ($P<.001$).[69] However, several studies showed that the fixed combination is inferior in IOP-lowering effect to the unfixed combination.[27,68] The fixed combination produced a less reduction in diurnal IOP of 1.1 mmHg than the unfixed combination.[68] Webers, in a meta-analysis of randomized controlled trials, showed that the concomitant use and fixed combination of latanoprost and timolol provided a decrease of 6.0 mmHg and 3.0 mmHg, respectively, at mean diurnal curve.[27]

There were several studies comparing the efficacy of the fixed combination of latanoprost/timolol and concomitant use of various drugs.[85-87] Shin et al. compared the efficacy of the fixed combinations of latanoprost/timolol and dorzolamide/timolol; Latanoprost/timolol provided a diurnal IOP reduction of 9.4±0.27 mmHg, where dorzolamide/ [85] Martinez-de-la-Casa et al. demonstrated that concomitant administration of travoprost and brinzolamide showed a greater efficacy than the fixed combination of latanoprost/timolol in IOL-lowering.[86] Stewart et al. showed no significant difference at each time point and for the diurnal curve for each therapy between the fixed combination of latanoprost/timolol and concomitant brimonidine and latanoprost.[87]

3) Bimatoprost/Timolol Combination

Hommer et al. showed that the fixed combination of bimatoprost/timolol and concomitant administration of its components produced mean diurnal IOP reductions of 8.7 mmHg and 9.0 mmHg, respectively; the fixed combination was not inferior to the unfixed combination.[72] Martinez and Sanchez demonstrated that the fixed combination of bimatoprost/timolol and latanoprost/timolol produced mean diurnal IOP reduction of 2.8±0.9 mmHg and 2.1±0.6 mmHg, respectively, and the fixed combination of bimatoprost/timolol provided a greater reduction ($p = 0.0214$).[73]

4) Travoprost/Timolol Combination

Hughes et al. reported that a fixed combination of travoprost/timolol provided a significant reduction that was comparable to concomitant therapy with its components.[75] The fixed combination of travoprost/timolol provided a slightly better IOP control compared with the fixed combination of latanoprost/timolol.[74,77,78] Toposzis et al showed that the combination of travoprost/timolol produced lower mean IOP values than latanoprost/timolol at some points in the morning, and mean IOP was 0.6 mmHg lower in patients with the fixed combination of travoprost/timolol compared with latanoprost/timolol.[77] Hyperemia was reported from a higher percentage of patients in patients with the fixed combination of travoprost/timolol. Denis et al. also showed in a retrospective, cross-sectional sectional study, that the combination of travoprost/timolol has longer-lasting residual effects than the combination of latanoprost/timolol when IOP is measured longer than 24 hours after instillation.[78] Schmir et al. compared visual field progression of patients with both fixed combinations and showed no significant difference in projected visual field progression between the two fixed combinations.[76]

5) Brimonidine/Timolol Combination

The fixed combination of brimonidine/timolol fixed combination and monotherapy with timolol or brimonidine provided a reduction of 4.4 to 7.6 mmHg, 3.9 to 6.2 mmHg and 2.7 to 5.5 mmHg, respectively; the fixed combination provided sustained IOP lowering superior to monotherapy with either timolol or brimonidine [80]

6) Pilocarpine/Timolol Combination

Diestelhorst et al. showed that mean diurnal pressure of the fixed combination of pilocarpine/timolol and latanoprost was 16.8±2.1 mmHg and 16.9±2.5 mmHg, respectively ($p = 0.60$), and the fixed combination of pilocarpine/timolol may be more effective in the late morning and may have a greater incidence of mild ocular side-effects.[81]

Limitations and Conclusion

This study has important limitations. The sample size of this study was small and therefore not powered to detect small differences. Small sample size also precluded an assessment of safety. Furthermore, a masked study design could have reduced observer bias.

Although the sample size in each group was small, the current study demonstrated that (1) the discontinuation of timolol XE or latanoprost provided a significant increase in intraocular pressure in patients who were already receiving timolol XE and latanoprost, (2) the discontinuation of timolol XE, latanoprost or brinzolamide produced a significant increase in intraocular pressure in patients who were already receiving the three drugs, (3) the discontinuation of latanoprost increased IOP significantly greater compared with the discontinuation of timolol XE or brinzolamide, and (4) the discontinuation of brinzolamide provided a significant increase of IOP compared with timolol. Future study of a large population is needed to verify this observation. However, this information may be clinically valuable when treating patients with open-angle glaucoma.

References

[1] United States Latanoprost Study Group, Camras CB. Comparison of latanoprost and timolol in patients with ocular hypertension and glaucoma: a six-month, masked, multicenter trial in the United States. *Ophthalmology.*1996;103:138–147.

[2] Diestelhorst M. The additive intraocular pressure-lowering effect of latanoprost 0.005% daily once and pilocarpine 2% t.i.d. in patients with open-angle glaucoma or ocular hypertension. A 6-month, randomized, multicenter study. German Latanoprost Study Group. *Graefes Arch. Clin. Exp. Ophthalmol.* 2000;238:433-439.

[3] Hoyng PF, Rulo A, Greve E, et al. The additive intraocular pressure-lowering effect of latanoprost in combined therapy with other ocular hypotensive agents. *Surv. Ophthalmol.* 1997;41 suppl 2:s93-s98.

[4] Simmons ST, Samuelson TW. Comparison of brimonidine with latanoprost in the adjunctive treatment of glaucoma. ALPHAGAN/XALATAN Study Group. *Clin. Ther.* 2000;22:388-399.

[5] Kimal AM, Topalkara A, Guler C. Additive effect of latanoprost and dorzolamide in patients with elevated intraocular pressure. *Int. Ophthalmol.* 1998;22:37-42.

[6] Kobayashi H, Kobayashi K, Okinami S. Efficacy of bunazosin hydrochloride 0.01% as adjunctive therapy of latanoprost or timolol. *J. Glaucoma.* 2004; 13:73-80.

[7] Kobayashi H, Kobayashi K. A comparison of efficacy of timolol XE, brinzolamide, and bunazosin as adjunctive therapy of latanoprost. Rinsho Ganka, in press.

[8] Rait JL, Adena MA. Persistency rates for prostaglandin and other hypotensive eyedrops: population-based study using pharmacy claims data. *Clin. Experiment. Ophthalmol.* 2007;35:602-11.

[9] Nordstrom BL, Friedman DS, Mozaffari E, et al. Persistence and adherence with topical glaucoma therapy. *Am. J. Ophthalmol.* 2005;140:598-606.

[10] Day DG, Schacknow PN, Sharpe ED, et al. A persistency and economic analysis of latanoprost, bimatoprost, or beta-blockers in patients with open-angle glaucoma or ocular hypertension. *J. Ocul. `Pharmacol. Ther.* 2004;20:383-92.

[11] Schwartz GF, Reardon G, Mozaffari E. Persistency with latanoprost or timolol in primary open-angle glaucoma suspects. *Am. J. Ophthalmol.* 2004;137 Suppl 1:S13 6.

[12] Reardon G, Schwartzs GF, Mozaffari E. Patient persistency with topical ocular hypotensive therapy in a managed care population. *Am. J. Ophthalmol.* 2004;137 Suppl 1:S3-12.

[13] Reardon G, Schwartz GF, Mozaffari E. Patient persistency with ocular prostaglandin therapy: a population-based, retrospective study. *Clin. Ther.* 2003;25:1172-85.

[14] The Japan Glaucoma Society guidelines for glaucoma (2nd edition). *Nippon Ganka Gakkai Zasshi.* 2006;110:777-815.

[15] Schwartz GF. Compliance and persistency in glaucoma follow-up treatment. *Curr. Opin. in Ophthalmol.* 2005;16:114-121.

[16] Stewart WC, Holmes KT, Johnson MA. Washout periods for brimonidine 0.2% and latanoprost 0.005%. *Am. J. Ophthalmol.* 2001;131:798-9.

[17] Linden C, Nuija E, Alm A. Effects on IOP restoration and blood-aqueous barrier after long-term treatment with latanoprost in open angle glaucoma and ocular hypertension. *Br. J. Ophthalmol.* 1997;81:370-2.

[18] Schuman JS. Effects of systemic beta-blocker therapy on the efficacy and safety of topical brimonidine and timolol. Brimonidine Study Groups 1 and 2. *Ophthalmology.* 2000;107:1171-7.

[19] Steinert RF, Thomas JV, Boger WP. Long-term drift and continued efficacy after multiyear timolol therapy. *Arch. Ophthalmol.* 1981;99:100-106.

[20] Boger WP, Puliafito CA, Steinert RF, et al. Long-term experience with timolol ophthalmic solution in patients with open-angle glaucoma. *Ophthalmology.* 1979;85:259-263.

[21] Brubaker RF, Nagasaki S, Bourne WM. Effect of chronically administered timolol on aqueous humor flow in patients with glaucoma. *Ophthalmology.* 1982;89:280-285.

[22] Stewart WC, Konstas AG, Nelson LA, Kruft B. Meta-analysis of 24-hour intraocular pressure studies evaluating the efficacy of glaucoma medicines. *Ophthalmology.* 2008;115:1117-1122.

[23] Rulo AH, Greve EL, Hoyng PF. Additive effect of latanoprost, a prostaglandin F2 alpha analogue, and timolol in patients with elevated intraocular pressure. *Br. J. Ophthalmol.* 1994;78:899-902.

[24] Villumsen J, Alm A. The effect of adding prostaglandin F2-alpha-isopropylester to timolol in patients with open angle glaucoma. *Arch. Ophthalmol.* 1990;108:1102.

[25] Lee PY, et al. Additivity of prostaglandin F2-alpha-isopropyl ester to timolol in glaucoma patients. *Ophthalmology.* 1991;98:1097.

[26] Alm A, et al. Latanoprost administration once daily caused a maintained reduction of intraocular pressure in glaucoma patients treated concomittanlly with timolol. *Br. J. Ophthalmol.* 1995;79:12.

[27] Webers CAB, van der Valk R, Schouten JAG, et al Intraocular pressure-lowering effect of adding dorzolamide or latanoprost to timolol. *Ophthalmology.* 2007;114:40-46.

[28] Wang RF, Serle JB, Gagliuso DJ, Podos SM. Comparison of the ocular hypotensive effect of brimonidine, dorzolamide, latanoprost, or artificial tears added to timolol in glaucomatous monkey eyes. *J. Glaucoma.* 2000;9:458-62.

[29] Stewart WC, Sharpe ED, Day DG, et al. Comparison of the efficacy and safety of latanoprost 0.005% compared to brimonidine 0.2% or dorzolamide 2% when added to a topical beta-adrenergic blocker in patients with primary open-angle glaucoma or ocular hypertension. *J. Ocul. Pharmacol. Ther.* 2000;16:251-9.

[30] Petounis A, Mylopoulos N, Kandarakis A, et al. Comparison of the additive intraocular pressure-lowering effect of latanoprost and dorzolamide when added to timolol in patients with open-angle glaucoma or ocular hypertension: a randomized, open-label, multicenter study in Greece. *J. Glaucoma.* 2001;10:316-24.

[31] Kimal Arici M, Topalkara A, Guler C. Additive effect of latanoprost and dorzolamide in patients with elevated intraocular pressure. *Int. Ophthalmol.* 1998;22(1):37-42.

[32] Shoji N, Ogata H, Suyama H, et al. Intraocular pressure lowering effect of brinzolamide 1.0% as adjunctive therapy to latanoprost 0.005% in patients with open angle glaucoma or ocular hypertension: an uncontrolled, open-label study. *Curr. Med. Res. Opin.* 2005;212:503-8.

[33] Tsukamoto H, Noma H, Matsuyama S, et al. The efficacy and safety of topical brinzolamide and dorzolamide when added to the combination therapy of latanoprost and a beta-blocker in patients with glaucoma. *J. Ocul. Pharmacol. Ther.* 2005;21:170-3.

[34] Nakamoto K, Yasuda N. Effect of concomitant use of latanoprost and brinzolamide on 24-hour variation of IOP in normal-tension glaucoma. *J. Glaucoma.* 2007;16:352-7.

[35] Erdogan H, Toker I, Arici Mk, et al. A short-term study of the additive effect of latanoprost 0.005% and brimonidine 0.2%. *Jpn. J. Ophthalmol.* 2003 ;47:473-8

[36] Mundorf T, Noecker RJ, Earl M. Ocular hypotensive efficacy of brimonidine 0.15% as adjunctive therapy with latanoprost 0.005% in patients with open-angle glaucoma or ocular hypertension. *Adv. Ther.* 2007;24:302-9.

[37] Barany EH. The mode of action of miotics on outflow resistance. A study of pilocarpine in the vervet monkey Cercopithecus ethiops. *Trans. Ophthalmol. Soc.* UK 1967;86:539-78.

[38] Alm A. The potential of prostaglandin derivates in glaucoma therapy. *Curr. Opin. Ophthalmol.* 1993;4:44–50.

[39] Frisrom B, Nielsson SE. Interaction of PhXA41, a new prostaglandin analogue, with pilocarpine: a study on patients with elevated pressure. *Arch. Ophthalmol.* 1993;111:662-5.

[40] Linden C, Alm A. Latanoprost and physostigmine have mostly additive ocular hypertensive effects in human eyes. *Arch. Ophthalmol.* 1997;115:857-61.

[41] Toris CB, Zhan G, Zhao J, et al. Potential mechanism for the additivity of pilocarpine and latanoprost. *Am. J. Ophthalmol.* 2001;131:722-8.

[42] Toris CB, Alm A, Camras CB. Latanoprost and cholinergic agonists in combination. *Surv. Ophthalmol.* 2002;47 Suppl 1:S141-7.

[43] Miura K, Ito K, Okawa C, et al. Comparison of ocular hypotensive effect and safety of brinzolamide and timolol added to latanoprost. *J. Glaucoma.* 2008;17:233-7.

[44] O'Conner DJ, Martone JF, Mead A. Additive intraocular pressure lowering effect of various medications with latanoprost. *Am. J. Ophthalmol.* 2002;133:836-7.

[45] Sodhi PK, Pandey RM, Ratan SK. Efficacy and safety of brimonidine, dorzolamide and latanoprost as adjunctive therapy in primary open angle glaucoma. *Int. J. Clin. Pract.* 2003;57:875-8.

[46] Feldman RM, Tanna AP, Gross RL, et al. Comparison of the ocular hypotensive efficacy of adjunctive brimonidine 0.15% or brinzolamide 1% in combination with travoprost 0.004%. *Ophthalmology*. 2007;114:1248-54.

[47] Reis R, Queiros CF, Santos LC, et al. A randomized, investigator-masked, 4-week study comparing timolol maleate 0.5%, brinzolamide 1%, and brimonidine tartrate 0.2% as adjunctive therapies to travoprost 0.004% in adults with primary open-angle glaucoma or ocular hypertension. *Clin. Ther.* 2006;28:552-9.

[48] Hollo G, Chiselita D, Petkova N, et al. The efficacy and safety of timolol maleate versus brinzolamide each given twice daily added to travoprost in patients with ocular hypertension or primary open-angle glaucoma. *Eur. J. Ophthalmol.* 2006;16:816-23.

[49] Simmons ST, Earl ML; Alphagan/Xalatan Study Group Three-month comparison of brimonidine and latanoprost as adjunctive therapy in glaucoma and ocular hypertension patients uncontrolled on beta-blockers: tolerance and peak intraocular pressure lowering. *Ophthamology*. 2002;109:307-14.

[50] Netland PA, Michael M, Rosner SA, et al. Brimonidine Purite and bimatoprost compared with timolol and latanoprost in patients with glaucoma and ocular hypertension. *Adv. Ther.* 2003;20:20-30.

[51] Patel SC, Spaeth GL. Compliance in patients prescribed eye-drops for glaucoma. *Ophthal. Surg.* 1995;26:233-6.

[52] Robin AL, Covert D. Does adjunctive glaucoma therapy affect adherence to the initial primary therapy? *Ophthalmology.* 2005;112:863-8.

[53] Robin AL, Novack GD, Covert DW, et al. Adherence in glaucoma: objective measurements of once-daily and adjunctive medication use. *Am. J. Ophthalmology.* 2007;144:533-40.

[54] Weinreb RN. Compliance with medical treatment in glaucoma. *J. Glaucoma.* 1992;1:134-6.

[55] Hutzelmann J, Owens S, Shedden A, et al. Comparison of the safety and efficacy of the fixed combination of dorzolamide/timolol and the concomitant administration of dorzolamide and timolol: a clinical equivalent study. International Clinical Equivalent Study Group. *Br. J. Ophthalmol.* 1998;82:1249-53.

[56] Polo V, Larrosa JM, Gomez ML, et al. Latanoprost versus combined therapy with timolol plus dorzolamide: IOP-lowering effect in open-angle glaucoma. *Acta Ophthalmol. Scand.* 2001;79:6-9.

[57] Bron AM, Emmerich KH. Latanoprost versus combined timolol and dorzolamide. *Surv. Ophthalmol.* 2002;47 Suppl 1:S148-54.

[58] Francis BA, Du LT, Breke S, et al. Comparing the fixed combination dorzolamide-timolol (Cosopt) to concomitant administration of 2% dorzolamide (Trusopt) and 0.5% timolol – a randomized controlled trial and a replacement study. *J. Clin. Pharm. Ther.* 2004;29:375-80.

[59] Fechtner RD, Airaksinen PJ, Getson AJ et al. Efficacy and tolerability of the dorzolamide 2%/timolol 0.5% combination (COSOPT) versus 0.005% (XALATAN) in the treatment of ocular hypertension or glaucoma: results from two randomized clinical trials. *Acta Ophthalmol. Scad.* 2004;82:42-8.

[60] Polo V, Larrosa JM, Ferreras A, Honrubia FM. Latanoprost vs combined therapy with timolol plus dorzolamide in open-angle glaucoma. A 24-month study. *Ann. Ophthalmol.* 2005;37:33-36.

[61] Fechtner RD, McCarroll KA, Lines CR, Adamsons IA. Efficacy of the dorzolamide/timolol fixed combination versus latanoprost in the treatment of ocular hypertension or glaucoma: combined analysis of pooled data from two large randomized observer and patient-masked studies. *J. Ocul. Pharmacol. Ther.* 2007;21:242-9.

[62] Sharma T, Salmon JF. Hypotony and choroidal detachment as a complication of topical combined timolol and dorzolamide. *J. Ocul. Pharmacol. Ther.* 2007;23:202-5.

[63] Lesk MR, Koulis T, Samplalis F, et al. Effectiveness and safety of dorzolamide-timolol alone or combined with latanoprost in open-angle glaucoma or ocular hypertension. *Ann. Pharmacother.* 2008;42:498-504.

[64] Shall KN, Greff LJ, Johnson-Pratt LR, et al. Dorzolamide/timolol combination versus concomitant administration of brinzolamide and timolol: six-month comparison of efficacy and tolerability. *Ophthalmology.* 2003;110:615-24.

[65] Larsson LI. Effect on intraocular pressure during 24 hours after repeated administration of the fixed combination of latanoprost 0.005% and timolol 0.5% in patients with ocular hypertension. *J. Glaucoma.* 2001;10:109-14.

[66] Higginbotham EJ, Feldman R, Stiles M, Dubiner H. Latanoprost and timolol combination therapy vs monotherapy: one-year randomized trial. *Arch. Opthalmol.* 2002;120:915-22

[67] Pfeiffer N. A comparison of the fixed combination of latanoprost and timolol with its individual components. *Graefes Arch. Clin. Exp. Ophthalmol.* 2002;240:893-9.

[68] Diestelnorst M, Larsson LI. A 12 week study comparing the fixed combination of latanoprost and timolol with the concomitant use of the individual components in patients with open angle glaucoma and ocular hypertension. *Br. J. Ophthalmol.* 2004;88:199-203.

[69] Konstas AG, Boboridis K, Tzetzi D, et al. Twenty-four-hour control with latanoprost-timolol-fixed combination therapy vs latanoprost therapy. *Arch. Ophthalmol.* 2005;123:898-902.

[70] Magacho L, Reis R, Shetty RK, et al. Efficacy of latanoprost or fixed combination of latanoprost-timolol in patients switched from a combination of a nonprostaglandin medication. *Ophthalmology.* 2006;113:442-5.

[71] Tabet R, Stewart WC, Feldman R, Konstas AG. A review of additivity to prostaglandin analogs: fixed and unfixed combinations. *Surv. Ophthalmol.* 2008;53 Suppl 6:S85-92.

[72] Hommer A. A double-masked, randomized, parallel comparison of a fixed combination of bimatoprost 0.03%/timolol 0.5% with non-fixed combination use in patients with glaucoma or ocular hypertension. *Eur. J. Ophthalmol.* 2007;17:53 62

[73] Martinez A, Sanchez M. A comparison of the safety and intraocular pressure lowering of bimatoprost/timolol fixed combination versus latanoprost/timolol fixed combination in patients with open-angle glaucoma. *Curr. Med. Res. Opin.* 2007;23:1025-32.

[74] Martinez de la Casa JM, Wieland H, Wells D, Sullivan K. Comparative efficacy and safety of fixed combinations of travoprost 0.004%/timolol 0.5% and latanoprost 0.005%/timolol 0.5% in patients with open-angle glaucoma or ocular hypertension. World Glaucoma Congress, Vienna, June6-9, 2005.

[75] Hughes BA, Bacharrach J, Craven R, et al. A three-month, multicenter, double-masked study of the safety and efficacy of travoprost 0.004%/timolol 0.5% ophthalmic solution compared to travoprost 0.004% ophthalmic solution and timolol 0.5% dosed concomitantly in subjects with open angle glaucoma or ocular hypertension. *J. Glaucoma.* 2005;12392-399.

[76] Schmier JK, Halpern MT, Covert DW, et al. Travoprost versus latanoprost combinations in glaucoma: economic evaluation based on visual field deficit progression. *Cur. Med. Res. Opin.* 2006;22:1737-43.

[77] Toposzis F, Mealmed S, Danesh-Meyer H, et al. A 1-year study to compare the efficacy and safety of once-daily travoprost 0.004%/timolol 0.5% to once-daily latanoprost

0.005%/timolol 0.5% in patients with open-angle glaucoma or ocular hypertension. *Eur. J. Ophthalmol.* 2007;17:183-90.

[78] Denis P, Lafuma A, Jeanbat V, et al. Intraocular pressure control with latanoprost/timolol and travoprost/timolol fixed combinations : a retrospective, multicentre, cross-sectional study. *Clin. Drug Investig.* 2008;28(12):767-76.

[79] Crichton ACS. Timolol/brimonidine combination therapy in glaucoma management. *Clin. Surg. J. Ophthalmol.* 2005;23:356-9.

[80] Sherwood MB, Craven ER, Chou C, et al. Twice-daily 0.2% brimonidine-0.5% timolol fixed combination therapy vs monotherapy with timolol or brimonidine in patients with glaucoma or ocular hypertension. A 12-month randomized trial. *Arch. Ophthalmol.* 2006;124:1230-7.

[81] Diestelhorst M, Nordmann JP, Toris CB. Combined therapy of pilocarpine or latanoprost with timolol versus latanoprost monotherapy. *Surv. Ophthalmol.* 2002;47 Suppl 1:S155-61.

[82] Konstas AG, Mikropulos D, Dimopoulos AT, et al. Second-line therapy with dorzolamide/timolol or latanoprost/timolol fixed combination versus adding dorzolamide/timolol fixed combination to latanoprost monotherapy. *Br. J. Ophthalmol.* 2008;92:1498-502.

[83] Susanna R Jr, Nicolela MT, Oga E. Additive effect of latanoprost to the combination of timolol and dorzolamide. *J. Glaucoma.* 2000;9:183-6.

[84] Akman A, Centinkaya A, Akova YA, Ertan A. Comparison of additional intraocular pressure-lowering effects of latanoprost vs brimonidine in primary open-angle glaucoma patients with intraocular pressure uncontrolled by timolol-dorzolamide combination. *Eye.* 2005;19:145-51.

[85] Shin DH, Feldman RM, Sheu WP; Fixed combination latanoprost/timolol study group. Efficacy and safety of the fixed combinations latanoprost/timolol versus dorzolamide/timolol in patients with elevated intraocular pressure. *Ophthalmology.* 2004;111:276-82.

[86] Martinez-de-la-Casa JM, Castillo A, Garcia-Feijco J. Concomitant administration of travoprost and brinzolamide versus fixed latanoprost/timolol combined therapy: three-month comparison of efficacy and safety. *Cur. Med. Res. Opin.* 2004;9:1333-9.

[87] Stewart WC, Stewart JA, Day DG, et al. Efficacy and safety of the latanoprost/timolol maleate fixed combination vs concomitant brimonidine and latanoprost therapy. *Eye.* 2004;18:990-5.

In: Eye Research Developments
Editor: Alan N. Westerhouse

ISBN: 978-1-60741-177-2

Chapter V

Computer-Aided Detection of Glaucomatous Changes

***Pantelis A. Asvestas*[1], *Konstantinos K. Delibasis*[2] *and George K. Matsopoulos*[*2]**

[1] Department of Medical Instruments Technology,
Faculty of Technological Applications,
Technological Educational Institute of Athens,
Ag. Spyridonos Street, Egaleo 122 10, Athens, Greece
[2] Department of Electrical and Computer Engineering,
National Technical University of Athens, 9 Iroon Polytechniou Street,
157 80 Zografou, Athens, Greece

Abstract

Glaucoma, a leading cause of blindness worldwide, is a progressive optic neuropathy with characteristic structural changes in the optic nerve head and concomitant visual field defects. Ocular hypertension (i.e. elevated intraocular pressure without glaucoma) is the most important risk factor to develop glaucoma. Even though a number of variables, including various optic disc and visual field parameters, have been used in order to identify early glaucomatous damage, there is a need for computer-based methods that can detect early glaucomatous progression so that treatment to prevent further progression can be initiated. The chapter is mainly focused on the analytical description of a computer-based system that consists of two modules: a) the module for the calculation of quantitative parameters to define vessel deformation in glaucomatous images and the classification of subjects based on these parameters, and b) the module for visualizing ophthalmologic data. Qualitative and quantitative results are presented to verify the usefulness of the developed computer-based system towards the discrimination of patients with ocular hypertension who developed glaucomatous damage and patients with ocular hypertension who remain stable.

[*] Corresponding Author: Name: George K. Matsopoulos; National Technical University of Athens; Mailing address: 9, Iroon Polytechniou Str, Zografos, 15780, Athens, Greece; Tel.: +302107722288; Fax: +302107723557; E-mail: gmatso@esd.ece.ntua.gr

Introduction

Glaucoma is a disease of the eye that is mainly associated with an increase in intraocular pressure. A build-up of fluid within the eye eventually leads to damage in the optic nerve fibres and a gradual loss of a patient's visual field. Diagnosis may be based on a combination of a number of parameters [1] and [2], but the most dependable single index is probably the identification of a characteristic pattern of visual field defects. There have been numerous studies towards the quantification of parameters that can be used for the discrimination of normal against glaucomatous retinal data.

The clinical detection of structural damage to the optic nerve head is central to the diagnosis of chronic glaucoma. Characteristic optic nerve cupping, visual field loss, and increased intraocular pressure (IOP) constitute a classic triad of findings, though glaucoma is often diagnosed in the absence of increased pressure. Careful evaluation of the optic disc can usually identify early glaucomatous damage before detectable visual loss occurs. The usual method used to evaluate the state of the optic disc in patients with glaucoma is the cup/disc ratio [3]. The reproducibility of the method, however, is only moderate [4] whereas the reliability is not high [5]. That is, some patients have small c/d ratios but significant visual field loss, whereas some have large c/d ratios with little visual field loss. In [6], the Disc Damage Likelihood Scale (DDLS), describing the appearance of the neuroretinal rim of the optic disc into eight stages, extending from no damage to far advanced damage, was used as a method of estimating the amount of optic disc damage in patients with glaucoma. The intraobserver and interobserver reproducibility was better using the DDLS than the c/d ratio (98% versus 85% for intraobserver of reproducibility, and 85% versus 74% for interobserver reproducibility).

In [7], a cross-sectional study has been performed to determine if optical coherence tomography (OCT) measurements of nerve fibre layer thickness can be used to predict the presence of visual field defects associated with glaucoma. According to this study, if nerve fibre layer damage occurs prior to the development of a visual field defect, then perhaps OCT-measured nerve fibre layer thickness values could predict the future development of visual field defects in subjects with glaucoma. Nevertheless, OCT may need higher resolution and better reproducibility to enhance its sensitivity and specificity for population screening. Also, in [8], a study was carried out in order to determine the reproducibility of the assessment for glaucomatous change in serial optic disc stereo-slides from 40 patients showing excellent results.

Recently, computerized systems based on image processing techniques have been used to identify and quantify measurements of glaucoma progression that will help guiding medical and surgical treatment. In [9], the optic nerve head has been automatically analyzed for patients with glaucomatous visual field damage heads and normal volunteers. The analysis was based on the modelling of the optic nerve head by a smooth two-dimensional surface with a shape described by 10 free parameters, including the degree of surface curvature of the disc region surrounding the cup, the steepness of the cup walls, the goodness-of-fit of the model to the image in the cup region, and measures of cup width and cup depth. These parameters, plus others derived from the image using the model as a basis, were used to discriminate between normal and abnormal images achieving overall classification accuracy up to 92%. In [10], a combination of innovative image processing and data mining techniques has been incorporated to detect abnormal symptoms such as abnormal optic disc to cup ratio, presence of exudates and tortuous blood vessels and to diagnose diabetic-related eye disease from the digitized retinal images. Also, the optic nerve heads of retina images have been used as a criterion in order to evaluate glaucoma disease status in [11]. The optic nerve head was measured automatically using an optical coherence tomography and a confocal scanning laser ophthalmoscopy and the measurements were then compared against the manual tracing method. The automatically obtained measurements using both devices showed a high correlation with glaucoma disease status against the manual method. A digital stereovision system for visualizing the topography of the optic nerve head from stereo optic disc images was also developed [12]. The system uses a semi-automatic method of obtaining 2-D as well as 3-D measures from a number of robust signal/image analysis approaches for feature extraction, registration and 3-D visualization of the optic nerve head from digital stereo fundus image. In a preliminary study of glaucoma patients, a strong correlation is found between the computer-generated quantitative cup/disc volume metrics and manual metrics commonly used in a clinic.

Furthermore, in [13], image processing techniques have been applied to digitized stereochronoscopical optic verve images acquired at two separate points in time with and without glaucomatous optic disc progression. A developed software was used for accurate image alignment based on the manually placement of corresponding points in these pairs and the application of a non-rigid polynomial warping algorithm to warp the later image into registration with the earlier image. Changes in vessels position and optic disc have been evaluated between glaucomatous patients and normal controls from independent observers, by viewing the registered images on a monitor, which allows rapid alternation (flickered rendering) of the two images. These evaluations were based on decisions from the observers and they were not quantitatively recorded. Recently, in [14], machine trained classifiers have been employed in order to improve differentiation between glaucomatous and non-glaucomatous eyes, from the standard automated perimetry. The machine learning algorithms studied included multilayer perceptron, support vector machine, and linear and quadratic discriminant analysis, Parzen window, mixture of Gaussian, and mixture of generalized Gaussian. Results show an improved performance of these classifiers over the best indexes from STATPAC, a specialized statistical analyses package employed by clinicians to interpret standard automated perimetry.

Nevertheless, the techniques actually available to discriminate between normal and glaucomatous discs are not sensitive and specific enough; thus significant changes might be detected after two-three years. Since treatment of glaucoma is more successful when started early, it is extremely important to develop new techniques that will allow earlier documentation of beginning glaucomatous optic disc alterations and disc progression. Consequently, reliably detecting glaucomatous progression remains challenging. Validated techniques with which to detect changes at the optic disc using the instruments described above are not yet available. Monitoring vessel deformation is the hallmark to detect glaucomatous progression when looking at optic disc stereo photographs. This is based on the concept that elevated intraocular pressure damages the ganglion cells and the supporting tissue of the optic disc vessels causing deformation of the vessels.

This chapter is mainly focused on the analytical description of an image processing system comprises of two modules: a module for the estimation of quantitative parameters to define vessel deformation in glaucomatous images and the classification of subjects into two classes: patients with ocular hypertension who develop early glaucoma (called hereafter *converters*) and patients with ocular hypertension who remain stable (called hereafter *non-converters*) and the module for visualizing ophthalmologic data, based on NURBS. Results on clinical ophthalmologic data are finally presented to verify the usefulness of the developed techniques towards the analysis of glaucomatous patients. In particular, an analytical description of the computer-based system design is presented along with the algorithmic implementation details used in the specific application. Qualitative results in terms of the application of image processing and visualization techniques along with quantitative results in terms of classification are then presented for discriminating between converters and non-converters patients.

2. Computer-Based System for Detecting Glaucomatous Changes

The computer-based system for detecting glaucomatous changes comprises of two modules: a) the 2D parameter estimation of vessels deformation / classification module and b) the VRML production and retinal image visualization module.

2.1. 2D Parameter Estimation of Vessels Deformation / Classification Module

This specific module is based on the combination of image processing techniques for estimating vessel deformation of ophthalmologic images. A number of patients with ocular hypertension who converted to early glaucoma (converters) and patients with ocular hypertension who remain stable (non-converters) were imaged with a fundus camera at regular intervals. The first acquired image serves as the reference image, while each acquired image at a later examination serves as the image to be compared with the reference image. Corresponding vessel segments between the reference image and subsequent images are compared by means of shape descriptors and classified as converters or non-converters. In the former case, the subsequent images were selected from the list of acquired images after the date of diagnosed conversion to glaucoma. A block diagram of the specific module is shown in figure 1. As can be seen from this figure, the module is an independent computer-based system comprising from the following techniques:

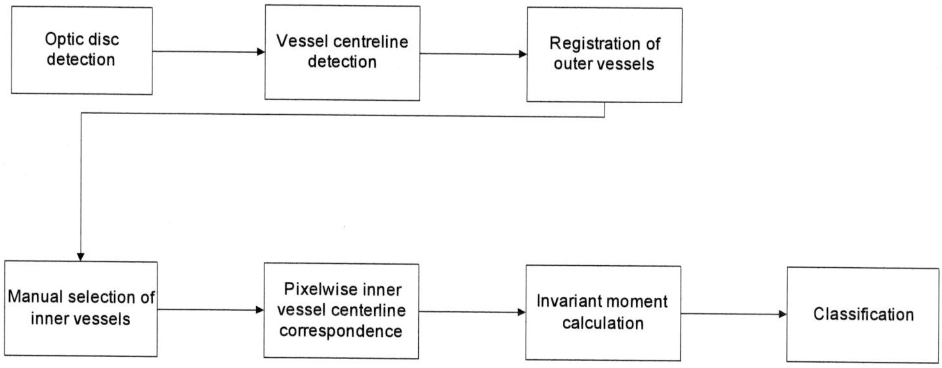

Figure 1. Block diagram of the "2D parameter estimation of vessels deformation / classification module".

2.1.1. Optic Disc Detection

The optic disc was automatically extracted as follows: a) a gray-level morphological closing operation is performed: $I_{closing} = I \bullet B$, using a 35 × 35 rectangular structuring element, B [15]. The closing operation results in the suppression of the vessels within the optic disc. b) The Canny edge detector is then applied [16], and after appropriate selection of the threshold level, points belonging to the contour of the optic disc are obtained. c) Finally, a best fitting circle to those points has been used resulting in the detection of the optic disc (figure 2). This process is applied in order to exclude the inner vessels during the subsequent registration process.

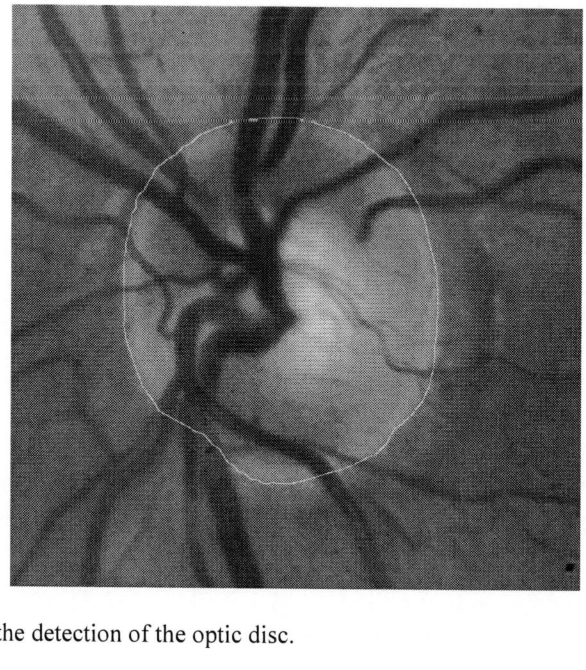

Figure 2. Example of the detection of the optic disc.

2.1.2. Vessel Centreline Detection

The vessel centrelines of a gray level retinal image $I(x,y)$ consist of the ridge points of the surface $S=\{(x,y,I(x,y))\}$. The detection of the ridge points can be accomplished as follows: Firstly, the second order derivatives, $I_{xx}(x_0,y_0)$, $I_{xy}(x_0,y_0)$ and $I_{yy}(x_0,y_0)$, of the image with respect to x and y at each pixel position (x_0,y_0) are estimated by convolving the image with the appropriate 2D Gaussian kernels [17]. Then, the eigenvalues and eigenvectors of the Hessian matrix are calculated using the Jacobi method [18].

$$\mathbf{H}(x_0,y_0)=\begin{bmatrix} I_{xx}(x_0,y_0) & I_{xy}(x_0,y_0) \\ I_{xy}(x_0,y_0) & I_{yy}(x_0,y_0) \end{bmatrix} \tag{1}$$

Let $\mathbf{u}=(u_x,u_y)$, $u_x^2+u_y^2=1$, be the eigenvector corresponding to the eigenvalue of maximum negative (positive) value. Then, the point (x_0,y_0) is a ridge (gorge) point if the first directional derivative across the direction of $\mathbf{u}$ at (x_0,y_0) vanishes, namely:

$$\langle \nabla I(x_0,y_0),\mathbf{u}\rangle = 0 \tag{2}$$

where $\langle\ \rangle$ denotes the inner product.

It can be shown [17] that if the following relation holds:

$$(tu_x,tu_y)\in[-0.5,0.5]\times[-0.5,0.5] \tag{3}$$

where

$$t=-\frac{u_xI_x(x_0,y_0)+u_yI_y(x_0,y_0)}{u_x^2I_{xx}(x_0,y_0)+2u_xu_yI_{xy}(x_0,y_0)+u_y^2I_{yy}(x_0,y_0)} \tag{4}$$

and I_x, I_y are the first derivatives of I with respect to x and y, then the pixel (x_0,y_0) is marked as a ridge pixel with exact position (x_0+tu_x,y_0+tu_y). A pixel that belongs to two vessels at the same time is defined as a bifurcation pixel. The result of this process is a binary image, $BW(x,y)$, of the vessel centrelines (figure 3).

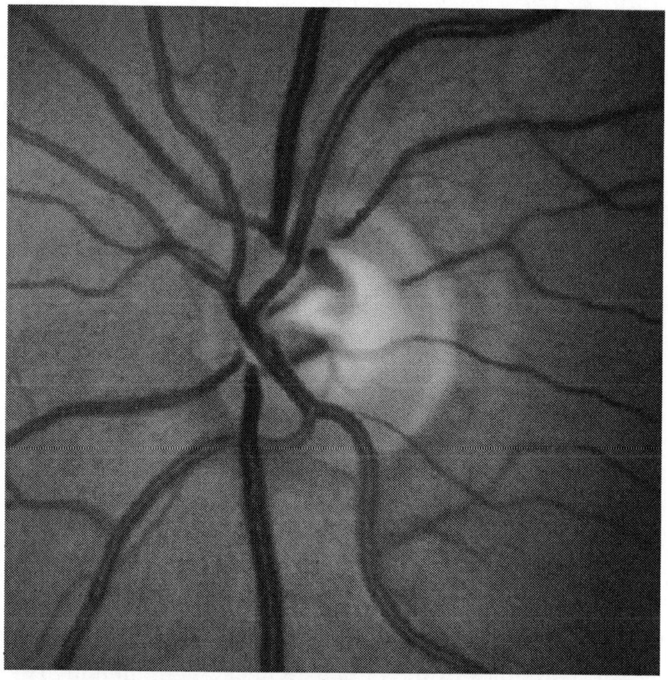

(a)

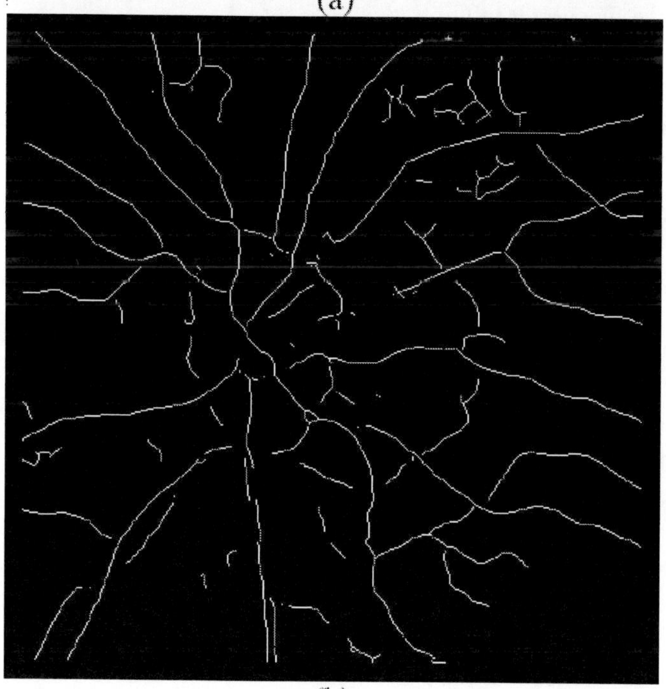

(b)

Figure 3. Detection of vessel centrelines. (a) Original retinal image. (b) Detected centrelines.

2.1.3. Registration of the Outer Vessels

This process aims to compensate displacement, rotation and scaling differences between two images, namely the reference and a subsequent image. These differences are due to the inconsistencies during the acquisition of the images and make the comparison of the two images difficult. However, the region inside the optic disc is also subject to (elastic) deformations due to the cardiac pulse. Therefore this region is excluded from the registration process. The following steps are followed for performing the registration:

a. The Distance Transform (DT) of the binary image of the vessel centrelines of the reference image is produced [19]. The DT provides the minimum distance of each pixel of the image from the nearest vessel centreline point (figure 4).
b. The parameters $\mathbf{a} = (a_{00}, a_{01}, b_0, a_{10}, a_{11}, b_1)$ of the affine geometric transform:

$$\begin{aligned} x' &= a_{00}x + a_{01}y + b_0 \\ y' &= a_{10}x + a_{11}y + b_1 \end{aligned} \tag{5}$$

that minimizes the distance between the transformed vessel centrelines of the subsequent image from the vessel centrelines of the reference image is minimum. Towards that end, the following objective function is minimised:

$$h(\mathbf{a}) = \frac{1}{N}\sum_x \sum_y DT(x', y') \tag{6}$$

where (x, y) denotes the position of a vessel centreline pixel on the subsequent image and N is the number of these pixels. The minimisation is performed by means of the Simulated Annealing (SA) algorithm [20], hybridized by the Powell's method [18]. Simulated annealing is a generic probabilistic meta-algorithm for the global optimization problem, namely locating a good approximation to the global minimum of a given function in a large search space. The name and inspiration come from annealing in metallurgy, a technique involving heating and controlled cooling of a material to increase the size of its crystals and reduce their defects. The heat causes the atoms to become unstuck from their initial positions (a local minimum of the internal energy) and wander randomly through states of higher energy; the slow cooling gives them more chances of finding configurations with lower internal energy than the initial one. By analogy with this physical process, each step of the SA algorithm replaces the current solution by a random "nearby" solution, chosen with a probability that depends on the difference between the corresponding function values and on a global parameter T (called the temperature), that is gradually decreased during the process. The dependency is such that the current solution changes almost randomly when T is large, but increasingly "downhill" as T goes to zero. The allowance for "uphill" moves saves the method from becoming stuck at local minima—which are the bane of greedier methods.

The result of the registration process is a transformed subsequent image (figure 5).

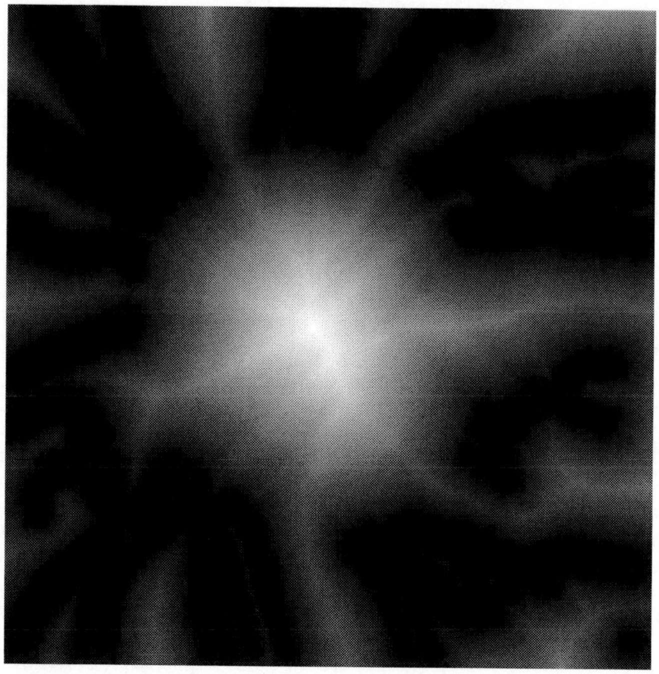

Figure 4. The Distance Transform of the image shown in figure 3(b).

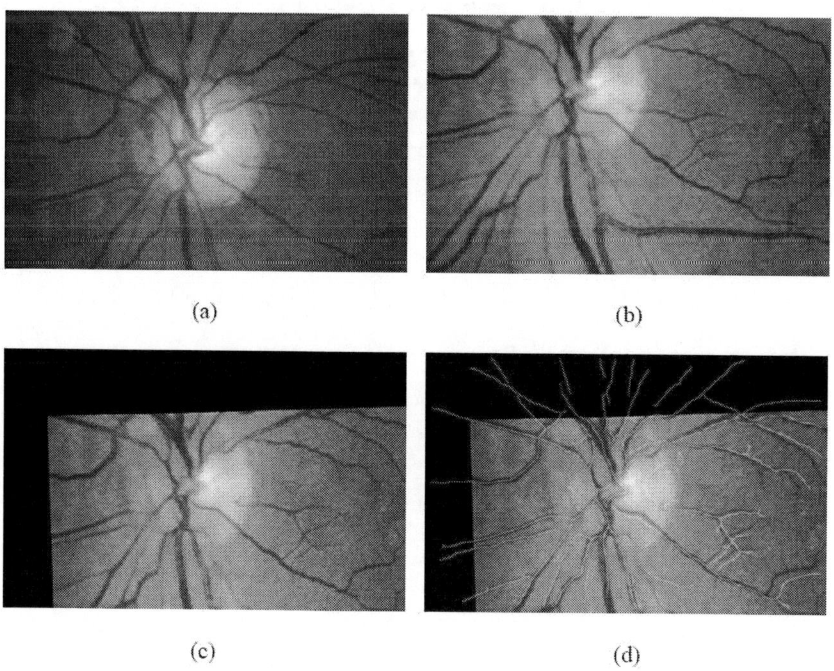

Figure 5. Example of registration. (a) Reference image. (b) Subsequent image to be registered. (c) Transformed image. (d) Superposition of the vessel centrelines from the reference image on the transformed image.

2.1.4. Manual Selection of Inner Vessels

The user selects corresponding pairs of vessels inside the optical disc from the reference image and the transformed subsequent image. The selection of a vessel is performed on the binary image of the vessel centrelines by clicking on a point on a vessel centreline. Then a region growing algorithm with seed point the selected one is used in order to form the vessel centreline.

2.1.5. Pixel-Wise Inner Vessel Centreline Correspondence

The Trimmed Iterative Closest Point (TrICP) algorithm [21] in conjunction with the Thin-Plate Spline (TPS) [22] is applied in order to define correspondence of the selected inner vessels centrelines. The TrICP is a variant of the well known Iterative Closest Point (ICP) algorithm [23] that is broadly used for allocating corresponding points, due to its robustness, simplicity and fast execution time. The TrICP has the capability to maximize the efficiency of the original ICP scheme. The innovation of this approach lies with the fact that it only considers a predefined number of points that have the minimum distances, instead of working with the entire sets. The Trimmed ICP starts with two sets of two-dimensional points, $P = \{\mathbf{p}_i\}_{i=1}^{N_p}$ and $Q = \{\mathbf{q}_i\}_{i=1}^{N_q}$, where $N_p \neq N_q$ are the number of points for the two sets. Then:

Step 1. For each point of $\mathbf{q}_i \left(i = 1, 2, \ldots, N_q\right)$ of Q, the closest point in P is found and the corresponding distance d_i is computed.

Step 2. The distances are sorted in descending order and the first N_{q0} distances are selected, where $N_{q0} = rN_q$ and $0 < r \leq 1$ is a user-supplied number.

Step 3. The sum of the selected distances, S_{TS}, is calculated.

Step 4. If any of the stopping conditions is satisfied, then the process stops.

Step 5. For the selected N_{q0} pairs of points, the optimal parameters of the selected transformation model that minimize S_{TS} are computed.

Step 6. The points of Q are transformed according to the computed parameters from Step 5 and the iteration starts over from Step 1.

The following stopping criteria are used:

1. The maximum number of iterations has been reached or
2. The Mean Square Error (MSE) $MSE = \dfrac{S_{TS}}{N_{q0}}$ is sufficiently small or
3. The difference of MSEs between two successive iterations is small enough.

The Trimmed Iterative Closest Point algorithm eventually converges to an optimal set of corresponding points, provided that a successful pre-registration stage is accommodated into the scheme.

The TrICP provides N_{q0} pairs of corresponding points $\left\{(\mathbf{p}_i,\mathbf{q}_i):\mathbf{p}_i \in P,\mathbf{q}_i \in Q\right\}_{i=1}^{N_{q0}}$ between the two sets. Thin-plate splines are a class of non-linear interpolation functions with several desirable properties for our application. They are globally smooth, easily computable and contain both affine and non-affine components. The TPS interpolation function $\mathbf{F}(\mathbf{r}):\Re^2 \rightarrow \Re^2$ with interpolant points $\{\mathbf{q}_i\}_{i=1}^{N_{q0}}$ has the following form:

$$\mathbf{F}(\mathbf{r}) = \sum_{i=1}^{N_{q0}} \mathbf{a}_i g\left(\|\mathbf{r}-\mathbf{q}_i\| + \lambda\right) + \mathbf{c}_0 + \mathbf{c}_1 x + \mathbf{c}_2 y \tag{7}$$

where $\mathbf{r}=(x,y)$, $\mathbf{a}_i=\left(a_i^x,a_i^y\right)$ $(i=1,2,\dots N_{q0})$ and $\mathbf{c}_0,\mathbf{c}_1,\mathbf{c}_2$ are the parameters of the TPS, $g(t)=\log\left(t^2+c^2\right)^{1/2}$ $(c^2>1)$ and $\lambda>0$ is the bending factor. The parameters $\mathbf{a}_i=\left(a_i^x,a_i^y\right)$ $(i=1,2,\dots N_{q0})$ and $\mathbf{c}_0,\mathbf{c}_1,\mathbf{c}_2$ are calculated by requiring:

$$\begin{gathered}\mathbf{F}(\mathbf{q}_i)=\mathbf{p}_i \\ \sum_{i=1}^{N_{q0}} \mathbf{a}_i = 0 \quad \sum_{i=1}^{N_{q0}} x_i a_i^x = 0 \quad \sum_{i=1}^{N_{q0}} y_i a_i^y = 0\end{gathered} \tag{8}$$

where $\left\{(\mathbf{p}_i,\mathbf{q}_i):\mathbf{p}_i \in P,\mathbf{q}_i \in Q\right\}_{i=1}^{N_{q0}}$ are pairs of corresponding points.

This is a system of $\left(N_{q0}+3\right)\times\left(N_{q0}+3\right)$ equations with $\left(N_{q0}+3\right)\times\left(N_{q0}+3\right)$ unknowns, which can be solved using for example LU decomposition [18].

The bending factor λ balances the requirement for exact matching of the interpolant points. When the bending factor is zero, $\lambda=0$, the calculated interpolation function **F** results in an exact match of the interpolant points at the expense of a possibly high total spatial bending measurement, of the image space. When λ approaches large positive values, the geometric transformation approaches the affine one. The value of the bending factor λ is estimated by visual inspection of the deformed image [24]. Figure 6 confirms these arguments for a synthetic grid image, containing six (6) interpolant points (crossed bullets in the figure). Four interpolant points remain fixed, whereas the other two interpolant points move towards each other, as shown in top left image. The warped images are shown in the top right image and in the two bottom images for increasing values of the bending factor λ corresponding from the pure RBF interpolation method (top right image) to the affine transformation approximation (bottom right image).

In figure 7(c), it is shown the result from applying the TrICP-TPS on the vessels shown in figure 7(a) and figure 7(b).

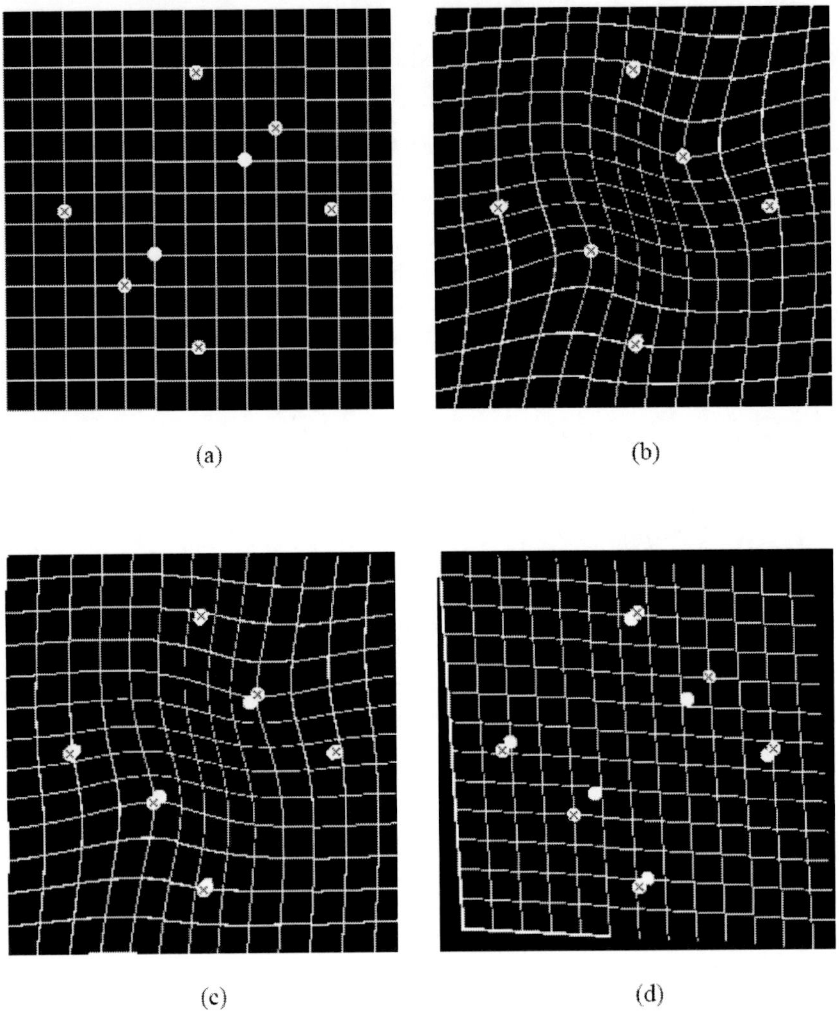

Figure 6. Effect of the bending factor λ on image warping. (a) The synthetic grid image showing initial (marked with 'x') and final position of the interpolant points. (b) for $\lambda=0.005$. (c) for $\lambda=0.05$. (d) for $\lambda=5$ (affine transformation approximation).

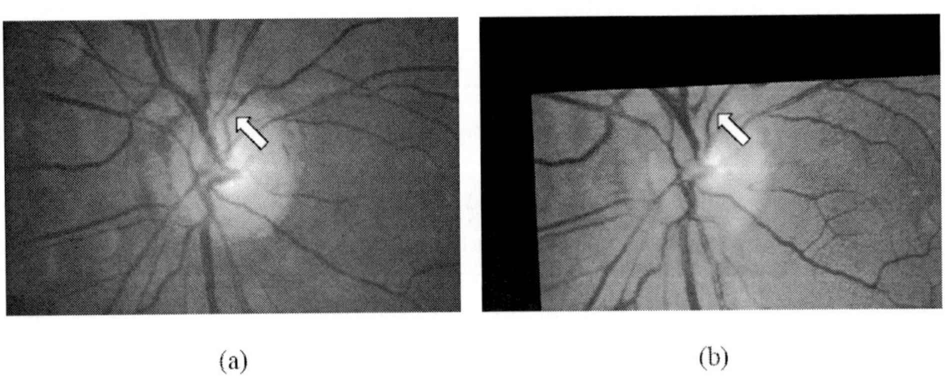

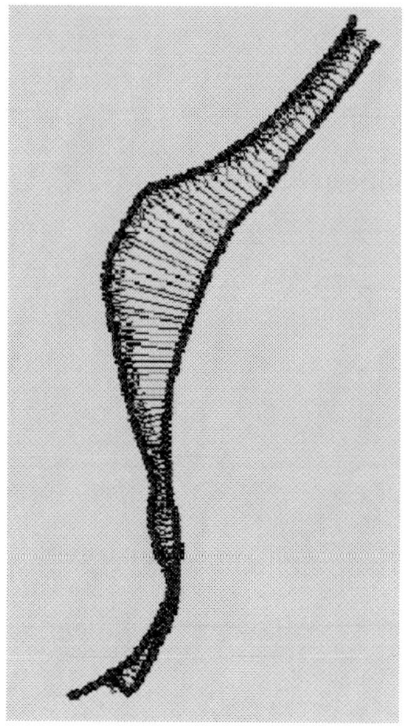

(c)

Figure 7. The vessel deformation scheme for a pair of images from a converter. (a) Reference image. (b) Transformed image. (c) Pixel-wise point correspondence of selected vessels (as indicated by the arrows in (a) and (b)).

2.1.6. Vessel Abnormality Indicator Calculation

In the case of glaucoma, the tissue beneath the retinal surface of the optic disc is being degenerated, which causes the retinal vessels inside the disc to move or deform. This motion is believed to be mostly visible mainly directly above or below ("12 o'clock" or "6 o'clock", respectively), midrange, without excluding other regions of the disc. The deformation motion is believed to vanish at the border of the disc (the sclera), which remains still with time. Retinal tissue degeneration, and therefore vessel deformation, is usually observed within a few months (typically six month intervals at most clinical protocols). To avoid confusion with vessel movement due to cardiac pulse, which is a normal finding, medium of small retinal vessels should be examined. The change in the vessel shape is identified with shape descriptors, applied to inner vessel's centreline, as determined previously. The invariant moments [16] have been selected as the appropriate shape descriptors, since:

- They are readily computed and well documented in the literature for similar applications
- They possess useful properties of invariability under transformations of rotation, translation and scaling.

For a vessel centreline that consists of the points (x_i, y_i) $(i = 1, 2, \ldots, N)$, the moment of order $p+q$ is defined as:

$$m_{q,p} = \sum_{i=1}^{N} x_i^p y_i^q \tag{9}$$

whereas the central moment definition of order $p+q$ is:

$$\mu_{q,p} = \sum_{i=1}^{N} (x_i - \bar{x})^p (y_i - \bar{y})^q \tag{10}$$

where $\bar{x} = \dfrac{m_{1,0}}{m_{0,0}}, \bar{y} = \dfrac{m_{0,1}}{m_{0,0}}$.

Then, the second order invariant moments can be defined as follows:

$$\begin{aligned} \phi_1 &= \mu_{2,0} + \mu_{0,2} \\ \phi_2 &= (\mu_{2,0} - \mu_{0,2})^2 + 4\mu_{1,1}^2 \end{aligned} \tag{11}$$

whereas the third order invariant moment, as follows:

$$\begin{aligned} \phi_3 &= (\mu_{3,0} - 3\mu_{1,2})^2 + (\mu_{3,0} - 3\mu_{2,1})^2 \\ \phi_4 &= (\mu_{3,0} + \mu_{1,2})^2 + (\mu_{3,0} + \mu_{1,2})^2 \\ \phi_5 &= (\mu_{3,0} - 3\mu_{1,2})(\mu_{3,0} + \mu_{1,2})\left((\mu_{3,0} + \mu_{1,2})^2 - 3(\mu_{2,1} - 3\mu_{0,3})^2\right) \\ &+ (\mu_{0,3} - 3\mu_{2,1})(\mu_{0,3} + 3\mu_{2,1})\left((\mu_{0,3} + \mu_{2,1})^2 - 3(\mu_{1,1} - 3\mu_{3,1})^2\right) \end{aligned} \tag{12}$$

In the present implementation, seven (7) second and third order invariant affine moments have been calculated. In order to reduce the dynamic range, the logarithm of the results. Finally, the relative change of the logarithm of the magnitude of the seven invariant moments of the retinal vessels between the reference and each subsequent registered image were employed as vessel shape attributes.

2.1.7. Classification

The purpose of this process is to utilize the inner vessel attributes defined above to correctly classify patients with ocular hypertension converting to glaucoma (converters) and patients with ocular hypertension who did not develop glaucoma (non-converters). In this specific implementation, the average classification rate over 50 runs was calculated, employing the Fuzzy C-Means algorithm [25]. In particular, FCM is an unsupervised clustering algorithm which allows one feature vector to belong to two or more clusters. It is based on minimization of the following objective function:

$$G_m = \sum_{i=1}^{N} \sum_{j=1}^{C} u_{ij}^m \left\| \mathbf{x}_i - \mathbf{c}_j \right\|^2 \tag{13}$$

where $\mathbf{x}_i$ is a n-dimensional feature vector, m is any real number greater than 1 (in our case, $m = 2$), u_{ij} is the degree of membership of $\mathbf{x}_i$ in the cluster j ($\sum_{j=1}^{c} u_{ij} = 1$), $\mathbf{c}_j$ is the n-dimensional center of the cluster, N and C are the number of data vectors and clusters, respectively and $\| \ \|$ is any norm expressing the similarity between any measured data and the center.

The algorithm is composed of the following steps:

1. Initialize matrix U randomly, $U^{(0)} = \left[u_{ij}^{(0)} \right]$ and set $G_m^{(0)} = 0$
2. For $k = 1, 2, \ldots$

$$\mathbf{c}_i^{(k)} = \frac{\sum_{i=1}^{N} \left(u_{ij}^{(k-1)} \right)^m \mathbf{x}_i}{\sum_{i=1}^{N} \left(u_{ij}^{(k-1)} \right)^m} \tag{14}$$

$$u_{ij}^{(k)} = \frac{1}{\sum_{p=1}^{C} \left(\frac{\left\| \mathbf{x}_i - \mathbf{c}_j^{(k)} \right\|}{\left\| \mathbf{x}_i - \mathbf{c}_p^{(k)} \right\|} \right)^{\frac{2}{m-1}}} \tag{15}$$

3. If $\left| G_m^{(k)} - G_m^{(k-1)} \right| < \varepsilon$ then STOP; otherwise return to step 2.

As already mentioned, data are bound to each cluster by means of a membership function, which represents the fuzzy behaviour of this algorithm. A data vector $\mathbf{x}_i$ is assigned to the cluster k using the following rule:

$$k = \arg\max_j \left\{ u_{ij} \right\} \tag{16}$$

In each run, 30% of the data were randomly selected as test set and the rest 70% as training set. In this way, the training and test set were not identical between any two runs and the available data set was fully exploited. The average values of the following parameters were computed:

- *Sensitivity:* True positives / Total positives
- *Specificity:* True negatives / Total negatives
- *Precision:* True positives / (True positives + False positives)
- *Accuracy:* (True positives + True negatives) / Total samples

The number of true positives is the number of converters that are correctly classified as converters. The number of false positives is the number of non-converters that are incorrectly classified as converters. The number of true negatives is the number of non-converters that are correctly classified as non-converters. The number of false negatives is the number of non-converters that are incorrectly classified as converters. Precision measures how consistent the results can be reproduced whereas accuracy reflects the overall correctness of the classifier.

2.2. Retinal Image Visualization

The specific module is a complementary module to the aforementioned 2D parameter estimation of vessels deformation / classification module and performs the visualization of the depth images as created by a reconstruction technique based on the Non Uniform Rational B Splines (NURBS). NURBS can be used for representation of arbitrarily complex shapes, while compressing the amount of data necessary for representing this shape [26].

Let us consider the case of curves represented by NURBS. The forward problem can be stated as following: Let us assume N points that control the shape of the curve:

$$\mathbf{p}_k = [x_k, y_k], \quad 0 \le k < N \tag{17}$$

NURBS is a curve **C** of order equal to d that consists of a blending of $N+d-1$ polynomial segments. The parametrization of the curve **C** is performed by a parameter u ranging in [0,1) for the whole curve, rather than for each individual curve segment: $\mathbf{C}(u) = [x(u), y(u)]$.

The boundaries of the parameter space u for each curve segment are defined by the knot vector **U**, formalized as following:

$$\mathbf{U} = [u_0, u_1, \ldots, u_{N+d-1}] \tag{18}$$

Since the knot need not be uniformly distributeded in the [0,1), parametrization of the B Splines is said to be "Non Uniform".

A NURBS curve of order d is parametrically defined as following:

$$\mathbf{C}(u)=\frac{\sum_{k=0}^{N-1} w_k B_{kd}(u)\mathbf{p}_k}{\sum_{k=0}^{N-1} w_k B_{kd}(u)} \quad \text{where} \quad \begin{array}{c} u_0 \le u \le u_{N+d-1} \\ 2 \le d \le N \end{array} \tag{19}$$

where B_{ij} is the basis function, recursively defined as:

$$B_{k,d}(u)=\frac{u-u_k}{u_{k+d-1}-u_k}B_{k,d-1}(u)+\frac{u_{k+d}-u}{u_{k+d}-u_{k+1}}B_{k+1,d-1}(u) \tag{20}$$

and $B_{k,1}(u)=\begin{cases} 1 & \text{if } u_k \le u \le u_{k+1} \\ 0 & \text{otherwise} \end{cases}$

Given a set of data points $\mathbf{Q}=\left[q_0,q_1,\ldots,q_{M-1}\right]^T$, the relevant knot vector and the appropriate parametrization: $\left(t_0,t_1,\ldots,t_{M-1}\right)$, the problem of NURBS encoding and curve generation is defined as deciding the set of control points to be used $\mathbf{P}=\left[p_0,p_1,\ldots,p_{N-1}\right]^T$.

Assuming that $w_k=1\ \forall k$, the definition of NURBS becomes:

$$\mathbf{P}(t_i)=\mathbf{c}_i \Rightarrow \sum_{k=0}^{N-1} B_{k,d}(t_i)\mathbf{p}_k=\mathbf{c}_i,\quad 0\le i<M \tag{21}$$

The above equation states three systems (one for each cartesian axes) of M linear equations (one for each data point) of N uknown parameters (one for each control point).

$$\underbrace{\begin{bmatrix} B_{0,d}(t_0) & B_{1,d}(t_0) & \cdots & B_{N-1,d}(t_0) \\ B_{0,d}(t_1) & B_{1,d}(t_1) & \cdots & B_{N-1,d}(t_1) \\ \vdots & \vdots & \cdots & \vdots \\ B_{0,d}(t_{M-1}) & B_{1,d}(t_{M-1}) & \cdots & B_{N-1,d}(t_{M-1}) \end{bmatrix}}_{\mathbf{B}} \times \underbrace{\begin{bmatrix} \mathbf{p}_0 \\ \mathbf{p}_1 \\ \vdots \\ \mathbf{p}_{N-1} \end{bmatrix}}_{\mathbf{P}} = \underbrace{\begin{bmatrix} \mathbf{c}_0 \\ \mathbf{c}_1 \\ \vdots \\ \mathbf{c}_{M-1} \end{bmatrix}}_{\mathbf{C}} \Leftrightarrow \mathbf{BP}=\mathbf{C} \tag{22}$$

If $M=N$ then the action is curve interpolation, if $M>N$ then curve approximation takes place.

The nontrivial case of $M>N$ is solved employing Least Squares Approximation (LSA) to minimize $\mathbf{e}^{\mathbf{T}}\mathbf{e}$; where $\mathbf{e}=\mathbf{BP}-\mathbf{C}$:

$$\mathbf{B}^T\mathbf{BP}=\mathbf{B}^T\mathbf{C} \tag{23}$$

while the transpose of $\mathbf{B}$, $\mathbf{B}^{\mathrm{T}}$, is calculated by Singular Value Decomposition.

Given a set of surface points: $\mathbf{f}_{i,j}\left(i=0,1,\ldots,m-1, j=0,1,\ldots,n-1\right)$, the parametrization of data points $\left(s_i,t_j\right)$ and the relevant knot vector, the problem of surface fitting is formulated as determining the surface control points $\mathbf{p}_{kl}$.

Under a similar assumtion as with curves ($w_{k,l}=1\ \forall k,l$), the NURBS surface equation can be rewritten separating the two independent parameters:

$$\mathbf{f}_{i,j}=\sum_{k=0}^{N_u-1} B_{k,d}\left(s_i\right)\sum_{l=0}^{N_v-1} B_{l,d}\left(t_j\right)\mathbf{p}_{k,l} \qquad (24)$$

where $0\le i<m, 0\le j<n$

Due to excesive memory requirements the surface fitting is performed as curve fitting problem sucesively along the two parameters of the surface *s, t.*

3. Results

3.1. Data Selection

Optic disc photographs from 67 subjects have been acquired with a Zeiss FF3 fundus camera (Carl Zeiss, Oberkochen, Germany) used for non-simultaneous stereoscopic imaging. For each subject, optic disc photos have been taken every six months for a period up to five years. The first image of the sequence served as the reference image. The data were provided by the optic disc reading centre of the European Glaucoma Prevention Study (EGPS) [27]. The data were divided into two groups (as determined by the optic disc reading centre of the EGPS): 25 subjects were characterized as optic disc converters and 42 subjects as non-converters. All images were digitized using a colour slide scanner (Minolta Dimage Dual III Film & Slide Scanner) with 8 bits per colour channel and 2,820 dpi resolution; thus producing coloured images of 24-bit-RGB in TIF format and initial size of 2,688 × 4,032 pixels. The digitized images were then down sampled to half size using an averaging process to speed up the execution process and they were further pre-processed using a cropping algorithm in order to exclude the film borders resulting in a final image resolution of 1,000 × 1,000 pixels. Furthermore, effort has been made by the experts to identify multiple corresponding inner vessels on the retinal pairs in order to finalize the training and testing sets during classification. Thus, 61 pairs of vessels were finally obtained from the converter group and 115 pairs of vessels from the non-converter group to be included in the classification process.

3.2. Experimental Results

In figure 6, typical results from the application of the proposed vessel deformation scheme are displayed. Figure 6(a) and (b) show the baseline image (reference image) of the left eye of a patient and the same image of the patient (image to be transformed) acquired after 6 months, respectively. Figure 6(c) shows the transformed image whereas the same image is displayed in figure 6(d) having superimposed the outer vessels centrelines of the reference image in order to demonstrate the performance of the registration process. Then, two corresponding vessels are manually selected, one vessel belonging to the reference image (see arrow in (a)) and the other to the transformed (see arrow in (c)). Figure 6(e) displays successful pixel-wise point correspondence of the two selected vessels (the red vessel corresponds to the reference and the green vessel to the transformed image).

As described so far, shape attributes are extracted and calculated at the level of vessels. The classification of a subject is based on the classification of the corresponding vessels, according to the following rule: *A subject is assigned to the non-converter group if all selected vessel pairs were found not glaucomatous; otherwise, the subject is assigned to the converter group.*

In table 1, results are presented in terms of number of subjects as well as in terms of number of corresponding vessels. In terms of number of subjects, only one subject was incorrectly classified for both converter and non-converter groups, respectively. In terms of number of corresponding vessels, three vessel pairs were incorrectly classified for both converter and non-converter groups, respectively. The ratio of misclassified cases can be explained by the aforementioned subject classification rule; if at least one vessel pair of a glaucomatous subject was classified as converter, then the subject was correctly classified, independently of the classification results on the other selected pairs of the same subject. On the other hand, for a subject to be correctly classified as non-converter, all vessel pairs have to be correctly classified.

Table1. The Confusion Matrix

Output	Desired Classification Results			
	Number of corresponding vessels		Number of subjects	
	Converter	Non-converter	Converter	Non-converter
Converter	15	3	7	1
Non-converter	3	32	1	12
Total Number	18	35	8	13

The values of the classification parameters based on the number of subjects are also given in table 2. As can be seen from table 2, the sensitivity and specificity of the system were 83.7% and 89.7%, respectively. The classification precision was 83.3% suggesting satisfactory reproducibility. Finally, the total classification accuracy in terms of number of subjects provided by the proposed system was 87.5%.

Table 2. The Values of Classification Parameters Based on the Number of Subjects

Classification parameters	Values (%)
Sensitivity	83.7
Specificity	89.7
Precision	83.3
Total Classification Accuracy	87.5

In figure 8, the optic disk of the images shown in figure 7(a) and (b) are shown.

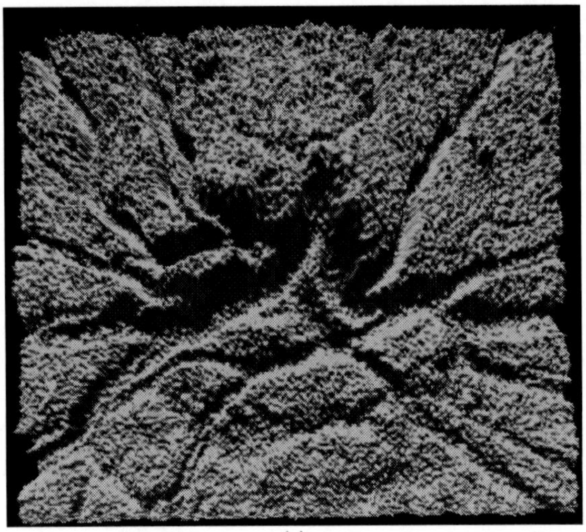

(a)

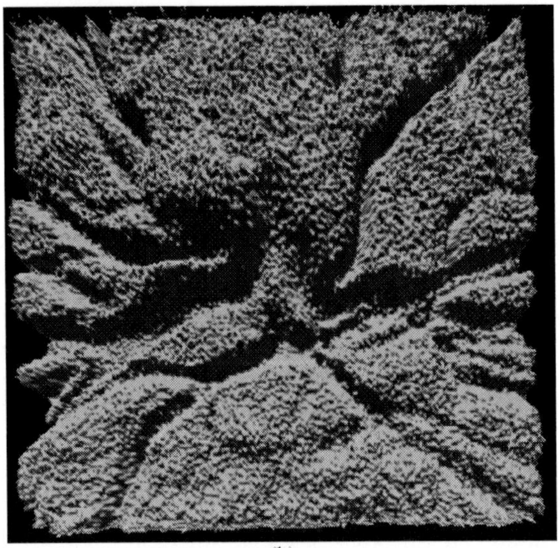

(b)

Figure 8. Surface reconstruction by means of Non Uniform Rational B-Splines. (a) Optic disc for the image in figure 7(a). (b) Optic disc for the image in figure 7(b).

4. Conclusion

In this chapter, a new methodology for identifying shape changes of optic disc vessels that are due to the presence of glaucoma is developed. High-quality images of the optic nerve head have been acquired using a fundus camera and the application of the proposed system on data, previously classified as converters and non-converters, provided an overall classification rate up to 87.5%. The principal findings of our study are twofold: First, that vessel segments possess diagnostic information capable for automatic identification of early glaucomatous change. Second, that the module of the proposed computer-based system, based on the implementation of image processing and classification techniques, can correctly classify the majority of the subjects; therefore seem to be well suited to a clinical environment.

Examination of the optic nerve head and measurement of the visual filed defects are fundamentals to the diagnosis of the glaucoma and to detection of the progression of the disease [2]. However, these visual field defects may only appear after optic disc damage has occurred. Several imaging technologies have been developed allowing more objective measurement of the optic nerve head. Scanning laser ophthalmoscopy, optical coherence tomography, and scanning laser polarimetry have been useful to discriminate between individuals with glaucoma and those without [29]-[30]. Validated techniques for the detection of glaucomatous change at the optic disc using these instruments are not yet available. The evaluation of the optic nerve head by stereoscopic imaging remains the gold standard by which new technologies are compared [31]-[32]. This was the first motive for our study to profit from existing and new retinal image data obtained with a standardized fundus camera. Furthermore, this type of retinal images can be obtained in most clinical environments compared to the other technologies used, including the stereoscopic imaging, which demand either specialized equipment or predefined geometry settings.

Existing image processing techniques applied on either stereoscopic or non-stereoscopic optic disc images in glaucoma using a fundus camera resulted in the estimation of various parameters including the cup and disc diameter, the cup and disc areas and the cup and disc volumes towards the evaluation of the optic disc deformation [12]-[13]. Our study is focused on the estimation of deformations of corresponding vessel segments within the optic disc occurred due to glaucoma. To our knowledge, there is no previously reported work related to the quantification of the deformation of retinal vessels towards automatic identification of early glaucomatous change. Nevertheless, retinal vessels diameter changes have been estimated in order to examine the relationship of these changes to the open-angle glaucoma [33]. According to this study, retinal arteriolar narrowing is associated with optic nerve damage caused by open-angle glaucoma. On the other hand, it was not clear if the retinal arteriolar change reflects an ischemic process or results from loss of retinal neurons due to glaucoma.

Furthermore, an intermediate step using the proposed system is the corresponding vessel segments selection. At the present, the selection is semi-automatic according to which the expert manually selects a vessel within the optic disc of the reference image and the system automatically identifies the corresponding vessel on the registered image based on the proximity criterion. The purpose of implementing this step in a semi-automatic way lies with the fact that only specific vessels were selected by the experts that were identified as suspicious located close to periphery of the optic disc and to the nasal retinal area. Thus, the main vessels within the optic disc were excluded since the deformations observed were more likely to be mainly due to cardiac pulsation. In the near future, a fully automatic process will be developed, where the criteria for the automatic vessel selection will be the diameter of the vessels as well as their relative location.

Nevertheless, the developed system could be used as a decision support system towards the detection of glaucomatous progression and not as a diagnostic tool. Even though image analysis gained more recognition from the ophthalmologists, the application of the system should always be incorporated with other ophthalmologic tests, clinical findings as well as other risk factors such as age, race and family history, according to a predefined clinical protocol. In the near future, a clinical evaluation of the system is scheduled involving a great number of retinal data.

Acknowledgment

The authors would like to thank all the key medical experts of the European Glaucoma Preservation Study Group (EGPS) for providing the tested retinal data. The authors would like to acknowledge their participation to the "Glaucoma Prevention by Computer Aided Diagnostics – *GLAUCAD*", an EC Funded Project – Quality of Life, where a substantial number of retinal data used in the present study had been acquired, and they would like to thank all partners within the project.

References

[1] H.A. Quigley (1993). Open angle glaucoma. *New England J. Med., 328,* 1097–1106.

[2] Sommer (1996). Glaucoma: facts and fancies. *Eye, 10,* 295–301.

[3] M. Armaly (1967). Genetic determination of cup/disc ratio of the optic nerve. *Arch. Ophthalmol. 78,* 35-43.

[4] R.C. Wolfs, R.S. Ramrattan, A. Hofman, et al. (1999). Cup-to-disc ratio: ophthalmoscopy versus automated measurement in a general population: the Rotterdam study. *Ophthalmology. 106,* 1597-1601.

[5] S. Miglior, L. Brigatti, C. Lonati, et al. (1995). Correlation between the progression of optic disc and visual field changes in glaucoma. *Curr. Eye Res. 14,* 145-149.

[6] G.L. Spaeth, J. Henderer, C. Liu, M. Kesen, U. Altangerel, A. Bayer, L.J. Katz, J. Myers, D. Rhee, and W. Steinmann (2002). The disc damage likelihood scale: Reproducibility of a new method of estimating the amount of optic nerve damage cause by glaucoma. *Trans. Am. Ophthalmol. Soc. 100,* 181-186.J.B.

[7] Z.Y. Williams, J.S. Schuman, L. Gamell, A. Nemi, E. Hertzmark, J.G. Fujimoto, C. Mattox, J. Simpson, G. Wollstein (2002). Optical Coherence Tomography Measurement of Nerve Fiber Layer Thickness and the Likelihood of a Visual Field Defect. *American Journal of Ophthalmology. 134,* 547-551.

[8] The European Glaucoma Prevention Study Group (EGPS) (2003). Reproducibility of Evaluation of Optic Disc Change for Glaucoma with Stereo Optic Disc Photographs. *Ophthalmology. 110,* 340–344.

[9] N.V. Swindale, G. Stjepanovic, A. Chin, F.S. Mikelberg (2000). Automated Analysis of Normal and Glaucomatous Optic Nerve Head Topography Images. *Investigative Ophthalmology & Visual Science. 41,* 1730-1742.

[10] K. Goh, W. Hsu, M. Li Lee, H. Wang (2001). ADRIS: an Automatic Diabetic Retinal Image Screening System. In Krzysztof Cios Editor. *Medical Data Mining and Knowledge Discovery*. Springer-Verlag; 2001; 181-210.

[11] J.S. Schuman, G. Wollstein, T. Farra, E. Hertzmark, A. Aydin, J.G. Fujimoto, L.A. Paunescu (2003). Comparison of Optic Nerve Head Measurements Obtained by Optical Coherence Tomography and Confocal Scanning Laser Ophthalmoscopy. *American Journal of Ophthalmology. 135,* 504-512.

[12] E. Corona, S. Mitra, M. Wilson, T. Krile, Y.H. Kwon, P. Soliz (2002). Digital Stereo Image Analyzer for Generating Automated 3-D Measures of Optic Disc Deformation in Glaucoma. *IEEE Trans. Medical Imaging. 21,* 1244-1253.

[13] J.W. Berger, T.R. Patel, D.S. Shin, J.R. Piltz, R.A. Stone (2000). Computerized Stereochronoscopy and Alternation Flicker to Detect Optic Nerve Head Contour Change. *Ophthalmology. 107,* 1316–1320.

[14] K. Chan, Te-Won Lee, P.A. Sample, M. H. Goldbaum, R. N. Weinreb, L. M. Zangwill, T.J. Sejnowski (2002). Comparison of Machine Learning and Traditional Classifiers in Glaucoma Diagnosis. *IEEE Trans. Biomedical Engineering. 49,* 963-974.

[15] J. Serra (1988). *Image Analysis and Mathematical Morphology. vol. 2*. Academic Press.

[16] R.C. Gonzalez, R.E. Woods (1993). *Digital image processing, Second Edition.* Addison Wesley.

[17] Steger (1998). An unbiased detector of curvilinear structures. *IEEE Trans. PAMI, 20,* 113-125.

[18] W.H. Press, S.A. Teukolsky, W.T. Vetterling, B.P. Flannery (1992). *Numerical Recipes in C: the art of scientific computing.* Cambridge University Press; U.K.

[19] G.K. Matsopoulos, K.K. Delibasis, N.A. Mouravliansky, P.A. Asvestas, K.S. Nikita, V.E. Kouloulias, N.K. Uzunoglu (2003). CT-MRI automatic surface-based registration schemes combining global and local optimization techniques. *Technology and Health Care: Official Journal of the European Society for Engineering and Medicine. 11,* 219-232.

[20] L. Ingber (1993). Simulated annealing: practice versus theory, *J. Math. Comput. Modelling. 18,* 29-57.

[21] Chetverikov, D. Stepanov, P. Krsek (2005). Robust Euclidean alignment of 3D point sets: the trimmed iterative closest point algorithm. *Image and Vision Computing. 23,* 299–309.

[22] F.L. Bookstein (1989). Principal warps: thin-plate splines and the decomposition of deformation. *IEEE Trans. PAMI, 11,* 567-585.

[23] P.J. Besl, N.D. McKay. (1992). A method of registration of 3-D shapes. *IEEE Trans Patt Anal Mach Intell. 14,* 239-256.

[24] K. Rohr, M. Fornett, H.S. Stiehl, Spline-based elastic image registration: integration of landmark errors and orientation attributes, *Comput. Vis. Imag. Under.* 90 (2003) 153-168.

[25] J.C. Bezdek "Pattern Recognition with Fuzzy Objective Function Algorithms", Plenum Press, New York, 1981.

[26] L.A. Piegl, W. Tiller (1997). *The NURBS book, 2nd ed.* New York: Springer.

[27] The European Glaucoma Prevention Study Group (2002). The European Glaucoma Prevention Study: Design and baseline description of the participants. *Ophthalmology. 109,* 1612-1621.

[28] The European Glaucoma Prevention Study Group (2005). Results of the European Glaucoma Prevention Study. *Ophthalmology. 112,* 366-375.

[29] J.S. Schuman, G. Wollstein, T. Farra, E. Hertzmark, A. Audin, J.G. Fujimoto, L.A. Paunescu (2003). Comparison of optic nerve head measurements obtained by Optical Coherence Tomography and Confocal Scanning Laser Ophthalmoscopy. *Am. J. Ophthalmol., 135,* 504-512.

[30] F.A. Medeiros, R. Jr. Susanna (2003). Comparison algorithms for detection of localized nerve fibre layer defects using scanning laser polarimetry. *Br. J. Ophthalmol., 87,* 413-419.

[31] A.J. Correnti, G. Wollstein, L.L. Price, J.S. Schuman (2003). Comparison of optic nerve head assessment with a Digital Stereoscopic Camera (Discam), Scanning Laser Ophthalmoscopy, and Stereophotography. *Ophthalmol., 110*, 1499-1505.

[32] J.E. Morgan, N.J.L. Sheen, R.V. North, R. Goyal, S. Morgan, E. Asari, J.M. Wild (2005). Discrimination of glaucomatous optic neuropathy by digital stereoscopic analysis. *Ophthalmol., 112*, 855-862.

[33] P. Mitchell, H. Leung, J.J. Wang, E. Rochtchina, A.J. Lee, T.Y. Wong, R. Klein (2005). Retinal vessel diameter and open-angle glaucoma – The Blue Mountains Eye Study. *Ophthalmology. 112*, 245-250.

In: Eye Research Developments
Editor: Alan N. Westerhouse
ISBN: 978-1-60741-177-2

Chapter VI

Corneal Endothelial Cells Stress During Acute Allogenic Graft Rejection

Jean-Louis Bourges and Francine Behar-Cohen
Paris Descartes University, Assistance Publique des Hopitaux de Paris, Hotel-Dieu Hospital, Paris, France
Centre de Recherche des Cordeliers, INSERM U 872 team 17.

Abstract

Good vision requires a perfect corneal transparency which is largely supported by endothelial cells (EC). Secondary endothelial failure is a common cause of vision loss and the major cause of corneal graft failure. Any corneal graft is exposed to metabolic stress from the day of the initial keratoplasty surgery to the cumulative consequences of graft ageing. Additionally, during the graft rejection process, an acute cell stress occurs, leading to EC death through both necrosis and apoptosis. Oxidative and nitrosative reactions combine to release highly reactive substances that are toxic to the biological microenvironment. As a consequence, ECs either engage cytoplasm cell defense mechanisms or initiate apoptosis cascade. We observed in animal models that inducible Nitric Oxide Synthase (iNOS) was overproduced during the rejection process in the corneal graft endothelium and that nitrosative EC stress could be caused by in situ formed peroxynitrite. To counterbalance this phenomenon, EC are overproducing anti-apoptotic proteins that can convert into proapoptotic proteins once the defense mechanisms are overwhelmed. Highly specific iNOS inhibitors have been tested in animal models to lower the graft's oxidative reactions and therefore protect graft ECs during acute rejection with encouraging results. Validation of these mechanisms remains to be confirmed in human. In the future however, new therapeutic perspectives could be further investigated to protect metabolically stressed corneal ECs, using focused anti-oxidative or anti-apoptotic drugs.

Introduction

Corneal grafts have a special status compared to other grafts. The corneal tissue differs among other tissues because it is not physiologically vascularized and is permanently exposed to natural radiations (photon, Ultraviolet) favoring transformation of oxygen dioxide (O_2) into free radicals. The precious corneal endothelial cells do not physiologically renew but critically contribute to the maintenance of corneal transparency. Such a transformation of molecular oxygen can contribute to irreversible alterations of the corneal endothelium under combined aggression of both ageing and alloimmune defenses of graft recipient.

Physiologically, oxygen derivatives (like superoxide anion) or nitrogen derivatives (like nitric oxide) generated by oxidation reaction have an essential role for cells. They act as intracellular signals, specifically to promote cell growth, cell differentiation, and to preserve homeostasis. They also demonstrate bactericidal or virucidal properties and allow for necessary apoptosis in immune cells. [1] A permanent consumption counterbalances the production of oxidative components. A positive oxidative imbalance is yet responsible for oxidative stress.

Oxidative stress is commonly used as a generic term pointing both oxidant stress with biological toxicity of oxygen (dioxide, O_2) decomposition and nitrosant stress due to the cross reaction of nitrogen components and oxygen. Thus, a maybe more appropriate term would be oxidative-nitrosative stress. In 2007, the consequences of the "*oxidative stress*" on biological tissues gave rise to more than 14000 review articles among hundred thousand scientific papers found on *Pubmed* database, underlining the exceptional attention paid by the scientific community on that topic.

There are growing arguments suggesting that oxidative and nitrosant stress could be responsible for the alteration of grafted tissues during slow or acute rejection processes in several organs such as kidney, liver, heart, lung or vessels as a consequence of oxidative stress. In this situation, oxidative and nitrosative elements are either generated by immune and phagocytic cells or result from the ischemia-reperfusion syndrome in vascularized organs. The nature and the concentration of oxidative components as well as the time course of tissue exposure modulate the biological toxicity that eventually can cause graft failure.

Although complex and still largely unknown, the toxic role of oxidative reactions taking place in corneal graft cells during the rejection process seems to play a crucial role so that targeted original treatments could protect corneal grafted cells from apoptosis and death.

Oxidative Reactions

An oxidative reaction is characterized be the electron transfert between reductor (giving n electons) and oxidant (catching n electron) as following:

reductor 1 ➔ oxidant1 + n electrons
n electrons + oxidant 2 ➔ reductor 2
The balance reaction is therefore: reductor 1 + oxidant 2 ➔ oxidant 1 + reductor 2

Biological tissues experiment oxidative stress when they face the chemical reaction of oxygen transformation at a toxic level. Two separated phenomenon occur while oxygen transforms: the oxidant reaction, leading to oxidant stress and the nistrosant reaction responsible for nitrosant stress. When the physiological balance between production and consumption of both reactive oxygen species (ROS) or reactive nitrogen species (RNS) of if anti-oxidative defense mechanisms are overwhelmed, organic molecules such as amino acid, fat acid, ose, nucleic acid as well as their biological compound (protein, lipid, sugar, DNA, RNA…) are denatured.

The Oxidant Reaction

Oxygen reduction transforms oxygen dioxide (O_2) into water (H_2O).(figure 1)

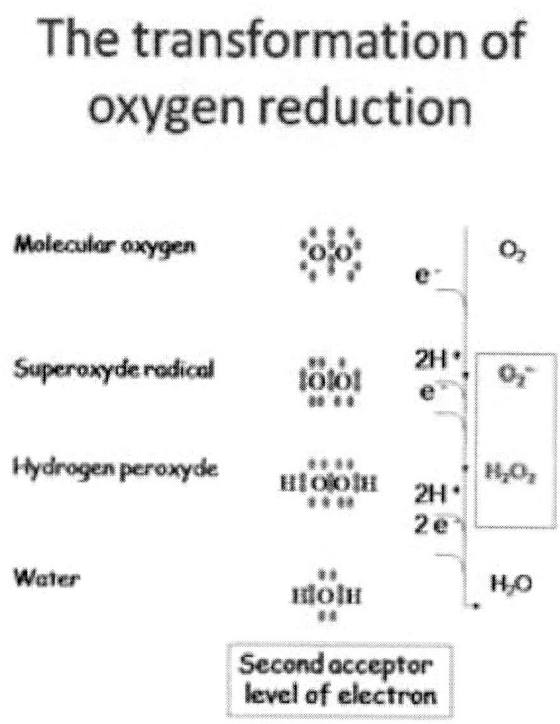

Figure 1. The oxidant reaction catches electrons and hydrogen atoms to generate water. Dots symbols correspond to electrons.

By this way in normal breathing condition, aerobic organisms reduce 1 to 5% of available O_2, producing transient reactive oxygen species (ROS). Some of them have free radicals (OFR) which are lacking a single electron at the second electron level, making them highly reactive to any surrounding environment that could possibly yield the missing electron.

The successive ROS involved in the oxidant reaction are superoxide anion (O2•-), hydrogen peroxide (H_2O_2) and hydroxyle radical (HO•).(table 1)

H_2O_2 is highly reactive with the environment and has strong oxidant properties. It is also highly diffusible through biological membranes and therefore can be active away from the site where it has been produced.

Although less diffusible due to an extremely short half-life (only few nanoseconds), HO• is probably the most reactive ROS in organic environment like proteins, lipids, polyoses and nucleic acids.

Table 1. Chemical entities derived from oxygen transformation or reactive oxygen species (ROS) including oxygen free radicals (OFR) and reactive nitrogen species (RNS)

oxygen free radicals (OFR)	reactive oxygen species (ROS) without free radical
superoxide anion ($O2•^{-}$)	singulet oxygen ($1O_2$)
hydroxyle radical (OH•)	hydrogen peroxide (H_2O_2)
peroxyle radical (R-OO•)	ozone or trioxygen (O_3)
radical alkoxyle (R-O•)	Lipid peroxide (L-OOH)
lipid peroxyle (L-OO•)	hypochloric acid (HOCl)
RNS	
Nitric oxide (NO•)	Nitrogen trioxide (N_2O_3)
nitrosyl cation (NO^{+})	nitroxyl anion (NO^{-})
Nitrite (NO_2•)	Peroxynitrite ($ONOO^{-}$)
nitric acide (HNO_2)	Peroxynitrate (O_2NOOH)
nitryl chloride (NO_2Cl)	

Physiological and Pathological Consequences of the Oxidative Reaction

Each cell in a redox micro environment [2] maintained in a steady state by enzymes [3, 4] as it has also been demonstrated in corneal cells. [5] A change of 30mV in the redox potential multiplies by ten times the cell ROS production. As the oxidant reaction is a part of the mitochondrial breathing chain, it contributes to cell energy production. [6] ROS interact with serine intracellular signalization pathways [7] to modulate cell replication as a function of their concentration. [3, 8-11] Thought the Fenton reaction, oxygen free radicals (OFR) are released, allowing organisms to efficiently fight against infections. [12]

The ROS action has extensively been studied on vascular endothelial cells. Although constantly renewing, the vascular endothelium demonstrates numerous similarities with corneal endothelium. They both share same histological features as a flat monocellular layer unified by and interacting through similar junctions and interestingly also both share similar microenvironments based on collagen matrix (either the tunica intima or the posterior stroma) at their basal side, with liquid bathing their apical side (either blood or aqueous humor). They also interestingly share a couple of identical protein productions(figure 2) ROS have vasoconstriction properties, control lifetime and cell proliferation. [13] they increase pericellular permeability by opening intercellular junctions [14] and/or oxidizing phospholipids. [15]

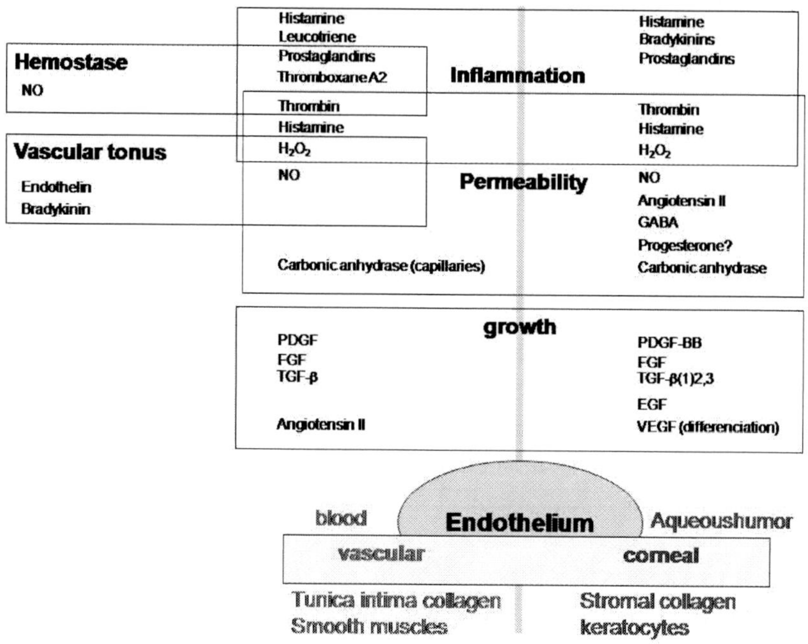

Figure 2. Similarities and differences in microenvironment and production between vascular and corneal endothelial cells.

Pathological conditions such as inflammation, infection, sepsis or hypertension generate ROS production in the microenvironment of vascular endothelial cells. Superoxyde anion induces vasoconstriction when produced at high concentration. [16] A H_2O_2 concentration ranged from 50 to 100 μM induces vascular endothelial apoptosis [17] and cytoskeleton conformational changes occur when H_2O_2 concentration exceeds 200 μM, further increasing intercellular vascular permeability and even leaks. [18] ROS can alter the extracellular matrix in such a way that non-adherent circulating vascular endothelial cells have been pointed out to be markers for vascular prognosis. [19]

Somewhere in between physiology and pathology, the cell ageing is now considered as a consequence of oxidant stress accumulation mediated by OFR. [20] This phenomenon is of particular importance in the cornea and other tissues that are permanently exposed to UV radiation. The ultraviolets generate OFR inducing cell differentiation, mitochondrial DNA deletions [21, 22] and triggering apoptosis cascade. [1, 23]

In the cornea, the transendothelial permeability dramatically increases when H_2O_2 is perfused in the anterior chamber[24] and worsens as a function of age. Additionally, the endothelial cell (EC) density decreases proportionally to age and intraocular inflammation in animals knock-out for extracellular superoxide dismutase (SOD), an key enzyme of the oxidative reaction chain.[25] Hydrogen peroxide is also responsible both for corneal edema and EC loss when accidentally applied on corneal surface by contact lens wearers using non neutralized decontaminant solutions. This emphasize the toxic role of H_2O_2 and O2•- on corneal EC vitality. The ROS could also take a part in the physiopathology of keratoconus as keratoconic cells produce more O2•-than normal ones, maybe due to an abnormal activity of

SOD.[26] They seems to be more sensitive to H_2O_2 toxicity and eventually experiment early apoptosis cascade compared to normal cells. [27]

Oxidant Stress and Organ Transplantation

Once transplanted, vascularized organs are susceptible to ischemia-reperfusion syndrome during which ROS are overproduced both by altered mitochondria and infiltrating inflammatory cells and where, in the end, OH• produced by Fenton reaction transforms lipid (including membrane phospholipids) in toxic peroxylipids. Such a transformation has been successfully inhibited with ROS inactivation. [28, 29] During acute rejection, the level of ROS and RNS in cellular microenvironment tin ten time increased by infiltrating monocytes/macrophages and other immune or inflammatory cells. [30, 31] Reversely, strategies inhibiting the activity of targeted enzymes [32] or administrating OFR scavengers [33-35] during the rejection process resulted in less inflammatory infiltrates, and improved the resistance to oxidant stress as well as preserved the function of rejected organs, thus clearly demonstrating the direct toxicity of ROS.

Nitrosative Reactions

Nitrogen derivatives react with biological environment according to their oxidation level. In fact, the nitrosative reaction can be approached as the interaction between nitric oxide (NO•) or reactive nitrogen species (RNS) and biological components. Schematically, the nitrosative reaction includes nitration responsible for the greater part of nitrosative stress, nitrosylation involved in intracellular signalization processes, nitrosation also contributing to nitrosative stress by nitrite production and finally nitratation transforming nitrite anion. The key substances of nitrosative stress are nitric oxide (NO•), nitric oxide synthases (NOS) and RNS with their own derivatives such as peroxynitrite ($ONOO^-$) or nitrites.

The nitric oxide, originally called "*endothelium derived relaxing factor*" by Furchgott *et coll.* in 1980[36, 37], diffuses in tissues 1.4 times faster than oxygen and only has 1 to 3 seconds of half-life. It reacts with L-arginin under the NOS enzyme activity. Combined with superoxide anion (O2•-), it transforms into peroxynitrite, a highly toxic component for organic environments. [38] The NOS are present in organisms through constitutive (endothelial and neuronal) and inducible (iNOS) isoforms. Interestingly, the endothelial isoform (eNOS) is expressed by corneal endothelium which therefore physiologically produces a basal level of NO•. (figure 3) Constitutive forms are permanently expressed at basal levels and use Ca^{2+} as a co-factor whether iNOS do not need Ca^{2+} as a co-factor but rather transcriptional expression to be produced under inflammatory signals from cytokines or infectious stimuli (IL1β, INF-γ, TNF-α, prostaglandins, bacterial LPS). Despite a delayed production when compared to constitutive NOS, the iNOS lasting activity prolongs for 4 to 24 hours and is that powerful that NO• concentrations can rise to 100 times from basal levels. Unlike constitutive NOS, iNOS is ubiquitary produced.

In combination with oxygen or ROS, NO transforms into ONOO• or nitrite, giving in turn RNS, strongly active in the nitrosative stress. (figure 4)

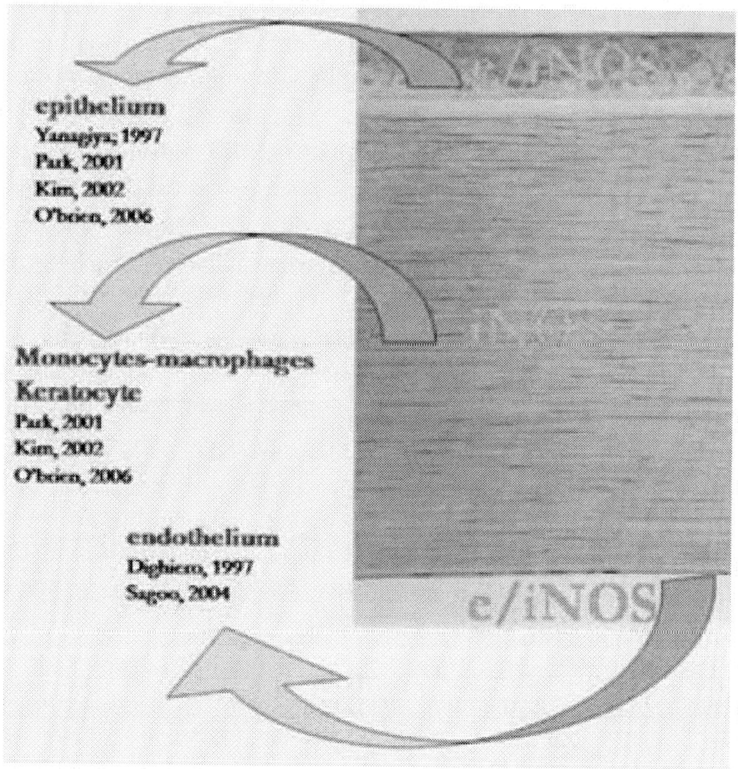

Figure 3. Nitric Oxide Synthase isoforms are produced by the three corneal cell layers, either constitutively (endothelial NOS or eNOS) or is induced by stimuli (inducible NOS or iNOS).

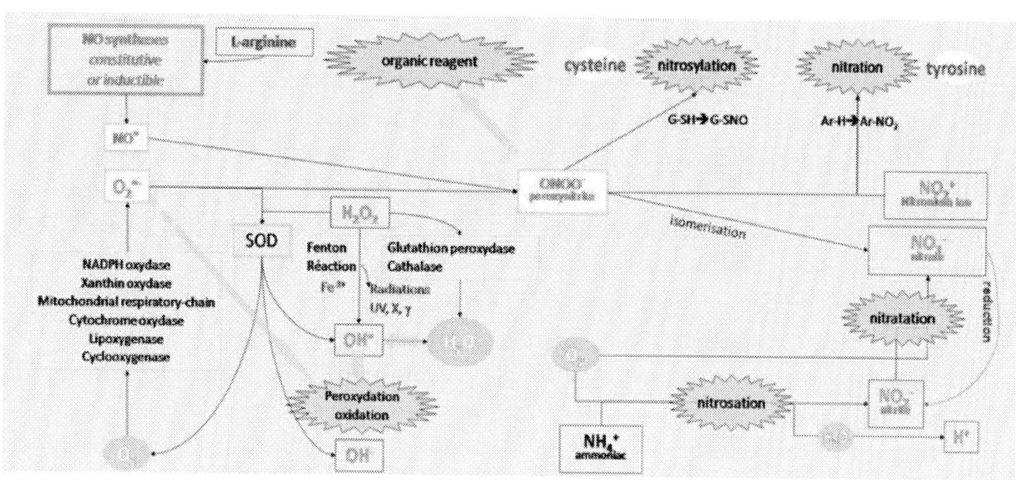

Figure 4. Oxidative and nitrosative reactions are not separated from each other and interact to transform oxygen and nitric oxide into highly reactive components.

Physiological and Pathological Consequences of the Nitrosative Reaction

The effects of NO• can be ambivalent and depend on concentration, duration of production and surrounding environment as well. [39] The basal production of NO• was initially identified to maintain a normal vascular tonus, acting on smooth muscular cells of vessels. Actually, it contributes to numerous signalization pathways. As an example, between 10 to 100nM of concentration, NO• demonstrates anti-apoptotic properties on freshly isolated kindney cells whereas more than 300 nM of concentration confers to NO• a pro-apoptotic activity. [40] More generally, when produced at basal levels through eNOS or nNOS activity, it activates Bcl-2 proteins protecting cells against apoptosis.[41] In the opposite, NO• is produced at high concentration when induced by iNOS and triggers the apoptosis cascade through multiple pathways. [39, 41-45]

In vascular endothelial cell layer, NO• seems to act as an inhibitor of cell proliferation [46] and to increase the endothelial layer permeability, but in a reversible manner when endothelial NOS (eNOS) is inhibited. [47] Nonetheless, a basal production of NO• catalysed by eNOS is necessary to prevent thrombocyte and leucocyte adhesion to the vascular EC wall, unless vessels would easily develop thrombosis. [48]

As non dividing cells in normal condition, neurons and corneal EC both have to face similar and very specific survival issues. It is therefore interesting to observe that some neurons, also called nitrergic neurons, are capable of neuronal NOS expression (nNOS) and have been described to play a significant role in neuromuscular relaxation. [49]

In critical conditions, under iNOS enzymatic activity, NO• level can dramatically surge in cells'microenvironment. During the infectious process, iNos is normally released by immune system cells or phagocytes to provide efficient shield against hostile microorganisms. This generates an overproduction of NO• and consequently a release of RNS, interfering with the mitochondrial respiratory chain of infectious elements or denaturing viruses through S-nitrosylation. [50]

Usually, the "*nitrosative stress*" term designs the toxicity of nitrosative reactions on biological tissues or on organic components. More generally, it induces cell apoptosis and accelerates tissue ageing. Monocytes, macrophages, natural killer cells, phagocytic cells, neutrophil granulocytes, carcinomatous cells and endothelial cells (in addition to eNOS) are well known to express iNOS under appropriate stimuli. Alone or in combination, ROS, NO• and RNS change biological functions of proteins by nitration of each single tyrosine or tryptophan residue so that protein conformation changes. This 3-dimentional transformation of proteins can be now precisely anticipated by computerized programs.

Among all RNS, the peroxynitrite ($ONOO^-$) is one of the most toxic for biological tissues despite it degrades is very fast (degradation constant=6 x 10^9 M/sec). It leads to both oxidation and nitration depending on pH and CO_2 levels in the environment. [51] In vascular EC, when appropriate conditions are set together to allow peroxinitrite formation, it consumes a part of the basal production of NO• (figure 4) and promotes apoptosis. [52]

In the cornea, eNOS is constitutively expressed by endothelium (figure 3) and a corneal thickening has been observed after experimental inhibition, assuming that one of the eNOS function would be to maintain watertightness in the corneal endothelial layer[53], although we rather would expect opposite effects from results obtained in vascular endothelium. On the other hand, corneal endothelium also produces iNOS, NO• and can generate nitrotyrosines when exposed to excessive stress such as infection, inflammation, organoculture or radiations. [54-57] An high concentration of NO• in aqueous humor results in corneal edema in rabbits[58]. Furthermore, in experimental inflammation, corneal thickness can be significantly reduced by iNOS inhibition alone. [59]

Oxidative-Nitrosative Stress and Cell Death

Schematically, cells undergo death through many different ways. Cell death can either be programmed or occurs following a sudden event. Programmed cell death can be seen as the opposite process of cell proliferation. It allows cells to disappear without any damage to their surrounding microenvironment. This process refers to type 1 cell death (apoptosis, paraptosis) and type 2 (autophagy). In the opposite, non programmed cell death (necrosis or type 3 cell death) suddenly occurs, associating cytoplasmic and lysosomial disorders. This type of cell death is often responsible for collateral damages to the cell vicinity.

The ROS H_2O_2 and $O^{2}•^{-}$ are able to trigger apoptosis by activating the mitochondrial pathway [60] usually in response to protein kinase signals, in a reversible manner by activation of Bcl-2 proteins. [61] However, at high concentrations, H_2O_2 directly induces necrosis. NO• also interfere with the apoptosis mitochondrial pathway through MAP kinases and RNS (especially peroxynitrite) activation of JNK pathway is decreased by inhibition of iNOS in vascular endothelial cells. [62] ROS and RNS are synergic to trigger apoptosis. Stimulated by oxidative-nitrosative stress, cells can trigger either caspase dependant or non-caspase dependant apoptosis pathways. As an example, the apoptosis Inducible Factor (AIF) pathway is engaged by $ONOO^-$ in neurons. [63] Interestingly in neurons, the ONOO- could originate both from $O^{2}•^{-}$ and the endogenous NO• produces under eNOS enzymatic activity. [64] This would strongly suggest that corneal endothelial cells, that are also able to produce endogenous NO•, could be subjected to some identical stress.

Nitrosative Stress and Organ Transplantation

During rejection, iNOS is overexpressed [65-70] largely by inflammatory cells[71] and resident endothelial cells. This results in an overproduction of RNS that both lead to oxidative stress by SOD nitration[72] and generates nitrotyrosines by protein degradation. Scabolz *et Al.* have demonstrated the responsibility of iNOS expression in the immune process of heart rejection and in apoptosis of cardiac muscle cells. [73] More generally, nitrate and nitrites can be used as markers to evaluate the time course of the rejection process when dosed in biological fluids. [68] It seems that peroxynitrite could also be involved in function failure of rejected organs as a normal function can be preserved in some part after rejection when peroxinitrite is inhibited. [74]

Oxidative-Nitrosative Stress During Corneal Graft Rejection

Does Oxidative-Nitrosative Stress Affect Corneal Grafted Endothelial Cell Death During Rejection?

Although oxidative and nitrosative stress should theoretically develop during acute phase of the rejection process which releases many inflammatory cytokines in corneal microenvironment, little was known about this until Strestikova et coll. [75] observed that iNOS was inhibited by FK506 (Tacrolimus ™), an effective immunosuppressor they used in grafted mice subjected to allogeneic rejection. They reported better survival curves for treated grafts, even once rejection has occurred. This first step led us to investigate the role of iNOS, NO• and peroxynitrite, one of the most biologically toxic NO derivate.

To address this question, we used a previously characterized experimental model of acute rejection in total thickness corneal grafts where Brown-Norway rat corneas were grafted on Lewis rat recipients. [76-78] This model allows to graft rejection usually on day 5 after keratoplasty and progress until day 13-14 where the acute inflammatory phase of rejection transforms into stable non inflammatory opacities and fibrosis.(figure 5) The corneal edema, the neovessel growing progression as well as the buttons' transparency can be observed and quantified with clinical scores. (table 2)

Table 2. Grading scale used to quantify clinical patterns of rejection

Clinical Score	Corneal transparency	Stromal Edema	Neovascularization
0	clear cornea	no edema	no observable growth of new vessels
1	slight opacity	slight edema	new vessels invading < 1/3 of the recipient bed
2	mild opacity with iris details visible	diffuse and moderate stromal edema	new vessels invading < 2/3 of the recipient bed
3	moderate, iris details not visible	diffuse and marked edema	new vessels growing up to the limiting ring
4	white cornea		new vessels invading the graft

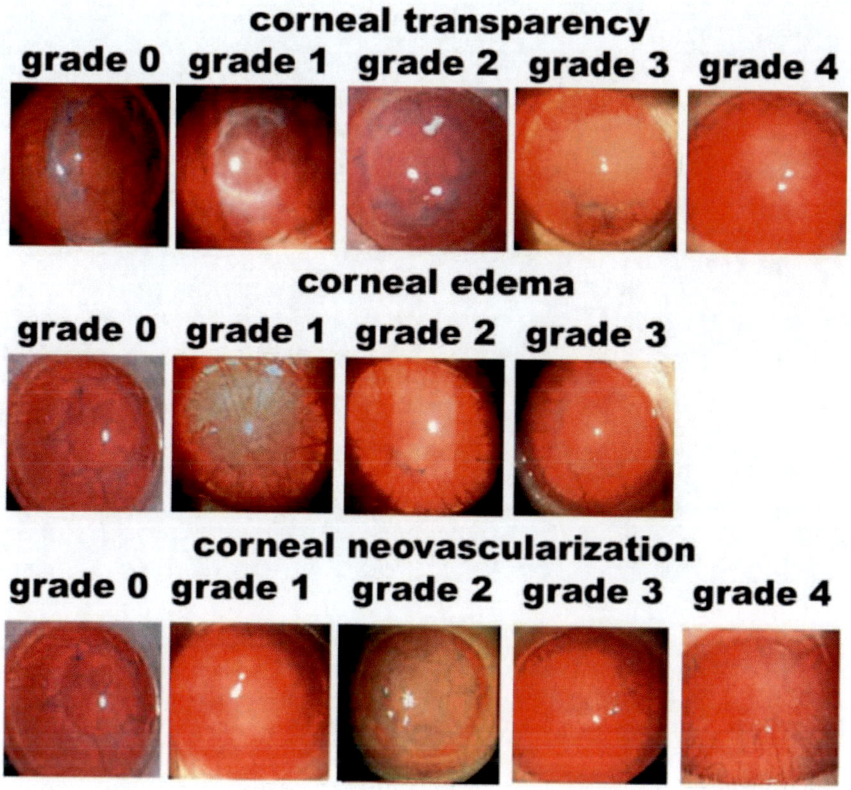

Figure 5. The experimental corneal graft model of acute allogeneic rejection is quantified with clinical scores of transparency, edema and neovascularization.

We used this model to analyze buttons and recipient beds at various critical time points (D5, D7, D10, D13 and D14) during the rejection time course. Corneas were immunostained with anti-iNOS, anti-nitrotyrosine (a marker of peroxynitrite toxicity on proteins), ED1 and OX42 (monocyte and macrophage cell lines) antibodies. As the rejection process progressed, we observed a co-staining of infiltrating monocyte-macrophages cells and iNOS or anti-nitrotyrosine in the corneal stroma or both recipients and buttons. After 5 days, only infiltrating cells were stained for iNOS and nitrotyrosine in the anterior stroma of both graft and recipient corneas, growing up in intensity as the rejection developed. No staining was seen in the endothelial cell layer until day 10 where iNOS and nitrotyrosine revealed in EC of buttons but not in recipient corneas. (figure 6) When the acute rejection phase resolved at day 14, ED1+/OX42+ cells density dramatically decreased in recipient bed whereas it increased markedly in grafted stroma. No staining could be identified as endothelial due to the extreme rarefaction of EC in the graft at that time point. We concluded that, through iNOS induction in infiltrating cells and in corneal endothelial cells, NO• and peroxynitrite formation could contribute to cell toxicity and more specifically graft EC cell death in the during corneal graft rejection in this animal model. [79, 80]

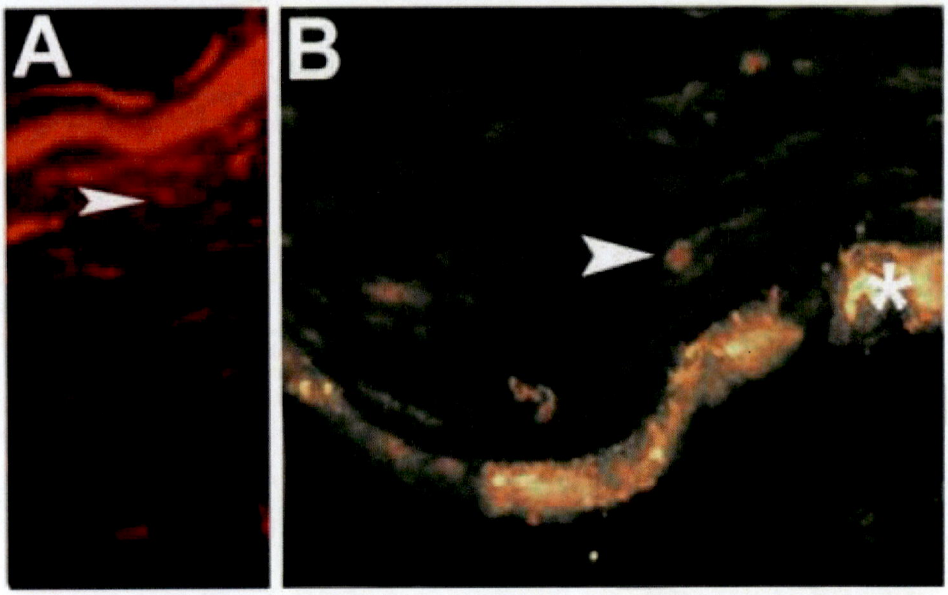

Figure 6. At day 10, iNOS is expressed in the recipient, mostly in the anterior stroma and associated to vessels (A, arrow head). In the graft (B), iNOS (green) is expressed in stromal infiltrating cells and in the endothelium (asterisk) or in cells adherent to the endothelium where nitrotyrosines (B; red, arrowhead) were also observed (red+green=orange).

We therefore aimed to further characterize the nitrosative toxicity on cornea and particularly corneal EC. To achieve this, we exposed corneal endothelia directly to peroxynitrite. As this component is extremely labile, it should be dissolved in low concentration of iced NaOH. Thus, we previously dosed the perxoxynitrite concentration in NaOH solution with spectrometry and controlled each experiment with both NaOH vehicle and denatured peroxynitrite.

We injected increasing concentration of peroxynitrite (from 50 to 500 μM $ONOO^-$)in the anterior chamber of rats and observed corneas at various time points from 10 min to 24 hours after injection with biomicroscopic direct examination, *in-vivo* confocal microscope (HRT II; Heidelberg Engineering, Dossenheim, Allemagne). We also performed tunnel assay (general maker for caspase-dependant apoptosis) and immunostaining with anti-nitrotyrosine and LEI/LDNAse II (marker for non-caspase dependant apoptosis) antibodies. Whatever the ONOO- concentration was, a corneal edema occurred immediately after injection and only resolved after 6 hours at the lowest concentration (50μM ONOO-) whereas controls did not induced any clinical change. (figure 7) After 24 hours, microhemorrhages and fibrin developed in the anterior chamber of 250 and 500 μM $ONOO^-$ injected rats. While 50 μM ONOO- shown some alterations of intercellular junctions (figure 8), significant increase in corneal thickness ($p<0.0001$) and decrease in EC density ($p<0.001$), higher concentration completely destroyed the EC layer. Immunochemistery showed no anti-nitrotyrosine staining in controls, which only expressed LEI in their cytoplasm. In the opposite, a strong staining of both anti-nitrotyrosine and intranuclear translocated LEI/DNAse II was observed in every exposed corneal endothelial cell, demonstrating the toxicity and the apoptosis triggering induced by the $ONOO^-$itself.[81] We further confirmed those results on human eye-banked corneas, demonstrating a significant decrease in EC vitality and density after exposure to peroxynitrite. [81] All those results taken together, it seems that during corneal graft rejection, iNOS is overexpressed by inflammatory infiltrating cells and, although it is still debated[82], possibly by endothelial cells, allowing L-arginine to transform into NO• at high concentration that further transform into $ONOO^-$. The latest, nitrating protein tyrosins, either exerts a direct toxicity on graft cells or triggers a programmed death in exposed cells.

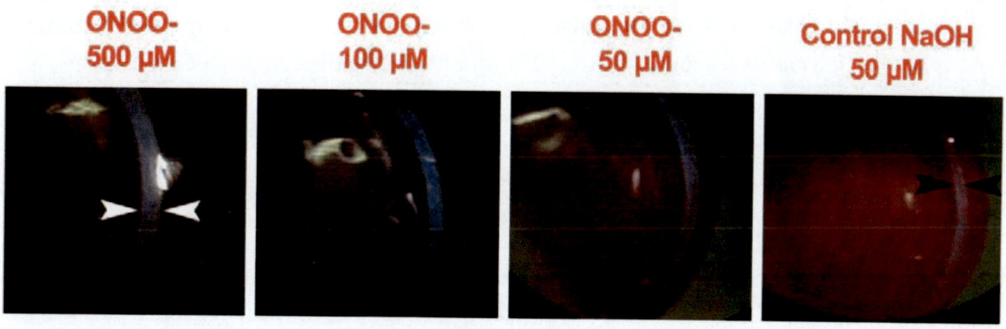

Figure 7. When injected at increasing concentrations in the anterior chamber of rats, $ONOO^-$ induced a corneal edema occurred immediately after injection, clinically seen as an increase in corneal thickness (between white arrow heads on slit lamp examination) and only resolved after 6 hours at the lowest $ONOO^-$ concentration (50μM), whereas controls did not induced any clinical change (between black arrow heads).

Fi

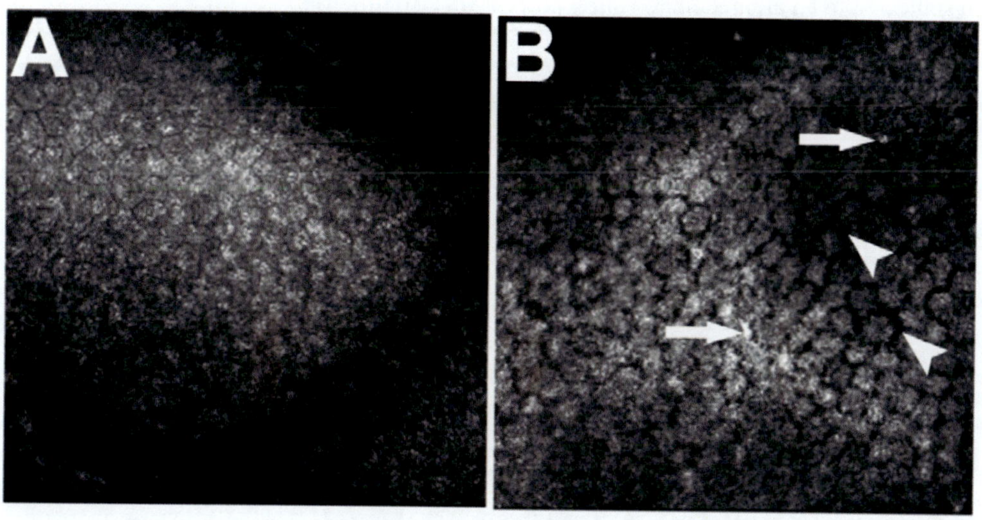

Figure 8. The vivo confocal microscope examination 24H after 50μM NaOH control (A) or 50 μM ONOO- (B) injection in the anterior chamber shows that non exposed endothelium remains normal (A) whereas alterations of intercellular endothelial cell junctions (B, arrow heads) developed in ONOO- exposed cells and adherent inflammatory cells were layed at the inner endothelial side(arrows).

How to Extrapolate the Rat Data to Human Situation?

One must consider that contrarily to the rat corneal endothelium, the human endothelium doesn't have mitotic activity. Because endothelial cells integrity is essential to vision, it is expected that very strong anti-oxidant mechanisms are effective in the human cornea to prevent oxidative damages. When endothelial anti-oxidant mechanisms are overstepped, phenomenon of oxidative damages are likely to be triggered as well, but probably at higher thresholds compared to what we observed in the rat, which could explain why endothelial failure is a very unusual outcome of chronic anterior segment inflammations.

Can Corneal Endothelial Cells Be Protected from the Oxidative-Nitrosative Stress?

To address this, our experiments focused on whether the nitrosative toxic cascade could be inflexed during and after rejection by protecting cells against nitrosative stress.

Once again, we used the animal model of acute corneal graft rejection to address this question. We systemically administrated to grafted animals a powerful selective inhibitor of iNOS, so-called 1400W and observed the effect on the endothelial cell layer versus saline controls. No effect was observed on the rejection rate as one would expect, but the EC density was statistically improved in every part of rejected buttons in treated animals, demonstrating the protective effect of nitrosative stress inhibitors on corneal endothelium when subjected to an allogeneic rejection process. [81](figure 9)

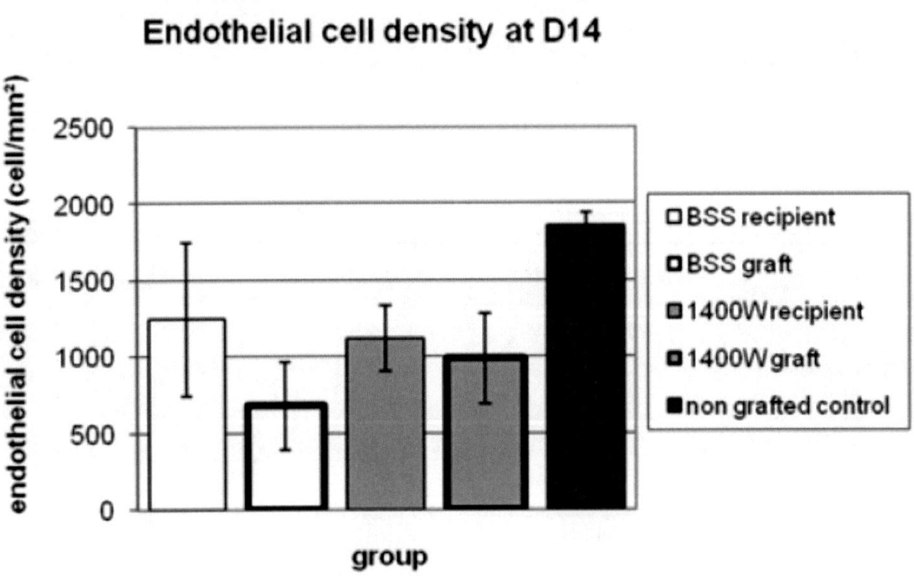

Figure 9. The EC density of rejected buttons can be improved in animals treated by systemic selective inhibitor of iNOS.

In conclusion, oxidative-nitrosative stress refers to chemical reactions and pathways with close relationships. Oxidative and nitrosative reactions can exert synergistic toxicities on tissues. Indeed, corneal rejection is a consequence of an alloimmune phenomenon and has to be treated as soon as possible accordingly. However, the final buttons' outcome could also depend on oxidative-nitrosative "collateral" damages that may contribute corneal graft failure even after successfully reversed rejections. It is an encouraging that endothelial cell density could be preserved during and after acute rejection by inhibitors of iNOS. This could be an interesting way to protect corneal grafts. We might therefore consider anti-oxidant drugs as possible therapies to administrate in grafted patients in addition to usual immunosuppressive and/or anti-inflammatory treatments.

References

[1] Valko M, Leibfritz D, Moncol J, Cronin MT, Mazur M, Telser J. Free radicals and antioxidants in normal physiological functions and human disease. *Int. J. Biochem. Cell. Biol.* 2007;39(1):44-84.

[2] Schafer FQ, Buettner GR. Redox environment of the cell as viewed through the redox state of the glutathione disulfide/glutathione couple. *Free Radic. Biol. Med.* 2001;30(11):1191-212.

[3] Droge W. Free radicals in the physiological control of cell function. *Physiol. Rev.* 2002;82(1):47-95.

[4] Thannickal VJ, Fanburg BL. Reactive oxygen species in cell signaling. *Am. J. Physiol. Lung Cell Mol. Physiol.* 2000;279(6):L1005-28.

[5] O'Brien WJ, Krema C, Heimann T, Zhao H. Expression of NADPH oxidase in rabbit corneal epithelial and stromal cells in culture. *Invest. Ophthalmol. Vis. Sci.* 2006;47(3):853-63.

[6] Adam-Vizi V, Chinopoulos C. Bioenergetics and the formation of mitochondrial reactive oxygen species. *Trends Pharmacol. Sci.* 2006;27(12):639-45.

[7] Gopalakrishna R, Jaken S. Protein kinase C signaling and oxidative stress. *Free Radic. Biol. Med.* 2000;28(9):1349-61.

[8] Galter D, Mihm S, Droge W. Distinct effects of glutathione disulphide on the nuclear transcription factor kappa B and the activator protein-1. *Eur. J. Biochem.* 1994;221(2):639-48.

[9] Kuge S, Jones N. YAP1 dependent activation of TRX2 is essential for the response of Saccharomyces cerevisiae to oxidative stress by hydroperoxides. *Embo J.* 1994;13(3):655-64.

[10] Aslund F, Zheng M, Beckwith J, Storz G. Regulation of the OxyR transcription factor by hydrogen peroxide and the cellular thiol-disulfide status. *Proc. Natl. Acad. Sci. U. S. A.* 1999;96(11):6161-5.

[11] Hehner SP, Breitkreutz R, Shubinsky G, Unsoeld H, Schulze-Osthoff K, Schmitz ML, et al. Enhancement of T cell receptor signaling by a mild oxidative shift in the intracellular thiol pool. *J. Immunol.* 2000;165(8):4319-28.

[12] Fialkow L, Wang Y, Downey GP. Reactive oxygen and nitrogen species as signaling molecules regulating neutrophil function. *Free Radic. Biol. Med.* 2007;42(2):153-64.

[13] Abid MR, Kachra Z, Spokes KC, Aird WC. NADPH oxidase activity is required for endothelial cell proliferation and migration. *FEBS Lett.* 2000;486(3):252-6.

[14] Lee HS, Namkoong K, Kim DH, Kim KJ, Cheong YH, Kim SS, et al. Hydrogen peroxide-induced alterations of tight junction proteins in bovine brain microvascular endothelial cells. *Microvasc. Res.* 2004;68(3):231-8.

[15] DeMaio L, Rouhanizadeh M, Reddy S, Sevanian A, Hwang J, Hsiai TK. Oxidized phospholipids mediate occludin expression and phosphorylation in vascular endothelial cells. *Am. J. Physiol. Heart Circ. Physiol.* 2006;290(2):H674-83.

[16] Didion SP, Faraci FM. Effects of NADH and NADPH on superoxide levels and cerebral vascular tone. *Am. J. Physiol. Heart Circ. Physiol.* 2002;282(2):H688-95.

[17] Thomas SR, Chen K, Keaney JF, Jr. Hydrogen peroxide activates endothelial nitric-oxide synthase through coordinated phosphorylation and dephosphorylation via a phosphoinositide 3-kinase-dependent signaling pathway. *J. Biol. Chem.* 2002;277(8):6017-24.

[18] Dudek SM, Garcia JG. Cytoskeletal regulation of pulmonary vascular permeability. *J. Appl. Physiol.* 2001;91(4):1487-500.

[19] Dignat-George F, Sampol J, Lip G, Blann AD. Circulating endothelial cells: realities and promises in vascular disorders. *Pathophysiol. Haemost. Thromb.* 2003;33(5-6):495-9.

[20] Balaban RS, Nemoto S, Finkel T. Mitochondria, oxidants, and aging. *Cell.* 2005;120(4):483-95.

[21] Wei YH, Lee HC. Oxidative stress, mitochondrial DNA mutation, and impairment of antioxidant enzymes in aging. *Exp. Biol. Med.* (Maywood) 2002;227(9):671-82.

[22] Terman A, Gustafsson B, Brunk UT. Mitochondrial damage and intralysosomal degradation in cellular aging. *Mol. Aspects Med.* 2006;27(5-6):471-82.

[23] Le Bras M, Clement MV, Pervaiz S, Brenner C. Reactive oxygen species and the mitochondrial signaling pathway of cell death. *Histol. Histopathol.* 2005;20(1):205-19.

[24] Hull DS. Oxygen free radicals and corneal endothelium: effect on fluxes and permeability. *Trans Am. Ophthalmol. Soc.* 1991;89:195-204; discussion 204-8.

[25] Behndig A, Karlsson K, Brannstrom T, Sentman ML, Marklund SL. Corneal endothelial integrity in mice lacking extracellular superoxide dismutase. *Invest. Ophthalmol. Vis. Sci.* 2001;42(12):2784-8.

[26] Behndig A, Karlsson K, Johansson BO, Brannstrom T, Marklund SL. Superoxide dismutase isoenzymes in the normal and diseased human cornea. *Invest. Ophthalmol. Vis. Sci.* 2001;42(10):2293-6.

[27] Chwa M, Atilano SR, Reddy V, Jordan N, Kim DW, Kenney MC. Increased stress-induced generation of reactive oxygen species and apoptosis in human keratoconus fibroblasts. *Invest. Ophthalmol. Vis. Sci.* 2006;47(5):1902-10.

[28] Bando K, Teramoto S, Tago M, Seno S, Murakami T, Nawa S, et al. Oxygenated perfluorocarbon, recombinant human superoxide dismutase, and catalase ameliorate free radical induced myocardial injury during heart preservation and transplantation. *J. Thorac. Cardiovasc. Surg.* 1988;96(6):930-8.

[29] Carrea FP, Lesnefsky EJ, Kaiser DG, Horwitz LD. The lazaroid U74006F, a 21-aminosteroid inhibitor of lipid peroxidation, attenuates myocardial injury from ischemia and reperfusion. *J. Cardiovasc. Pharmacol.* 1992;20(2):230-5.

[30] Rauen U, Viebahn R, Lauchart W, de Groot H. The potential role of reactive oxygen species in liver ischemia/reperfusion injury following liver surgery. *Hepatogastroenterology.* 1994;41(4):333-6.

[31] Jaeschke H. Reactive oxygen and ischemia/reperfusion injury of the liver. *Chem. Biol. Interact.* 1991;79(2):115-36.

[32] Olcott AP, Tocco G, Tian J, Zekzer D, Fukuto J, Ignarro L, et al. A salen-manganese catalytic free radical scavenger inhibits type 1 diabetes and islet allograft rejection. *Diabetes.* 2004;53(10):2574-80.

[33] Sepodes B, Maio R, Pinto R, Marques C, Mendes-do-Vale J, McDonald MC, et al. Tempol, an intracelullar free radical scavenger, reduces liver injury in hepatic ischemia-reperfusion in the rat. *Transplant. Proc.* 2004;36(4):849-53.

[34] He SQ, Zhang YH, Venugopal SK, Dicus CW, Perez RV, Ramsamooj R, et al. Delivery of antioxidative enzyme genes protects against ischemia/reperfusion-induced liver injury in mice. *Liver Transpl.* 2006;12(12):1869-79.

[35] Tocco G, Illigens BM, Malfroy B, Benichou G. Prolongation of alloskin graft survival by catalytic scavengers of reactive oxygen species. *Cell Immunol.* 2006;241(2):59-65.

[36] Furchgott RF, Zawadzki JV. The obligatory role of endothelial cells in the relaxation of arterial smooth muscle by acetylcholine. *Nature.* 1980;288(5789):373-6.

[37] Palmer RM, Ferrige AG, Moncada S. Nitric oxide release accounts for the biological activity of endothelium-derived relaxing factor. *Nature.* 1987;327(6122):524-6.

[38] Nathan C, Shiloh MU. Reactive oxygen and nitrogen intermediates in the relationship between mammalian hosts and microbial pathogens. *Proc. Natl. Acad. Sci. U. S. A.* 2000;97(16):8841-8.

[39] Hara MR, Agrawal N, Kim SF, Cascio MB, Fujimuro M, Ozeki Y, et al. S-nitrosylated GAPDH initiates apoptotic cell death by nuclear translocation following Siah1 binding. *Nat. Cell Biol.* 2005;7(7):665-74.

[40] Goligorsky MS, Brodsky SV, Noiri E. Nitric oxide in acute renal failure: NOS versus NOS. *Kidney Int.* 2002;61(3):855-61.

[41] Tamatani M, Ogawa S, Niitsu Y, Tohyama M. Involvement of Bcl-2 family and caspase-3-like protease in NO-mediated neuronal apoptosis. *J. Neurochem.* 1998;71(4):1588-96.

[42] Messmer UK, Brune B. Nitric oxide-induced apoptosis: p53-dependent and p53-independent signalling pathways. *Biochem. J.* 1996;319 (Pt 1):299-305.

[43] Glockzin S, von Knethen A, Scheffner M, Brune B. Activation of the cell death program by nitric oxide involves inhibition of the proteasome. *J. Biol. Chem.* 1999;274(28):19581-6.

[44] Kim KM, Kim PK, Kwon YG, Bai SK, Nam WD, Kim YM. Regulation of apoptosis by nitrosative stress. *J. Biochem. Mol. Biol.* 2002;35(1):127-33.

[45] Guikema B, Lu Q, Jourd'heuil D. Chemical considerations and biological selectivity of protein nitrosation: implications for NO-mediated signal transduction. *Antioxid. Redox. Signal.* 2005;7(5-6):593-606.

[46] Bayraktutan U. Nitric oxide synthase and NAD(P)H oxidase modulate coronary endothelial cell growth. *J. Mol. Cell Cardiol.* 2004;36(2):277-86.

[47] Schubert W, Frank PG, Woodman SE, Hyogo H, Cohen DE, Chow CW, et al. Microvascular hyperpermeability in caveolin-1 (-/-) knock-out mice. Treatment with a specific nitric-oxide synthase inhibitor, L-NAME, restores normal microvascular permeability in Cav-1 null mice. *J. Biol. Chem.* 2002;277(42):40091-8.

[48] Lee PC, Wang ZL, Qian S, Watkins SC, Lizonova A, Kovesdi I, et al. Endothelial nitric oxide synthase protects aortic allografts from the development of transplant arteriosclerosis. *Transplantation.* 2000;69(6):1186-92.

[49] Toda N, Okamura T. The pharmacology of nitric oxide in the peripheral nervous system of blood vessels. *Pharmacol. Rev.* 2003;55(2):271-324.

[50] Fang FC. Antimicrobial reactive oxygen and nitrogen species: concepts and controversies. *Nat. Rev. Microbiol.* 2004;2(10):820-32.

[51] Ducrocq C, Blanchard B, Pignatelli B, Ohshima H. Peroxynitrite: an endogenous oxidizing and nitrating agent. *Cell Mol. Life Sci.* 1999;55(8-9):1068-77.

[52] Szabo C, Cuzzocrea S, Zingarelli B, O'Connor M, Salzman AL. Endothelial dysfunction in a rat model of endotoxic shock. Importance of the activation of poly (ADP-ribose) synthetase by peroxynitrite. *J. Clin. Invest.* 1997;100(3):723-35.

[53] Yanagiya N, Akiba J, Kado M, Yoshida A, Kono T, Iwamoto J. Transient corneal edema induced by nitric oxide synthase inhibition. *Nitric. Oxide.* 1997;1(5):397-403.

[54] Dighiero P, Behar-Cohen F, Courtois Y, Goureau O. Expression of inducible nitric oxide synthase in bovine corneal endothelial cells and keratocytes in vitro after lipopolysaccharide and cytokines stimulation. *Invest. Ophthalmol. Vis. Sci.* 1997;38(10):2045-52.

[55] O'Brien WJ, Heimann T, Tsao LS, Seet BT, McFadden G, Taylor JL. Regulation of nitric oxide synthase 2 in rabbit corneal cells. *Invest. Ophthalmol. Vis. Sci.* 2001;42(3):713-9.

[56] Sagoo P, Chan G, Larkin DF, George AJ. Inflammatory cytokines induce apoptosis of corneal endothelium through nitric oxide. *Invest. Ophthalmol. Vis. Sci.* 2004;45(11):3964-73.

[57] Cejkova J, Ardan T, Cejka C, Kovaceva J, Zidek Z. Irradiation of the rabbit cornea with UVB rays stimulates the expression of nitric oxide synthases-generated nitric oxide and the formation of cytotoxic nitrogen-related oxidants. *Histol. Histopathol.* 2005;20(2):467-73.

[58] Yanagiya N, Akiba J, Kado M, Hikichi T, Yoshida A. Effects of peroxynitrite on rabbit cornea. *Graefes Arch. Clin. Exp. Ophthalmol.* 2000;238(7):584-8.

[59] Behar-Cohen FF, Savoldelli M, Parel JM, Goureau O, Thillaye-Goldenberg B, Courtois Y, et al. Reduction of corneal edema in endotoxin-induced uveitis after application of L-NAME as nitric oxide synthase inhibitor in rats by iontophoresis. *Invest. Ophthalmol. Vis. Sci.* 1998;39(6):897-904.

[60] Cooke JP, Dzau VJ. Nitric oxide synthase: role in the genesis of vascular disease. *Annu. Rev. Med.* 1997;48:489-509.

[61] Hockenbery DM, Oltvai ZN, Yin XM, Milliman CL, Korsmeyer SJ. Bcl-2 functions in an antioxidant pathway to prevent apoptosis. *Cell.* 1993;75(2):241-51.

[62] Go YM, Patel RP, Maland MC, Park H, Beckman JS, Darley-Usmar VM, et al. Evidence for peroxynitrite as a signaling molecule in flow-dependent activation of c-Jun NH(2)-terminal kinase. *Am. J. Physiol.* 1999;277(4 Pt 2):H1647-53.

[63] Zhang X, Chen J, Graham S, Du L, Kochanek P, Draviam R, et al. Intranuclear localization of apoptosis-inducing factor (AIF) and large scale DNA fragmentation after traumatic brain injury in rats and in neuronal cultures exposed to peroxynitrite. *J. Neurochem.* 2002;82:181-91.

[64] Li X, Nemoto M, Xu Z, Yu SW, Shimoji M, Andrabi SA, et al. Influence of duration of focal cerebral ischemia and neuronal nitric oxide synthase on translocation of apoptosis-inducing factor to the nucleus. *Neuroscience.* 2007;144(1):56-65.

[65] Yang X, Chowdhury N, Cai B, Brett J, Marboe C, Sciacca RR, et al. Induction of myocardial nitric oxide synthase by cardiac allograft rejection. *J. Clin. Invest.* 1994;94(2):714-21.

[66] Russell ME, Wallace AF, Wyner LR, Newell JB, Karnovsky MJ. Upregulation and modulation of inducible nitric oxide synthase in rat cardiac allografts with chronic rejection and transplant arteriosclerosis. *Circulation.* 1995;92(3):457-64.

[67] Smith SD, Wheeler MA, Zhang R, Weiss ED, Lorber MI, Sessa WC, et al. Nitric oxide synthase induction with renal transplant rejection or infection. *Kidney Int.* 1996;50(6):2088-93.

[68] Albrecht EW, van Goor H, Tiebosch AT, Moshage H, Tegzess AM, Stegeman CA. Nitric oxide production and nitric oxide synthase expression in acute human renal allograft rejection. *Transplantation.* 2000;70(11):1610-6.

[69] Diao TJ, Yuan TY, Li YL. Immunologic role of nitric oxide in acute rejection of golden hamster to rat liver xenotransplantation. *World J. Gastroenterol.* 2002;8(4):746-51.

[70] Joles JA, Vos IH, Grone HJ, Rabelink TJ. Inducible nitric oxide synthase in renal transplantation. *Kidney Int.* 2002;61(3):872-5.

[71] Guzik TJ, Korbut R, Adamek-Guzik T. Nitric oxide and superoxide in inflammation and immune regulation. *J. Physiol. Pharmacol.* 2003;54(4):469-87.

[72] Nilakantan V, Halligan NL, Nguyen TK, Hilton G, Khanna AK, Roza AM, et al. Post-translational modification of manganese superoxide dismutase in acutely rejecting cardiac transplants: role of inducible nitric oxide synthase. *J. Heart Lung Transplant.* 2005;24(10):1591-9.

[73] Szabolcs MJ, Ma N, Athan E, Zhong J, Ming M, Sciacca RR, et al. Acute cardiac allograft rejection in nitric oxide synthase-2(-/-) and nitric oxide synthase-2(+/+) mice: effects of cellular chimeras on myocardial inflammation and cardiomyocyte damage and apoptosis. *Circulation.* 2001;103(20):2514-20.

[74] Vos IH, Joles JA, Rabelink TJ. The role of nitric oxide in renal transplantation. *Semin. Nephrol.* 2004;24(4):379-88.

[75] Strestikova P, Plskova J, Filipec M, Farghali H. FK 506 and aminoguanidine suppress iNOS induction in orthotopic corneal allografts and prolong graft survival in mice. *Nitric Oxide.* 2003;9(2):111-7.

[76] Larkin DF, Calder VL, Lightman SL. Identification and characterization of cells infiltrating the graft and aqueous humour in rat corneal allograft rejection. *Clin. Exp. Immunol.* 1997;107(2):381-91.

[77] Behar-Cohen F, Bourges JL, Agla E, Lallemand F, Gurny R, Jean–Maurice D, et al. Kinetics of Cell Reactions and Death during Corneal Graft Rejection. *Invest. Ophthalmol. Vis. Sci.* 2003;44(E-Abstract):911.

[78] Bourges JL, Valamanesh F, Agla EK, Lallemand F, Gurny FR, Jean–Maurice D, et al. Topical hydrosoluble prodrug of cyclosporin A to prevent corneal graft rejection. *Ophthalmic Research.* 2004;36(S1):75.

[79] Bourges JL, Valamanesh F, Torriglia A, Jeanny JC, Savoldelli M, Renard G, et al. Cornea graft endothelial cells undergo apoptosis by way of an alternate (caspase-independent) pathway. *Transplantation.* 2004;78(3):316-23.

[80] Bourges JL, Valamanesh F, Torriglia A, Savoldelli M, Renard G, BenEzra D, et al. Apoptosis pathways and role of nitric oxide in corneal endothelial cell death during acute graft rejection. *Invest. Ophthalmol. Vis. Sci.* 2004;45(E-Abstract):602.

[81] Bourges JL, Torriglia A, Valamanesh F, Benezra D, Renard G, Behar-Cohen FF. Nitrosative stress and corneal transplant endothelial cell death during acute graft rejection. *Transplantation.* 2007;84(3):415-23.

[82] Nicholls SM, Dick AD. Lack of IFN-{gamma} synthesis in aqueous humor during corneal graft rejection correlates with suppressed nitric oxide production by macrophages. *Invest. Ophthalmol. Vis. Sci.* 2008.

In: Eye Research Developments: ...
Editor: Alan N. Westerhouse

ISBN: 978-1-60741-177-2

Chapter VII

Variational Approach to Stable Numerical Approximation of Optimal Dirichlet Boundary Controls for the Wave Equation*

Mikhail Potapov≠
Department of Computational Mathematics and Cybernetics,
Lomonosov Moscow State University, Moscow, Russia

Abstract

This chapter considers boundary control problem for the wave equation with boundary conditions of Dirichlet type, and control actions from L^2. To get numerical solutions to these problems we apply the stable variational method proposed earlier by the author. This method works well when original continuous system is controllable. Controllability property has a usual form $T > T^*$ and is supposed to be satisfied. We provide a detailed outline of the computational algorithm and give several numerical results obtained for data of varying smoothness and difference grids of varying densities. These results are compared with results of direct finite-difference approximation of initial continuous control problem via system of linear equations of high dimensionality.

Key words: wave equation, boundary control, controllability, variational method, finite difference approximation

1. Introduction

Multiple research results for the problem of numerical approximation of the optimal boundary controls for the wave equation are available (see e.g.,[1]--[8] and the references

---

* 2000 *Mathematics Subject Classification*. Primary 93B40; Secondary 35L05, 65M06.
This chapter was supported by RFBR, project No. 07-01-00416, and by the Program "Development of the High School Scientific Potential", project No. 2.1.1.1714.
≠ Associate Professor, Department of Computational Mathematics and Cybernetics, email: mpotapov@tochka.ru

therein). The main drawback of applying finite-dimensional approximation by either the standard discrete, semi-discrete difference, and projection-difference schemes or by the finite element method, even in combination with the Hilbert Uniqueness Method (HUM) by J.-L.Lions [9], to continuous processes, is that the strong convergence of resulting approximate controls cannot be guaranteed in natural norms of those spaces where the continuous system is controllable. In [1]--[8], authors use various methods to obtain stable approximate controls, such as: filtering of high frequencies, multi-grid methods, mixed finite elements, numerical viscosity, and Tikhonov regularization. The article [5] by E.Zuazua describes and analyzes these methods and is an *excellent review article* to quote [8, p.320].

A different approach, which we will call Variational Method (VM), was first introduced in [10, 11]. It's application to various boundary control and observation problems is described in [11]--[15]. Advantages of both Variational and Tikhonov [16, 17] methods are their universality with respect to the classes of problems being solved, and their unpretentiousness with respect to the kind of the finite-dimensional approximation being used. Under specific conditions both methods can be used for solving any linear operator equations using standard discrete schemes without any additional filtering of high frequencies or numerical viscosity, and without worrying about constants' uniformity in discrete observability inequalities. Let's specify the conditions of when Tikhonov regularization method can be applied to equations

$$Au = f \tag{1}$$

with linear bounded operator $A \in L(H \to F)$, acting in Hilbert spaces H,F. The existence of a solution is assumed. Instead of the exact data $A \in L(H \to F), f \in F$, some of their approximations $\tilde{A} \in L(H \to F), \tilde{f} \in F$ may be available, but in that case the corresponding error levels $\eta > 0, \delta > 0$ must be known as well:

$$\|\tilde{A} - A\| \le \eta, \qquad \|\tilde{f} - f\|_F \le \delta. \tag{2}$$

Then Tikhonov approximations $\tilde{u}$, being solutions to the equations

$$(\tilde{A}^* \tilde{A} + \alpha I)\tilde{u} = \tilde{f}, \quad \alpha > 0,$$

converge to the unique solution u_* of (1) with the minimal norm:

$$\|\tilde{u} - u_*\| \to 0 \quad as \quad \eta, \delta \to 0,$$

if regularization parameter $\alpha = \alpha(\eta, \delta)$ is consistent with error levels of both operator A and right hand side f.

In control problems for the wave equation the operator A to each control assigns a pair of final state and final velocity. In the majority of cases such operators are not compact. It is well known, that non-compact operators A cannot have a family of finite-dimensional approximations $\tilde{A}$ with uniform error $\eta \to 0$ in (2). Because of that, we consider all attempts to apply Tikhonov regularization to control problems with non-compact operators to be heuristic from mathematical standpoint. Of course, we don't deny the usefulness of such applications in practice. VM's applicability conditions are discussed in the next section.

2. Variational Method

In order to apply VM method to the equation (1) we need to have the following a priori information. We assume existence of a solution and relax requirements to the approximate data $\tilde{A} \in L(H \to F), \tilde{f} \in F$:

$$\|\tilde{A}u - Au\| \to 0 \ \forall u \in H, \quad \|\tilde{A}^* v - A^* v\| \to 0 \ \forall v \in F^*, \quad \|\tilde{f} - f\|_F \to 0. \tag{3}$$

Thus, in (2), the error level η in A does not have to tend to zero, and the error level δ in f does not have to be known though it has to be infinitely small. On the other hand, we add a strong requirement of a source-wise representability of the normal solution:

$$u_* = J_H A^* v_*, \quad v_* \in F^*, \quad \|v_*\|_{F^*} \le r, \tag{4}$$

and assume that the value of r in (4) is known. The adjoint operator $A^* \in L(F^* \to H^*)$ maps into H^*, therefore we use the Riesz isomorphism $J_H : H^* \to H$ in (4).

Let $\tilde{F}$ be an arbitrary subspace of F, $R(\tilde{A}) \subset \tilde{F}$, and $\tilde{F}^* = J_F^{-1}(\tilde{F})$, where $J_F^{-1} : F \to F^*$ is the inverse operator of Riesz isomorphism $J_F : F^* \to F$. Let $B(r)$ defined by

$$B(r) = \{v \in \tilde{F}^* \ \|v\|_{F^*} \le r\} \tag{5}$$

be a ball of radius r in the subspace $\tilde{F}^*$ of Hilbert space F^*. Then we set elements

$$\tilde{u} = J_H \tilde{A}^* \tilde{v}, \qquad \tilde{v} \in \tilde{F}^*, \tag{6}$$

as approximations of the exact normal solution u_* of equation (1). Source elements $\tilde{v}$ in (6) are ε-optimal solutions of the following quadratic minimization problem on the ball $B(r)$:

$$\tilde{v} \in B(r), \quad I(\tilde{v}) \le \min_{v \in B(r)} I(v) + \varepsilon, \qquad I(v) = \|\tilde{A}^* v\|^2_{H^*} - 2\langle \tilde{f}, v \rangle. \tag{7}$$

Theorem 1 Let conditions (3),(4) be satisfied, and let elements $\tilde{u}$ be chosen by the rule (5)--(7). Then the following estimate holds true:

$$\|\tilde{u} - u_*\|^2_H \le (\|\tilde{A}^* v_*\|^2_{H^*} - \|A^* v_*\|^2_{H^*}) + \tag{8}$$

$$2r(3\|Au_* - \tilde{A} u_*\|_F + 2\|\tilde{f} - f\|_F) + \varepsilon \to 0 \quad as \quad \varepsilon \to 0.$$

Proof. Let us transform the deviation we need to estimate:

$$\|\tilde{u} - u_*\|^2_H = \|J_H \tilde{A}^* \tilde{v}\|^2_H - 2\langle J_H \tilde{A}^* \tilde{v}, u_* \rangle_H + \|u_*\|^2_H = I(\tilde{v}) + 2\langle \tilde{v}, \tilde{f} - \tilde{A} u_* \rangle + \|u_*\|^2_H. \tag{9}$$

By $\tilde{v}_*$ denote the orthogonal projection of the source element v_* on the subspace $\tilde{F}^*$. This projection satisfies the following conditions:

$$\tilde{v}_* \in \tilde{F}^*, \quad \|\tilde{v}_*\|_{F^*} \le \|v_*\|_{F^*} \le r, \quad \langle v_*, \tilde{g} \rangle = \langle \tilde{v}_*, \tilde{g} \rangle \ \forall \tilde{g} \in \tilde{F}. \tag{10}$$

Using (10), we estimate the value of $I(\tilde{v})$:

$$I(\tilde v) \le I(\tilde v_*) + \varepsilon = \|\tilde A^* \tilde v_*\|^2_{H^*} - 2\langle \tilde v_*, \tilde f\rangle + \varepsilon =$$

$$\|\tilde A^* v_*\|^2_{H^*} - 2\langle v_*, \tilde f\rangle + 2\langle \tilde v_* - v_*, \tilde A u_* - \tilde f\rangle + \varepsilon =$$

$$\|A^* v_*\|^2_{H^*} + (\|\tilde A^* v_*\|^2_{H^*} - \|A^* v_*\|^2_{H^*}) - 2\langle v_*, Au_*\rangle +$$

$$2\langle v_*, Au_* - \tilde A^* u_*\rangle + 2\langle \tilde v_*, \tilde A^* u_* - \tilde f\rangle + \varepsilon \le$$

$$-\|u_*\|^2_H + (\|\tilde A^* v_*\|^2_{H^*} - \|A^* v_*\|^2_{H^*}) + 2r(2\|Au_* - \tilde A u_*\|_F + \|\tilde f - f\|_F) + \varepsilon.$$

Substituting this estimation and the following inequality

$$2\langle \tilde v, \tilde f - \tilde A u_*\rangle \le 2r(\|Au_* - \tilde A u_*\|_F + \|\tilde f - f\|_F),$$

in (9), we get (8). The proof is complete.

Remark 1 Estimate (8) has a quite natural look and shows how exactly the inaccuracy in control $\|\tilde u - u_*\|_H$ depends on: the approximate data $\tilde A, \tilde A^*, \tilde f$, the exact solution u_*, the source element v_*, the radius r, and the parameter ε which is chosen as an acceptable error level for solving variational problem (5)--(7).

Remark 2 Controllability property of the original boundary control problem can be expressed in the observability inequality form:

$$\|A^* v\|^2_{H^*} \ge \mu \|v\|^2_{F^*} \quad \forall v \in F^* \quad (\mu = const > 0). \tag{11}$$

If the observability constant μ in (11) is known the upper bound r in (4) can be found explicitly:

$$\|v_*\|_{F^*} \le \frac{\|f\|_F}{\mu} \le \frac{\|\tilde f\|_F + \delta}{\mu}. \tag{12}$$

According to (12) we can take either any $r \geq \mu^{-1}\|f\|_F$ or any $r \geq \mu^{-1}(\|\tilde{f}\|_F + \delta)$ as a value of r. The choice depends on what is actually known: the exact f or its approximation $\tilde{f}$ with corresponding error level δ.

The convex quadratic minimization problem (5)--(7) can be solved by various methods in a finite number of steps. The number of steps can be calculated in advance based on the required accuracy level ε in (7) and the information available on the values of $r, \|\tilde{f}\|,$ and $\|\tilde{A}\|$. In particular, we can apply the iterative algorithm suggested in [10]. This algorithm is based on the Lagrange principle and the fact that the norm $\|\tilde{v}(\lambda)\|_{\tilde{F}^*}$ is a continuous monotone function of $\lambda > 0$ decreasing to 0 as $\lambda \to +\infty$. Here $\tilde{v}(\lambda)$ is a unique solution to the Euler equation for the Lagrange function $I(v) + \lambda(\|v\|^2 - r^2)$. Elements v are chosen from the subspace $\tilde{F}^*$ according to (6) and therefore can be represented as $v = \tilde{Q}^* \varphi, \varphi \in F^*$, where $\tilde{Q}^* : F^* \to \tilde{F}^*$ is the orthogonal projection operator. Then Euler equation for $\tilde{v}(\lambda) \in \tilde{F}^*$ becomes

$$(\tilde{A} J_H \tilde{A}^* + \lambda I)\tilde{v}(\lambda) = \tilde{Q}\tilde{f}, \qquad \tilde{v}(\lambda) \in \tilde{F}^*, \qquad \lambda > 0, \tag{13}$$

where $\tilde{Q} : F \to \tilde{F}$ is an adjoint to $\tilde{Q}^*$ operator of the orthogonal projection from F onto its subspace $\tilde{F}$.

Algorithm

Step 1. Choose two parameters $\tilde{\lambda}_0 > 0$ and $\tilde{\varepsilon} > 0$. Theoretically, both of them have to be consistent with approximate data $\tilde{A}, \tilde{f}$ satisfying (3) so that $\tilde{\lambda}_0 \to 0, \tilde{\varepsilon} \to 0$.

Step 2. Set $\lambda = \vec{\lambda}_0$ and compute the solution $\vec{v}(\vec{\lambda}_0)$ of (13). If $\|\vec{v}(\vec{\lambda}_0)\|_{F^*} \leq r + \vec{\varepsilon}$ then set output $\vec{v} = \vec{v}(\vec{\lambda}_0)$ and stop the process.

Step 3. If $\|\vec{v}(\vec{\lambda}_0)\|_{F^*} > r + \vec{\varepsilon}$ then use the iteration dichotomy method and find the first λ satisfying the following bilateral inequality:

$$r - \vec{\varepsilon} \leq \|\vec{v}(\vec{\lambda})\|_{F^*} \leq r + \vec{\varepsilon}.$$

Set $\vec{v} = \vec{v}(\vec{\lambda})$ as final output and stop computations. The original estimation of the ε-inaccuracy in (7) which we get when applying this algorithm was given in [10]. We provide an improved version of it below.

For convenience let us simplify some notations in the formulation of the minimization problem (7). Let X be a Hilbert space. Consider the following quadratic minimization problem on the ball of radius r in X:

$$g(x) = \langle Cx, x\rangle_X - 2\langle b, x\rangle_X \to \inf, \qquad \|x\|_X \leq r. \tag{14}$$

Here $C \in L(X \to X), C^* = C \geq 0,$ is a linear bounded symmetrical nonnegative operator, and $b \in X, b \neq 0, r > 0$. According to Lagrange principle for an exact solution x_* of (14) there exists a multiplier $\lambda_* \geq 0$ such that

$$(C + \lambda_* I)x_* = b, \qquad \lambda_*(\|x_*\|_X^2 - r^2) = 0, \qquad \|x_*\|_X^2 \leq r^2.$$

By $x(\lambda)$ denote the solutions of Euler equation

$$(C + \lambda I)x(\lambda) = b, \qquad \lambda \geq 0. \tag{15}$$

Notice that equation (15) has a unique solution when $\lambda > 0$ and may have non-unique solution in case of $\lambda = 0$. In either case the function $\gamma(\lambda) = g(x(\lambda))$ is one-valued at each point $\lambda \geq 0$.

Lemma 1 *Suppose that x_* is an exact solution of (14), $\lambda_* \geq 0$ is the value of Lagrange multiplier corresponding to x_*, and $\gamma(\lambda_*) = g(x(\lambda_*)) = g(x_*)$ is the optimal value of $g(x)$. Let $\lambda > 0$ and corresponding solution $x(\lambda)$ of (15) be the output values of* *algorithm applied to problem (14) with input values* $\tilde{\lambda}_0 > 0$ *and* $\tilde{\varepsilon} > 0$. *Then the following estimation holds true:*

$$\gamma(\lambda) - \gamma(\lambda_*) \le \max\{2r^2 \tilde{\lambda}_0, 4(r - \tilde{\varepsilon})^{-1} r(\|C\|r + \|b\|)\tilde{\varepsilon}\}. \tag{16}$$

Proof. The only case when estimation (16) is not trivial is $\lambda > \lambda_*$. This is due to the fact that $\gamma(\lambda) = g(x(\lambda))$ is a continuous increasing function of $\lambda \ge 0$. Let us take arbitrary $\lambda > \lambda_*$. Using (15) and the commutative property of operators $(C + \lambda I), (C + \lambda I)^{-1}, (C + \lambda_* I)$ let's transform the difference $\gamma(\lambda) - \gamma(\lambda_*)$ as follows:

$$\gamma(\lambda) - \gamma(\lambda_*) = \langle (C + \lambda_* I)x(\lambda_*), x(\lambda_*) - x(\lambda)\rangle + \lambda_* \|x(\lambda_*)\|^2 - \lambda\|x(\lambda)\|^2. \tag{17}$$

Taking into account that

$$x(\lambda) = (C + \lambda I)^{-1}(C + \lambda_* I)x(\lambda_*), \qquad (C + \lambda I)^{-1}(C + \lambda I) = I, \tag{18}$$

we go on with transformations in (17):

$$\begin{aligned} &\gamma(\lambda) - \gamma(\lambda_*) = (\lambda - \lambda_*)\langle (C + \lambda_* I)(C + \lambda I)^{-1} x(\lambda_*), x(\lambda_*)\rangle + \\ &\langle (C + \lambda I)^{-2}(\lambda_*(C + \lambda I)^2 - \lambda(C + \lambda_* I)^2)x(\lambda_*), x(\lambda_*)\rangle = \\ &(\lambda - \lambda_*)\langle (C + \lambda I)^{-2}((\lambda + \lambda_*)C + 2\lambda\lambda_* I)x(\lambda_*), x(\lambda_*)\rangle. \end{aligned} \tag{19}$$

Under the assumptions $C \ge 0, \lambda > \lambda_* \ge 0$ we have

$$\lambda I \le C + \lambda I, \quad \lambda + \lambda_* < 2\lambda, \quad 2\lambda\lambda_* < 2\lambda^2.$$

Substituting these to (19) we come to the following conclusion:

$$\gamma(\lambda) - \gamma(\lambda_*) \le 2(\lambda - \lambda_*)\|x(\lambda_*)\|^2 \le 2r^2(\lambda - \lambda_*). \tag{20}$$

If $\lambda_* = 0$ the algorithm must stop at Step 2 with output value $\lambda = \tilde{\lambda}_0 > 0$, in which case, from (20) it follows that

$$\gamma(\lambda) - \gamma(\lambda_*) = \gamma(\tilde{\lambda}_0) - \gamma(0) \le 2r^2 \tilde{\lambda}_0. \tag{21}$$

If $\lambda_* > 0$, the algorithm can stop at either Step 2 or Step 3. If it stops at Step 2 with value $\lambda = \tilde{\lambda}_0 > \lambda_* > 0$, we apply (20) again an get

$$\gamma(\lambda) - \gamma(\lambda_*) = \gamma(\tilde{\lambda}_0) - \gamma(\lambda_*) \le 2r^2(\tilde{\lambda}_0 - \lambda_*) < 2r^2\tilde{\lambda}_0. \tag{22}$$

If $\lambda_* > 0$ and the algorithm stops at Step 3, the following conditions are necessarily true:

$$\|x(\lambda_*)\| = r, \qquad r - \tilde{\varepsilon} \le \|x(\lambda)\| \le r + \tilde{\varepsilon}. \tag{23}$$

From (23) it follows at once that

$$\|x(\lambda_*)\|^2 - \|x(\lambda)\|^2 \le (2r - \tilde{\varepsilon})\tilde{\varepsilon} \le 2r\tilde{\varepsilon} \tag{24}$$

To define an upper bound of the difference $\lambda - \lambda_*$ in (20) let us estimate the difference $\|x(\lambda_*)\|^2 - \|x(\lambda)\|^2$. We do it taking into account (18) and using elementary inequalities

$$2C \ge C, \quad (C + \lambda I)^{-1} \ge (\|C\| + \lambda)^{-1} I, \quad \lambda + \lambda_* > \lambda.$$

Then we have

$$\|x(\lambda_*)\|^2 - \|x(\lambda)\|^2 = (\lambda - \lambda_*)\langle (C + \lambda I)^{-2}(2C + (\lambda + \lambda_*)I)x(\lambda_*), x(\lambda_*)\rangle \ge$$
$$(\|C\| + \lambda)^{-1}\|x(\lambda_*)\|^2(\lambda - \lambda_*) = (\|C\| + \lambda)^{-1} r^2 (\lambda - \lambda_*). \tag{25}$$

Combining (24) and (25) we get

$$0 < \lambda - \lambda_* \le 2r^{-1}(\|C\| + \lambda)\tilde{\varepsilon}. \tag{26}$$

Substituting estimate (26) in (20) we arrive to conclusion

$$\gamma(\lambda) - \gamma(\lambda_*) \le 4r(\|C\| + \lambda)\tilde{\varepsilon}. \tag{27}$$

Now we need to show that λ has an upper bound. Let us multiply Euler equation (15) by $x(\lambda)$ and take into account that operator C is non-negative:

$$\langle Cx(\lambda), x(\lambda)\rangle + \lambda\langle x(\lambda), x(\lambda)\rangle = \langle b, x(\lambda)\rangle \quad \Rightarrow \quad \lambda \le \|x(\lambda)\|^{-1}\|b\|. \tag{28}$$

Using (28) and the lower bound for $\|x(\lambda)\|$ from (23) we come to

$$\lambda \le (r - \tilde{\varepsilon})^{-1}\|b\|.$$

After this from (27) we get the final estimate

$$\gamma(\lambda) - \gamma(\lambda_*) \le 4r(\|\tilde{C}\| + (r-\tilde{\varepsilon})^{-1}\|b\|)\tilde{\varepsilon} \le 4(r-\tilde{\varepsilon})^{-1} r(\|C\|r + \|b\|)\tilde{\varepsilon}. \tag{29}$$

The statement (16) follows from (21),(22), and (29). The lemma is proved.
Now we are ready to estimate the error level ε in (7) caused by the algorithm. We set

$$X = F^*, \quad b = J_F^{-1}\tilde{Q}\tilde{f} \in F^*, \quad C = J_F^{-1}\tilde{A}J_H\tilde{A}^* \in L(F^* \to F^*), \quad x(\lambda) = \tilde{v}(\lambda) \in F^*,$$

and derive the following explicit estimation from Lemma 1:

$$\varepsilon \le \max\{2r^2\tilde{\lambda}_0, 4(r-\tilde{\varepsilon})^{-1} r(\|\tilde{A}\|^2 r + \|\tilde{f}\|_F)\tilde{\varepsilon}\}. \tag{30}$$

Estimation (30) shows that ε-inaccuracy in (7) has the same order of smallness as parameters $\tilde{\lambda}_0$ and $\tilde{\varepsilon}$.

3. Wave Equation With Dirichlet Boundary Control

Consider the following Dirichlet boundary control problem for the wave equation with variable coefficients:

$$\begin{aligned} &\rho(x)y_{tt} = (k(x)y_x)_x, && 0<t<T, \quad 0<x<l, \\ &y|_{x=0} = u_0(t), \qquad y|_{x=l} = u_1(t), && 0<t<T, \\ &y|_{t=0} = 0, \qquad y_t|_{t=0} = 0, && 0<x<l. \end{aligned} \tag{31}$$

We want to find controls $u = u(t) = (u_0(t), u_1(t))$ that would take our system (31) from the initial state of rest to a desired final state

$$y|_{t=T} = f^0(x), \qquad y_t|_{t=T} = f^1(x), \qquad 0 < x < l. \tag{32}$$

Coefficients $\rho(x)$ and $k(x)$ are given positive continuously differentiable functions of x.

If we set up a formally adjoint problem to problem (31),(32) with Dirichlet controls, we obtain the following problem with Neumann observations:

$$\rho(x)p_{tt} = (k(x)p_x)_x, \qquad 0 < t < T, \quad 0 < x < l,$$

$$p|_{x=0} = 0, \qquad p|_{x=l} = 0, \qquad 0 < t < T, \tag{33}$$

$$p|_{t=T} = v^0(x), \qquad p_t|_{t=T} = -v^1(x), \qquad 0 < x < l.$$

In this new observation problem, we need to find the final state $v = v(x) = (v^0(x), v^1(x))$ of proccss (33) from given Neumann boundary data $g = g(t) = (g_0(t), g_1(t))$:

$$kp_x|_{x=0} = g_0(t), \qquad -kp_x|_{x=l} = g_1(t), \qquad 0 < t < T. \tag{34}$$

Let us specify functional spaces of controls u, observations g, and solutions y and p of boundary valuc problems (31) and (33). Consider a well studied case [9, 18] when controls $u \in H = L^2(0,T) \times L^2(0,T)$. Solutions y corresponding to those controls u, possess the following properties [19, 20]:

$$y(t,x) \in C([0,T]; L^2_\rho(0,l)), \qquad y_t(t,x) \in C([0,T]; H^{-1}(0,l)),$$

where $H^{-1}(0,l) = (H^1_0(0,l))^*$ is the adjoint space of $H^1_0(0,l)$. Each of three spaces $H^1_0(0,l)$, $L^2_\rho(0,l)$, $L^2(0,T)$ is a Hilbert space with its own scalar product

$$\langle f, g \rangle_{H^1_0(0,l)} = \int_0^l k(x) f'(x) g'(x) dx, \quad \langle f, g \rangle_{L^2_\rho(0,l)} = \int_0^l \rho(x) f(x) g(x) dx,$$

$$\langle f, g \rangle_{L^2(0,T)} = \int_0^T f(t) g(t) dt.$$

It is important that we identify the adjoint and basic spaces $(L^2(0,T))^*$ and $L^2(0,T)$, as well as $(L^2_\rho(0,l))^*$ and $L^2_\rho(0,l)$, by the Riesz theorem. Let us introduce the Hilbert space $F = L^2_\rho(0,l)\times H^{-1}(0,l)$ of target states $f=(f^0(x),f^1(x))$ with components $f^0(x),f^1(x)$ taken from (32) and define operator $A:H\to F$ by

$$Au=(y(T,x),y_t(T,x)),\qquad 0<x<l. \tag{35}$$

This mapping $A\in L(H\to F)$ is a linear bounded operator and has a unique adjoint operator $A^*\in L(F^*\to H^*)$ acting through the conjugate system (33) as follows:

$$A^*v=(k(0)p_x(t,0),-k(l)p_x(t,l)),\qquad 0<t<T. \tag{36}$$

Regularity properties of solutions p corresponding to given data $v=(v^0(x),v^1(x))\in F^* = H^1_0(0,l)\times L^2_\rho(0,l)$ in (33) are also well known [19, 20]:

$$\begin{aligned} &p(t,x)\in C([0,T];H^1_0(0,l)), && p_t(t,x)\in C([0,T];L^2_\rho(0,l)),\\ &p(t,x)\in C([0,l];H^1(0,T)), && p_x(t,x)\in C([0,l];L^2(0,T)). \end{aligned} \tag{37}$$

According to (37) the adjoint operator $A^*:H^1_0(0,l)\times L^2_\rho(0,l)\to L^2(0,T)\times L^2(0,T)$ is well defined in (36). In the case (33),(34), observability inequality mentioned above in (11) takes the form

$$\begin{aligned} \|A^*v\|^2_{H^*} &= \|k(0)p_x(\cdot,0)\|^2_{L^2(0,T)}+\|k(l)p_x(\cdot,l)\|^2_{L^2(0,T)} \ge \\ &\mu(\|v^0\|^2_{H^1_0(0,l)}+\|v^1\|^2_{L^2_\rho(0,l)}) = \mu\|v\|^2_{F^*}. \end{aligned} \tag{38}$$

To get the estimation (38) it is sufficient to apply the well developed multiplier technique [9, 18] tuned to variable coefficients by L.F.Ho in [21]. Take a point $\xi\in[0,l]$ and define the multiplier $m(x)=m(x,\xi)$ by

$$m'(x)=1+a(x)m(x),\quad 0<x<l,\qquad m(\xi)=0,$$

$$a(x) = \min\left\{-\frac{\rho'(x)}{\rho(x)}, \frac{k'(x)}{k(x)}\right\} \quad as \quad 0 \le x \le \xi, \tag{39}$$

$$a(x) = \max\left\{-\frac{\rho'(x)}{\rho(x)}, \frac{k'(x)}{k(x)}\right\} \quad as \quad \xi \le x \le l.$$

Let $T_*(\xi)$ be a function of ξ defined as

$$T_*(\xi) = 2\max_{0\le x\le l}\left(|\, m(x,\xi)\,|\sqrt{\frac{\rho(x)}{k(x)}}\right),$$

and let $\xi_* \in [0,l]$ be a minimum point of $T_*(\xi)$ on $[0,l]$:

$$T_* = T_*(\xi_*) = \min_{0\le\xi\le l} T_*(\xi_*). \tag{40}$$

Using a special multiplier $m_*(x) = m(x,\xi_*)$, we get the final estimate

$$\frac{|\, m_*(0)\,|}{k(0)}\int_0^T (k(0)p_x(t,0))^2\,dt + \frac{|\, m_*(l)\,|}{k(l)}\int_0^T (k(l)p_x(t,l))^2\,dt \ge \tag{41}$$

$$\ge (T - T_*)\left(\int_0^l (k(x)\,|\,(v^0(x))'\,|^2 + \rho(x)\,|\,v^1(x)\,|^2)\,dx\right).$$

This is exactly the observability inequality (38) with

$$\mu = \frac{T - T_*}{M}, \qquad where \qquad M = \max\{\frac{|\, m_*(0)\,|}{k(0)}, \frac{|\, m_*(l)\,|}{k(l)}\}. \tag{42}$$

Remark 3 *The value of* T_* *in (40) plays a role of the threshold controllability-observability moment in dual control and observation problems (31)--(32) and (33)--(34). Note that if coefficients are constants:* $\rho(x) \equiv 1, k(x) \equiv 1,$ *we have* $\xi_* = l/2, m_*(x) = x - l/2, |\, m_*(0)\,| = m_*(l) = l/2,$ *and the threshold moment becomes equal to its optimal value* $T_* = l$. *In any case, from (39),(40),(42) it is clear that the value of* μ *can be found constructively: either analytically or numerically. This* μ *can be used to find the radius* r *which is an important parameter of the variational algorithm (see Remark 2 in section 2).*

4. Finite-Difference Approximation

We introduce uniform grids $t_j = j\tau,\ j = 0,1,\dots,M$, and $x_i = ih,\ i = 0,1,\dots,N$, on $[0,T]$ and $[0,l]$ with step sizes $\tau = T/M$ and $h = l/N$. We approximate solutions y and p of the differential problems (31) and (33) by the grid functions $y = y_i^j$ and p_i^j. To approximate the coefficients ρ and k we make a simple choice $\rho_i = \rho(x_i),\ k_i = k(x_i - h/2),\ i = 1,2,\dots,N-1$. Introduce the following common notations:

$$y_t = y_{t,i}^j = \frac{y_i^{j+1} - y_i^j}{\tau}, \quad y_{\bar{t}} = y_{\bar{t},i}^j = \frac{y_i^j - y_i^{j-1}}{\tau}, \quad y_{\bar{t}t} = y_{\bar{t}t,i}^j = \frac{y_{t,i}^j - y_{\bar{t},i}^j}{\tau},$$

$$y_x = y_{x,i}^j = \frac{y_{i+1}^j - y_i^j}{h}, \quad y_{\bar{x}} = y_{\bar{x},i}^j = \frac{y_i^j - y_{i-1}^j}{h}, \quad (ky_{\bar{x}})_x = (ky_{\bar{x}})_{x,i}^j = \frac{k_{i+1}y_{x,i}^j - k_i y_{\bar{x},i}^j}{h}.$$

Let's approximate the initial boundary value problems (31) and (33) by the simplest explicit difference schemes as follows:

$$\begin{gathered}\rho_i y_{\bar{t}t,i}^j = (ky_{\bar{x}})_{x,i}^j, \quad i = 1,2,\dots,N-1, \quad j = 1,2,\dots,M-1; \\ y_i^j\,|_{i=0} = u_0^j, \quad y_i^j\,|_{i=N} = u_1^j, \quad j = 1,2,\dots,M-1; \\ y_i^j\,|_{j=0} = 0, \quad y_{t,i}^j\,|_{j=0} = 0, \quad i = 1,2,\dots,N-1;\end{gathered} \tag{43}$$

and

$$\begin{gathered}\rho_i p_{\bar{t}t,i}^j = (kp_{\bar{x}})_{x,i}^j, \quad i = 1,2,\dots,N-1, \quad j = 1,2,\dots,M-1; \\ p_i^j\,|_{i=0} = 0, \quad p_i^j\,|_{i=N} = 0, \quad j = 1,2,\dots,M-1; \\ p_i^j\,|_{j=M} = v_i^0, \quad p_{\bar{t},i}^j\,|_{j=M} = -v_i^1, \quad i = 1,2,\dots,N-1.\end{gathered} \tag{44}$$

Of course, we assume that the step sizes satisfy the common consistency condition

$$\frac{\tau}{h} \le \alpha c_2, \qquad c_2 = \min_{1\le i\le N}\min\{\sqrt{\frac{\rho_i}{k_i}}, \sqrt{\frac{\rho_{i-1}}{k_i}}\}, \quad 0 < \alpha < 1, \tag{45}$$

as well as an additional condition

$$c_1 \le \frac{\tau}{h}. \tag{46}$$

Theoretically, any values of $\alpha \in (0,1)$ and $c_1 \in (0,c_2]$ are acceptable in (45),(46). However, small values of the ratio τ/h are inconvenient in practice. Discrete systems (43) and (44) are mutually adjoint in a sense of the following identity:

$$\sum_{i=1}^{N-1}\rho_i y_i^M v_i^1 h + \sum_{i=1}^{N-1}\rho_i y_{\bar{t},i}^M v_i^0 h = \sum_{j=1}^{M-1} u_0^j k_1 p_{\bar{x},1}^j \tau + \sum_{j=1}^{M-1} u_1^j (-k_N p_{\bar{x},N}^j)\tau \tag{47}$$

which holds true for all grid functions $u=(u_0,u_1)$ and $v=(v^0,v^1)$. Using difference schemes (43) and (44), we form finite-dimensional mutually adjoint mappings $\overset{\square}{A}$ and $\overset{\square}{A}{}^*$ acting in the same spaces as original operators A and A^*. The structure of $\overset{\square}{A}$ and $\overset{\square}{A}{}^*$ is almost identical to the one we used earlier in [11]. Let $e_i(x), i=1,2,\ldots,N-1$, be step functions equal to 1 within interval $[x_i-h/2, x_i+h/2]$ and equal to 0 outside this interval. Let $e_j(t), j=1,2,\ldots,M-1$, be the same step functions equal to 1 on time intervals $[t_j-\tau/2, t_j+\tau/2]$. We also use the Dirac delta functions $\delta(x-x_i)$ concentrated at the mesh nodes x_i. Above, we chose ρ-weighted $L_\rho^2(0,l)$ as the basic space for functions of variable x and decided to accept the Riesz identity $(L_\rho^2(0,l))^* \simeq L_\rho^2(0,l)$. Therefore, it is convenient for us to consider that delta functions are also ρ-weighted:

$$\langle \delta(x-x_i),\varphi\rangle = \rho(x_i)\varphi(x_i), \quad \forall\varphi(x)\in C[0,l], \quad i=1,2,\ldots,N-1.$$

Operator $\overset{\square}{A}$ acts on arbitrary functions $u=(u_0(t),u_1(t))\in H = L^2(0,T)\times L^2(0,T)$. These functions are processed into the discrete controls $u=(u_0,u_1)$ as follows:

$$u_0^j = \frac{1}{\tau}\langle u_0,e_j\rangle, \quad u_1^j = \frac{1}{\tau}\langle u_1,e_j\rangle, \quad where \tag{48}$$

$$\langle \psi,e_j\rangle = \int_{t_j-\tau/2}^{t_j+\tau/2}\psi(t)e_j(t)dt, \quad \psi(t)\in L^2(0,T), \quad j=1,2,\ldots,M-1.$$

Using the discrete controls $u=(u_0,u_1)$ defined in (48) as boundary values in (43) we solve the difference problem (43) and set the output of $\overset{\square}{A}$ as

$$\hat{A}u = \left(\sum_{i=1}^{N-1} y_i^M e_i(x), \sum_{i=1}^{N-1} y_{\bar{t},i}^M \delta(x - x_i)h \right) \quad \forall u \in H. \tag{49}$$

The operator $\hat{A}^*$ is applied to arbitrary pair $v = (v^0(x), v^1(x)) \in F^* = H_0^1(0,l) \times L_\rho^2(0,l)$. First, $\hat{A}^*$ transforms it into the grid pair $v = (v^0, v^1)$ with components

$$v_i^0 = \frac{1}{\rho_i h} \langle v^0, \delta(x - x_i)h \rangle = v^0(x_i), \quad \forall v^0(x) \in H_0^1(0,l),$$

$$v_i^1 = \frac{1}{\rho_i h} \langle v^1, e_i \rangle = \frac{1}{\rho_i h} \int_{x_i - h/2}^{x_i + h/2} \rho(x) v^1(x) e_i(x) dx \quad \forall v^1(x) \in L_\rho^2(0,l), \tag{50}$$

$i = 1, 2, \ldots, N-1.$

Using the discrete functions $v = (v^0, v^1)$ defined in (50) as final states in (44) we solve the difference problem (44) and set the output of $\hat{A}^*$ as

$$\hat{A}^* v = \left(\sum_{j=1}^{M-1} k_1 p_{\bar{x},1}^j e_j(t), \sum_{j=1}^{M-1} (-k_N p_{\bar{x},N}^j) e_j(t) \right) \quad \forall v \in F^*. \tag{51}$$

Lemma 2 *Operators $\hat{A} \in L(H \to F)$ and $\hat{A}^* \in L(F^* \to H^*)$ are linear bounded and mutually adjoint.*

The boundedness property follows from the finite dimensionality of $\hat{A}$ and $\hat{A}^*$. The statement that $\hat{A}^*$ is an adjoint operator to $\hat{A}$ is true because we defined these operators in (49),(51) consistently with the discrete duality identity (47).

Lemma 3 *Operators $\hat{A} \in L(H \to F)$ and $\hat{A}^* \in L(F^* \to H^*)$ are uniformly bounded as $\tau, h \to 0$.*

We can prove Lemma 3 using an energy estimation for the solution $z = z_i^j$ of the following completely inhomogeneous difference scheme having the same type as (43),(44):

$$\rho_i z^j_{\bar{t}t,i} = (k z_{\bar{x}})^j_{x,i} + w^j_i, \quad i = 1,2,\ldots,N-1, \quad j = 1,2,\ldots,M-1;$$

$$z^j_i\,|_{i=0} = u^j_0, \quad z^j_i\,|_{i=N} = u^j_1, \quad j = 1,2,\ldots,M-1;$$

$$z^j_i\,|_{j=0} = v^0_i, \quad z^j_{t,i}\,|_{j=0} = v^1_i, \quad i = 1,2,\ldots,N-1.$$

This energy estimation can be represented in the form

$$\max_{1\le j\le M}\Big(\sum_{i=1}^{N} | z^j_{\bar{x},i} |^2 h + \sum_{i=1}^{N-1} | z^j_{\bar{t},i} |^2 h\Big) + \max_{1\le i\le N} \sum_{j=1}^{M-1} | z^j_{\bar{x},i} |^2 \tau \le \tag{52}$$

$$C\left(\sum_{i=1}^{N} | v^0_{\bar{x},i} |^2 h + \sum_{i=1}^{N-1} | v^1_i |^2 h + \sum_{j=1}^{M} (| u^j_{0\bar{t}} |^2 + | u^j_{0\bar{t}} |^2)\tau + \Big| \sum_{j=1}^{M-1} \Big(\sum_{i=1}^{N-1} | w^j_i |^2 h\Big)^{1/2} \tau \Big|^2 \right),$$

where constant $C > 0$ doesn't depend on grid steps τ and h. When needed, the dependence that C has on coefficients $\rho(x), k(x)$, values l, T, and parameters c_1, c_2 from (46),(48) can be expressed explicitly. The uniform boundedness of operators $\tilde{A}^*$ or the uniform boundedness of their norms $\|\tilde{A}^*\|$ follows from the definition (51) of these operators and from (52) with zero data u_0, u_1, w. Then due to the equality of the norms $\|\tilde{A}\| = \|\tilde{A}^*\|$ operators $\tilde{A}$ are also uniformly bounded.

Lemma 4 *Operators* $\tilde{A}$ *and* $\tilde{A}^*$ *strongly point-wise converge to* A *and* A^* *as* τ, $h \to 0$:

$$\|\tilde{A}u - Au\|_F \to 0 \quad \forall u \in H, \qquad \|\tilde{A}^* v - A^* v\|_{H^*} \to 0 \quad \forall v \in F^*. \tag{53}$$

To prove Lemma 4 we use Lemma 3 and the Uniform Boundedness Principle [22, 23]. This principle allows us to prove point-wise convergence (53) for all u and v from certain dense subspaces of H and F^* which consist of sufficiently smooth functions. For example, as $u_0(t), u_1(t)$ we can take infinitely differentiable functions with compact supports in $(0, T)$, and as $v^0(x), v^1(x)$ we can take the same functions of $x \in (0, l)$.

5. Application of the Variational Method

In sections 3,4 we verified all conditions when VM (5)--(7) can be successfully applied to the boundary control problem (31),(32). The only question that is still open is: how to choose the subspace $\overset{\square}{F}^{*}$ in (5),(6). Recall that $\overset{\square}{F}^{*} = J_F^{-1}(\overset{\square}{F})$, where $\overset{\square}{F}$ is an arbitrary extension of the $R(\overset{\square}{A})$. As it follows from (49), one of the possibilities is to take

$$\overset{\square}{F} = L_h^2 \times H_h^{-1}, \quad L_h^2 = span\{e_i(x)\}_{i=1}^{N-1}, \quad H_h^{-1} = span\{\delta(x-x_i)\}_{i=1}^{N-1}. \tag{54}$$

Then taking into account the Riesz identity $(L_\rho^2(0,l))^* \simeq L_\rho^2(0,l)$ accepted above we set

$$\overset{\square}{F}^{*} = H_h^1 \times L_h^2, \quad H_h^1 = span\{z_i^*(x)\}_{i=1}^{N-1}, \tag{55}$$

$$z_i^*(x) = J_{H^{-1}(0,l)}^{-1}\delta(x-x_i) = J_{H_0^1(0,l)}\delta(x-x_i).$$

The Riesz image $z(x) = J_{H_0^1(0,l)} f(x) \in H_0^1(0,l)$ and its pre-image $f(x) \in H^{-1}(0,l)$ are connected by the following Riesz boundary value problem:

$$-(k(x)z'(x))' = \rho(x)f(x), \; 0 < x < l, \qquad z(0) = 0, \; z(l) = 0. \tag{56}$$

In case of $f(x) = \delta(x-x_i)$ the problem (56) can be solved analytically:

$$z_i^*(x) = \frac{\rho(x_i)k(x_i)}{I(l)}(I(l) - I(x_i))I(x) \quad as \quad x \in [0, x_i], \tag{57}$$

$$z_i^*(x) = \frac{\rho(x_i)k(x_i)}{I(l)} I(x_i)(I(l) - I(x)) \quad as \quad x \in [x_i, l],$$

where $I(x) = \int_0^x \frac{d\xi}{k(\xi)}$, $x \in [0,l]$. In specific terms of the control problem (31),(32) general Theorem 1 takes the following form.

Theorem 2 *Let the Dirichlet control problem (31),(32) be stated in the classes of boundary controls* $u = (u_0(t), u_1(t)) \in H = L^2(0,T) \times L^2(0,T)$ *and target states*

$f = (f^0(x), f^1(x)) \in F = L^2_\rho(0,l) \times H^{-1}(0,l)$, *and let the controllability condition* $T > T_*$ *be satisfied with value of the threshold moment* T_* *from (40). Let* $u_* = (u_{*0}(t), u_{*1}(t))$ *be an optimal boundary control with minimal* H*-norm. Let approximate solution* $\tilde{u}$ *be computed according to (5)--(7), where the subspaces* $\tilde{F}, \tilde{F}^*$ *are described in (54),(55),*

$$\|\tilde{u} - u_*\|^2_H = \|\tilde{u}_0 - u_{*0}\|^2_{L^2(0,T)} + \|\tilde{u}_1 - u_{*1}\|^2_{L^2(0,T)} \to 0 \quad as \quad \tau, h \to 0. \tag{58}$$

Convergence (58) is still valid in case of approximate data $\tilde{f} = (\tilde{f}^0(x), \tilde{f}^1(x)) \in F = L^2_\rho(0,l) \times H^{-1}(0,l)$ if $\|\tilde{f} - f\|_F \to 0$ as $\tau, h \to 0$.

Remark 4 *A similar convergence result for approximate solutions of dual observation problem (33)-(34) is valid in the space* $F^* = H^1_0(0,l) \times L^2_\rho(0,l)$. *Some results for approximation of observation problems are available in [11]--[15].*

Let's discuss some of the computational aspects. From (5)--(7) we see that the unknown function is a source pair $\tilde{v} = (\tilde{v}^0, \tilde{v}^1)$. Its components $\tilde{v}^0$ and $\tilde{v}^1$ are chosen from the subspaces

$$\tilde{v}^0(x) \subset H^1_h, \qquad \tilde{v}^1(x) \subset L^2_h.$$

The subspace H^1_h spans basis functions $z^*_i(x), i = 1,2,\ldots,N-1,$ from (57) which have nonlocal supports on $[0,l]$. Basis functions with local supports would be preferred from the computational viewpoint. We suggest to take the following piece-wise smooth functions $z_i(x) \in H^1_0(0,l)$ with local supports $[x_{i-1}, x_{i+1}]$:

$$z_i(x) = 0 \quad as \quad x \in [0, x_{i-1}] \cup [x_{i+1}, l],$$

$$z_i(x) = \frac{I(x) - I(x_{i-1})}{I(x_i) - I(x_{i-1})} \quad as \quad x \in [x_{i-1}, x_i], \tag{59}$$

$$z_i(x) = \frac{I(x_{i+1}) - I(x)}{I(x_{i+1}) - I(x_i)} \quad as \quad x \in [x_i, x_{i+1}], \quad i = 1,2,\ldots,N-1,$$

where $I(x)=\int_0^x \frac{d\xi}{k(\xi)}$, $x\in[0,l]$, as is the case in (57). Note that

$$H_h^1 = span\{z_i^*(x)\}_{i=1}^{N-1} = span\{z_i(x)\}_{i=1}^{N-1}, \tag{60}$$

and that the Gram matrix of functions $z_i(x)$ with elements $\langle z_i, z_j\rangle_{H_0^1(0,l)}$ is tridiagonal due to the support locality property of $z_i(x)$, while the Gram matrix of $z_i^*(x)$ is not sparse. Then we expand the unknown function $\vec{v}=(\vec{v}^{\,0}(x),\vec{v}^{\,1}(x))\in H_h^1\times L_h^2$ in a sum

$$\vec{v}^{\,0}(x)=\sum_{i=1}^{N-1}\alpha_i z_i(x), \qquad \vec{v}^{\,1}(x)=\sum_{i=1}^{N-1}\beta_i e_i(x) \tag{61}$$

of functions $z_i(x)$ from (59) and step functions $e_i(x)$ with supports $[x_i-h/2, x_i+h/2]$. The coefficients $\alpha=(\alpha_1,\alpha_2,\ldots,\alpha_{N-1})$ and $\beta=(\beta_1,\beta_2,\ldots,\beta_{N-1})$ of expansion (61) become the new unknown variables. If we substitute the sum (61) for $\vec{v}(\lambda)$ in (13), and scalarly multiply both sides of (13) by basis pairs $(z_i(x),0), i=1,2,\ldots,N-1$, and $(0,e_i(x)), i=1,2,\ldots,N-1$, we get a system of linear equations for $(\alpha,\beta)=(\alpha(\lambda),\beta(\lambda))$. Next we use the three-step Algorithm described in section 2 to find an optimal value of λ. Then taking corresponding values of $(\alpha,\beta)=(\alpha(\lambda),\beta(\lambda))$ we compute the source element $\vec{v}=\vec{v}(\lambda)$ using (61). According to (6),(50),(51) we set $\vec{u}=\vec{A}^{*}\vec{v}(\lambda)$ as a final approximation to the exact normal optimal control u_*.

6. Numerical Results

In this section, we present a numerical implementation of our VM and compare its results with results obtained by Discrete Hilbert Uniqueness Method (DHUM). Let's clarify what exactly DHUM means.

Applying HUM [9] to the continuous boundary control problem (31),(32) in spaces of controls $u\in H=L^2(0,T)\times L^2(0,T)$ and targets $f\in F=L_\rho^2(0,l)\times H^{-1}(0,l)$ we can reformulate this problem as a linear operator equation $Au=f$ with operator $A:H\to F$ from (35) and right side $f=(f^0(x),f^1(x))$ from (32). A unique normal solution u_* to this equation is found according to HUM in the source-wise form

$$u_* = A^* v_*, \qquad where \quad AA^* v_* = f, \tag{62}$$

and the adjoint operator $A^* : F^* \to H^* \simeq H$ is defined by (33),(36). We will be looking for the HUM approximate solution $\breve{u}_\Diamond$ to the equation $Au = f$ in the form (6) without taking into account any a priori information on the value of r which is used explicitly by the variational method (5)--(7). Thus, we have

$$\breve{u}_\Diamond = \breve{A}^* \breve{v}_\Diamond, \qquad \breve{A}\breve{A}^* \breve{v}_\Diamond = \breve{Q}\breve{f}, \qquad \breve{v}_\Diamond \in \breve{F}^* . \tag{63}$$

As in (61) we can expand unknown elements $\breve{v}_\Diamond = (\overset{0}{\breve{v}}_\Diamond(x), \overset{1}{\breve{v}}_\Diamond(x)) \in \breve{F}^*$ in a sum

$$\overset{0}{\breve{v}}_\Diamond(x) = \sum_{i=1}^{N-1} \alpha_{\Diamond i} z_i(x), \qquad \overset{1}{\breve{v}}_\Diamond(x) = \sum_{i=1}^{N-1} \beta_{\Diamond i} e_i(x). \tag{64}$$

We transform the equation $\breve{A}\breve{A}^* \breve{v}_\Diamond = \breve{Q}\breve{f}$ into a system of linear equations for coefficients $(\alpha_\Diamond, \beta_\Diamond)$ by scalar multiplication. We solve this system and first find $\breve{v}_\Diamond$ from (64) and then find $\breve{u}_\Diamond$ from (63). From now on we will call the control $\breve{u}_\Diamond$ a DHUM-control, and the result $\breve{u}$ produced by VM a VM-control.

We present three numerical examples for the boundary control problem (31),(32) with constant coefficients $\rho(x) \equiv 1, k(x) \equiv 1$, and $l = 1$. In each of these examples we monitor the ratio errors in control and target state

$$\frac{\|\breve{u} - u_*\|_H}{\|u_*\|_H}, \qquad \frac{\|\breve{u}_\Diamond - u_*\|_H}{\|u_*\|_H}, \qquad \frac{\|\breve{A}\breve{u} - f\|_F}{\|f\|_F}, \qquad \frac{\|\breve{A}\breve{u}_\Diamond - f\|_F}{\|f\|_F},$$

which appear when applying VM and DHUM, while we vary target states f, time duration T, radius r, step sizes τ, h, and add some artificial noise to target f. We also report the number of iterations executed by the Algorithm from section 2 to find the suitable value of λ.

Example 1: Smooth target pair Consider the following homogeneous boundary value problem without any initial conditions:

$$p_{tt} = p_{xx}, \quad 0 < t < T, \; 0 < x < 1, \quad p|_{x=0} = 0, \; p|_{x=1} = 0, \; 0 < t < T, \tag{65}$$

and take one of its solutions

$$p = p(t,x) = \sin(3\pi t)\sin(3\pi x).$$

Choose $T = 2$ satisfying the controllability condition: $T = 2 > T_* = l = 1$. Find the source pair $v_* = (v_*^0, v_*^1)$:

$$v_*^0(x) = p\,|_{t=2} = 0, \qquad v_*^1(x) = -p_t\,|_{t=2} = -3\pi\sin(3\pi x), \qquad 0 < x < 1,$$

and calculate its norm:

$$\|v_*\|_{F^*} = \sqrt{\|v^0\|^2_{H_0^1(0,l)} + \|v_*^1\|^2_{L_\rho^2(0,l)}} = 3\pi/\sqrt{2}. \tag{66}$$

Now using (36),(62) find normal optimal boundary controls:

$$u_{*0}(t) = p_x\,|_{x=0} = 3\pi\sin(3\pi t), \;\; u_{*1}(t) = -p_x\,|_{x=1} = 3\pi\sin(3\pi t), \;\; 0 < t < 2. \tag{67}$$

Then we need to solve the following nonhomogeneous initial boundary value problem with constant coefficients:

$$\begin{aligned}
&y_{tt} = y_{xx}, \qquad 0 < t < T,\; 0 < x < l,\\
&y\,|_{x=0} = u_{*0}(t), \quad y\,|_{x=l} = u_{*1}(t), \qquad 0 < t < T,\\
&y\,|_{t=0} = 0, \quad y_t\,|_{t=0} = 0, \qquad 0 < x < l.
\end{aligned} \tag{68}$$

Using a suitable formula from the ready-to-use set of analytical solutions provided in [24] we find the final state and velocity:

$$f^0(x) = -12\pi\sin(3\pi x), \qquad f^1(x) = 0, \quad 0 < x < 1. \tag{69}$$

Tables 1, 2, and 3 show numerical results obtained by applying DHUM and VM. The symbol u means either a DHUM-control $\overset{\square}{u}_{\diamond}$ or a VM-control $\overset{\square}{u}$ depending on the method. A noisy target is denoted by $\overset{\square}{f}$. We vary artificial noise amplitude and step sizes τ, h consistently. The last column contains the number of iterations executed by Algorithm which is built into VM to find the value of Lagrange multiplier λ. In all cases the Algorithm started from $\lambda = \overset{\square}{\lambda}_0 = h/10$ and stopped at step 2 or step 3 if certain $\overset{\square}{\varepsilon}$-inequalities are satisfied with $\tilde{\varepsilon} = h$. We use two different values of the VM's input parameter r. We take the first $r = 7 > 3\pi/\sqrt{2}$ directly from (66). To choose another value of r we use observability inequality (41), find values of $\mu = \dfrac{2-1}{1/2} = 2$ from (42) and $\|f\|_F = 6\pi\sqrt{2}$ from (69), and then looking at (12) take $r = 14 > 3\pi\sqrt{2} = \|f\|_F/\mu$.

Table 1. Example 1. Results of DHUM and VM for $T = 2$, $h = 1/50$, and $\tau/h = 5/6$.

Method	r	$\dfrac{\|\tilde{f} - f\|_F}{\|f\|_F}$	$\dfrac{\|u - u_*\|_H}{\|u_*\|_H}$	$\dfrac{\|\tilde{A}u - f\|_F}{\|f\|_F}$	# of iters
DHUM		0	0.08741	$5.1\cdot 10^{-15}$	
VM	7	0	0.08679	$5.1\cdot 10^{-4}$	1
VM	14	0	0.08679	$5.1\cdot 10^{-4}$	1
DHUM		0.02535	0.63658	0.02535	
VM	7	0.02535	0.09661	0.02829	8
VM	14	0.02535	0.11015	0.02465	13
DHUM		0.10038	2.51716	0.10038	
VM	7	0.10038	0.15992	0.10429	8
VM	14	0.10038	0.21449	0.09436	11

Table 2. Example 1. Results of DHUM and VM for $T = 2$, $h = 1/100$, and $\tau/h = 5/6$.

Method	r	$\dfrac{\|\tilde{f} - f\|_F}{\|f\|_F}$	$\dfrac{\|u - u_*\|_H}{\|u_*\|_H}$	$\dfrac{\|\tilde{A}u - f\|_F}{\|f\|_F}$	# of iters
DHUM		0	0.04235	$8.6\cdot 10^{-13}$	
VM	7	0	0.04176	$2.5\cdot 10^{-4}$	1
VM	14	0	0.04176	$2.5\cdot 10^{-4}$	1
DHUM		0.01001	120.062	0.01001	
VM	7	0.01001	0.04555	0.01223	8
VM	14	0.01001	0.04795	0.00989	14
DHUM		0.10433	1251.18	0.10433	
VM	7	0.10433	0.15707	0.11320	8
VM	14	0.10433	0.18954	0.09887	7

In the example we just discussed both DHUM and VM work equally well when smooth target f is known exactly. However, the situation changes drastically as soon as any noise appears in data f. The results of DHUM become unusable, while the results of VM stay adequate to the noise level and grid density.

Table 3. Example 1. Results of DHUM and VM for $T=2$, $h=1/200$, and $\tau/h=5/6$.

Method	r	$\frac{\lVert \tilde{f}-f\rVert_F}{\lVert f\rVert_F}$	$\frac{\lVert u-u_*\rVert_H}{\lVert u_*\rVert_H}$	$\frac{\lVert A\tilde{u}-f\rVert_F}{\lVert f\rVert_F}$	# of iters
DHUM		0	0.02079	$1.1\cdot 10^{-9}$	
VM	7	0	0.02048	$1.2\cdot 10^{-4}$	1
VM	14	0	0.02048	$1.2\cdot 10^{-4}$	1
DHUM		0.00506	66659.9	0.07588	
VM	7	0.00506	0.02236	0.00624	10
VM	14	0.00506	0.02258	0.00486	12
DHUM		0.05006	659583	0.7405	
VM	7	0.05006	0.07848	0.05586	10
VM	14	0.05006	0.08729	0.04687	13

Fig. 1 shows a graphical representation of the results given in Table 2 with noise $\frac{\lVert \tilde{f}-f\rVert_F}{\lVert f\rVert_F}=1\%$. In this case DHUM-error $\frac{\lVert u_\diamond-u_*\rVert_H}{\lVert u_*\rVert_H}=1200\%$ becomes too big, therefore Fig. 1 contains two graphs: of exact control $u_*(t)$ and its VM-approximation $\tilde{u}(t)$ obtained for $r=14$ with VM-error $\frac{\lVert \tilde{u}-u_*\rVert_H}{\lVert u_*\rVert_H}=4.8\%$. Because of (67) the situation at the left and right end points $x=0$ and $x=l$ is just the same, therefore on Fig. 1 only left side controls $u_{*0}(t)$ and $\tilde{u}_0(t)$ are plotted.

Example 2: Continuous non-smooth target state Here we take another solution of (65):

$$p=p(t,x)=\sin(\pi t)\sin(\pi x),$$

and another $T=3/2$ which also satisfies the controllability condition: $T=3/2>T_*=l=1$. Find the source pair $v_*=(v_*^0,v_*^1)$:

$$v_*^0(x)=p\,|_{t=3/2}=-\sin(\pi x),\qquad v_*^1(x)=-p_t\,|_{t=3/2}=0,\qquad 0<x<1.$$

and calculate its norm:

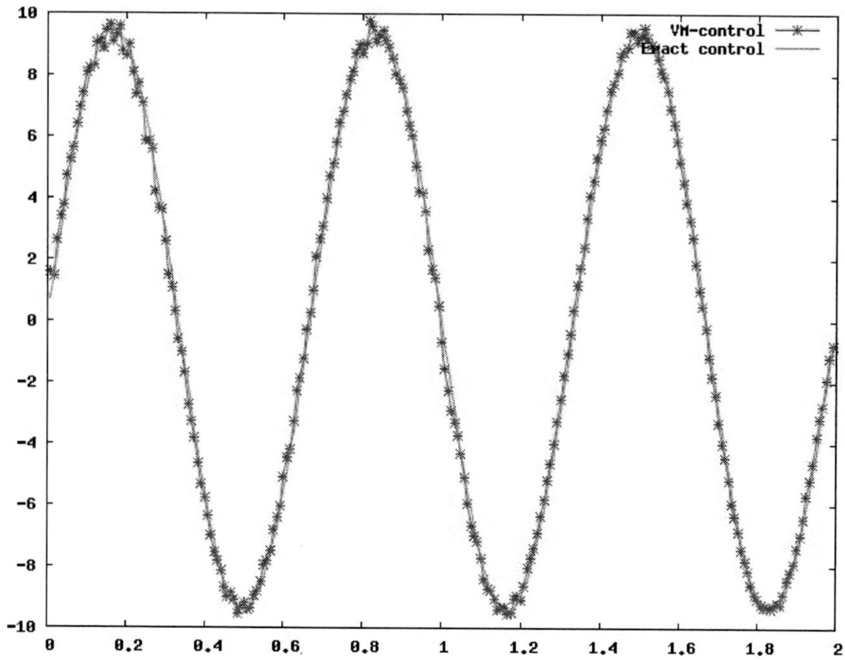

Figure 1. Example 1: Smooth target pair. $T=2,\ h=1/100,\ \tau/h=5/6$, noise=1%, exact control=u_{*0}, VM-control=$\tilde{u}_0$, $r=14$, VM-error=$\dfrac{\|\tilde{u}-u_*\|_H}{\|u_*\|_H}=4.8\%$.

$$\|v_*\|_{F^*}=\sqrt{\|v^0_*\|^2_{H^1_0(0,l)}+\|v^1_*\|^2_{L^2_\rho(0,l)}}=\pi/\sqrt{2}. \tag{70}$$

Equality (70) allows us to take the value $r=3\geq \pi/\sqrt{2}$. Using (36) find normal optimal boundary controls:

$$u_{*0}(t)=u_{*1}(t)=\pi\sin(\pi t),\ \ 0<t<3/2. \tag{71}$$

Then using the analytical formulae provided in [24] we find the solution y to the problem (68) with boundary data (71) and define the final state and velocity:

$$f^0(x)=-\pi\,|\cos(\pi x)|,\qquad f^1(x)=-3\pi^2\sin(\pi x),\quad 0<x<1.$$

The graph of the target state $f^0(x)$ is provided on Fig. 2 for convenience. Calculate the norm of the target:

$$\|f\|_F = \sqrt{\|f^0\|^2_{L^2_\rho(0,l)} + \|f^1\|^2_{H^{-1}(0,l)}} = \sqrt{\pi^2/2 + 9\pi^2/2} = \pi\sqrt{5}. \tag{72}$$

Using observability inequality (41) with μ defined by (42), the estimation (12), and the norm of the target (72), find the following lower bound for r:

$$\mu = \frac{3/2-1}{1/2} = 1, \qquad r \geq \frac{\|f\|_F}{\mu} = \pi\sqrt{5}. \tag{73}$$

As shown by (73) we can take $r = 10 > \pi\sqrt{5}$.

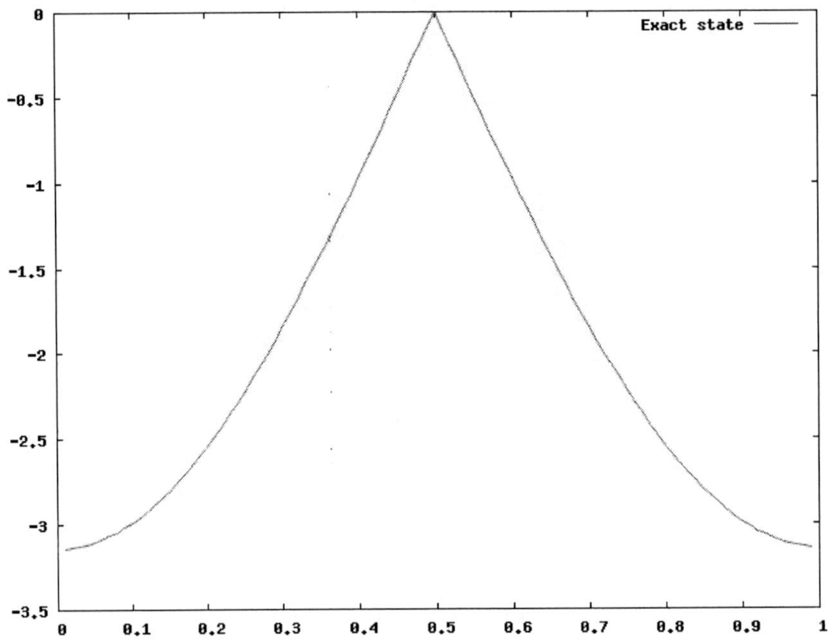

Figure 2. Example 2: Exact non-smooth target state $f^0(x) = -\pi\,|\cos(\pi x)| \in H^1_0(0,l)$.

Tables 4, 5, and 6 show numerical results obtained by applying DHUM and VM when $T = 3/2$.

To illustrate results contained in Table 5 we provide a graph of DHUM-control with exact target data on Fig. 3 and a graph of VM-control with noisy data on Fig. 4.

In the Example 2 DHUM could not handle even exact input data f, while VM proved to be reliable and robust in processing both exact and noisy data.

Table 4. Example 2. Results of DHUM and VM for $T = 3/2, h = 1/50,$ **and** $\tau/h = 15/16.$

Method	r	$\frac{\|\tilde{f}-f\|_F}{\|f\|_F}$	$\frac{\|u-u_*\|_H}{\|u_*\|_H}$	$\frac{\|\tilde{A}u-f\|_F}{\|f\|_F}$	# of iters
DHUM		0	0.13562	$3.7\cdot10^{-14}$	
VM	3	0	0.01410	$7.3\cdot10^{-4}$	1
VM	10	0	0.01410	$7.3\cdot10^{-4}$	1
DHUM		0.02514	0.69664	0.02514	
VM	3	0.02514	0.06349	0.02392	7
VM	10	0.02514	0.11610	0.02438	14
DHUM		0.10004	2.51501	0.10004	
VM	3	0.10004	0.16019	0.08990	8
VM	10	0.10004	0.26801	0.09369	13

Table 5. Example 2. Results of DHUM and VM for $T = 3/2, h = 1/100,$ **and** $\tau/h = 15/16.$

Method	r	$\frac{\|\tilde{f}-f\|_F}{\|f\|_F}$	$\frac{\|u-u_*\|_H}{\|u_*\|_H}$	$\frac{\|\tilde{A}u-f\|_F}{\|f\|_F}$	# of iters
DHUM		0	5.8785	$3.5\cdot10^{-10}$	
VM	3	0	0.00665	$3.5\cdot10^{-4}$	1
VM	10	0	0.00665	$3.5\cdot10^{-4}$	1
DHUM		0.01007	19.0811	0.01007	
VM	3	0.01007	0.02385	0.01004	11
VM	10	0.01007	0.03820	0.00986	16
DHUM		0.10086	165.496	0.10086	
VM	3	0.10086	0.15534	0.09553	7
VM	10	0.10086	0.18954	0.09887	11

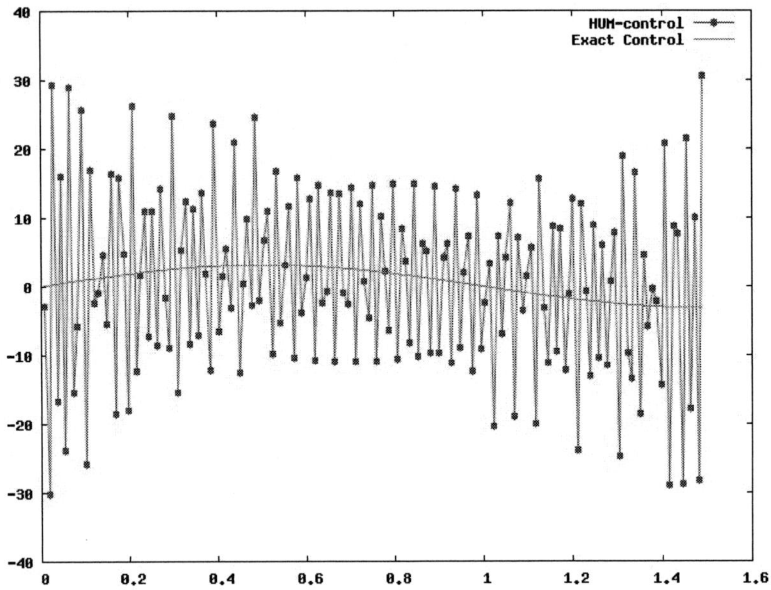

Figure 3. Example 2: Non-smooth target state. $T = 3/2,\ h = 1/100,\ \tau/h = 15/16,$ noise=0%, exact control= u_{*0}, DHUM-control= $u_{\diamond 0}$, DHUM-error= $\frac{\|u_{\diamond} - u_{*}\|_H}{\|u_{*}\|_H} = 588\%.$

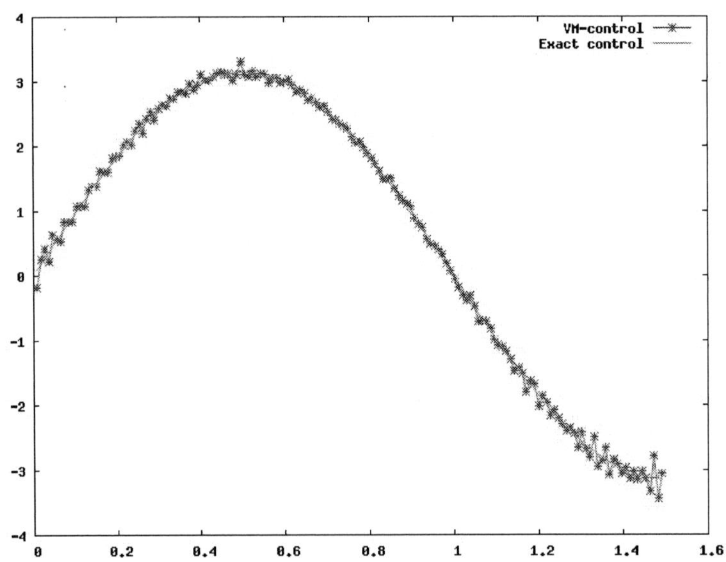

Figure 4. Example 2: Non-smooth target state. $T = 3/2,\ h = 1/100,\ \tau/h = 15/16,$ noise=1%, exact control= u_{*0}, VM-control= u_0, $r = 10,$ VM-error= $\frac{\|u - u_{*}\|_H}{\|u_{*}\|_H} = 3.8\%.$

Table 6. Example 2. Results of DHUM and VM for $T = 3/2,\ h = 1/200,$ and $\tau/h = 15/16.$

Method	r	$\frac{\|\tilde{f} - f\|_F}{\|f\|_F}$	$\frac{\|u - u_*\|_H}{\|u_*\|_H}$	$\frac{\|\tilde{A}u - f\|_F}{\|f\|_F}$	# of iters
DHUM		0	5137	0.00522	
VM	3	0	0.00299	0.00017	1
VM	10	0	0.00299	0.00017	1
DHUM		0.00519	15124.1	0.01093	
VM	3	0.00519	0.01499	0.00518	12
VM	10	0.00519	0.02477	0.00507	18
DHUM		0.05084	126552	0.11453	
VM	3	0.05084	0.09463	0.04892	9
VM	10	0.05084	0.12475	0.04810	14

Example 3: Discontinuous target velocity Let's take $T = 3/2$ and the following solution of (65):

$$p = p(t,x) = \sin(2\pi t)\sin(2\pi x).$$

Find the source pair $v_* = (v_*^0, v_*^1)$:

$$v_*^0(x) = p\,|_{t=3/2} = 0, \qquad v_*^1(x) = -p_t\,|_{t=3/2} = 2\pi\sin(2\pi x), \qquad 0 < x < 1.$$

and calculate its norm:

$$\|v_*\|_{F^*} = \sqrt{\|v^0\|^2_{H_0^1(0,l)} + \|v_*^1\|^2_{L^2_\rho(0,l)}} = \pi\sqrt{2}.$$

This allows us to use the value $r = 5 > \pi\sqrt{2}$. Using (36) find normal optimal boundary controls:

$$u_{*0}(t) = -u_{*1}(t) = 2\pi\sin(2\pi t),\ \ 0 < t < 3/2. \tag{74}$$

Then find the final state and velocity corresponding to (74):

$$f^0(x) = 6\pi\sin(2\pi x), \quad 0 < x < 1,$$

$$f^1(x) = -8\pi^2\cos(2\pi x),\ 0 < x < 1/2, \quad f^1(x) = f^1(x - 1/2),\ 1/2 < x < 1,$$

and calculate the norm

$$\|f\|_F = \sqrt{\|f^0\|^2_{L^2_\rho(0,l)} + \|f^1\|^2_{H^{-1}(0,l)}} = \tag{75}$$

$$\sqrt{18\pi^2 + (8\pi^2 - 64)} = \sqrt{26\pi^2 - 64} < 14.$$

Using (75) and the same value of $\mu = 1$ as in the Example 2 we choose another value $r = 15 > \|f\|_F / \mu$ for numerical experiments.

Fig. 5 illustrates the discontinuous target velocity $f^1(x)$. Tables 7, 8, and 9 show numerical results produced by DHUM and VM.

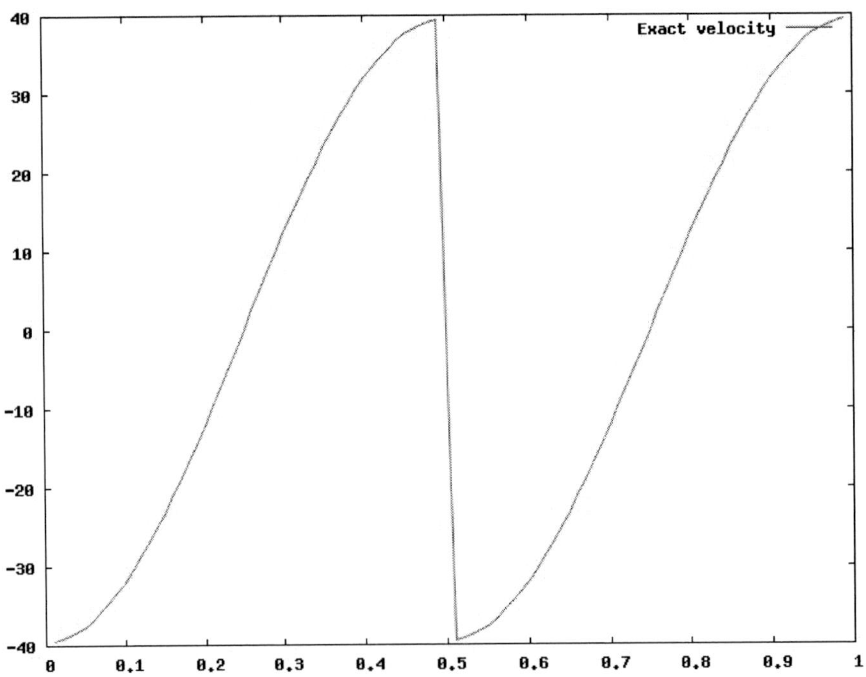

Figure 5. Example 3: Exact discontinuous target velocity $f^1(x)$ defined in (??).

To illustrate results contained in Table 8 we provide a graph of DHUM-control for noise level 1% on Fig. 6 and a graph of VM-control for noise level 5% on Fig. 7.

Table 7. Example 3. Results of DHUM and VM for $T = 3/2, h = 1/50,$ and $\tau/h = 15/16.$

Method	r	$\frac{\|\tilde{f}-f\|_F}{\|f\|_F}$	$\frac{\|u-u_*\|_H}{\|u_*\|_H}$	$\frac{\|A\tilde{u}-f\|_F}{\|f\|_F}$	# of iters
DHUM		0	0.06419	$4.0\cdot10^{-15}$	
VM	5	0	0.06391	$6.7\cdot10^{-4}$	1
VM	15	0	0.06391	$6.7\cdot10^{-4}$	1
DHUM		0.02519	0.50903	0.02519	
VM	5	0.02519	0.08045	0.02641	9
VM	15	0.02519	0.12636	0.02429	15
DHUM		0.10031	1.99126	0.10031	
VM	5	0.10031	0.15885	0.09975	6
VM	15	0.10031	0.24058	0.09281	13

Table 8. Example 3. Results of DHUM and VM for $T = 3/2, h = 1/100,$ and $\tau/h = 15/16.$

Method	r	$\frac{\|\tilde{f}-f\|_F}{\|f\|_F}$	$\frac{\|u-u_*\|_H}{\|u_*\|_H}$	$\frac{\|A\tilde{u}-f\|_F}{\|f\|_F}$	# of iters
DHUM		0	0.08211	$6.6\cdot10^{-13}$	
VM	5	0	0.03173	$3.3\cdot10^{-4}$	1
VM	15	0	0.03173	$3.3\cdot10^{-4}$	1
DHUM		0.01042	22.6703	0.01042	
VM	5	0.01042	0.03838	0.01085	9
VM	15	0.01042	0.04605	0.01019	17
DHUM		0.05000	108.864	0.04999	
VM	5	0.05000	0.08368	0.05077	7
VM	15	0.05000	0.10846	0.04835	15

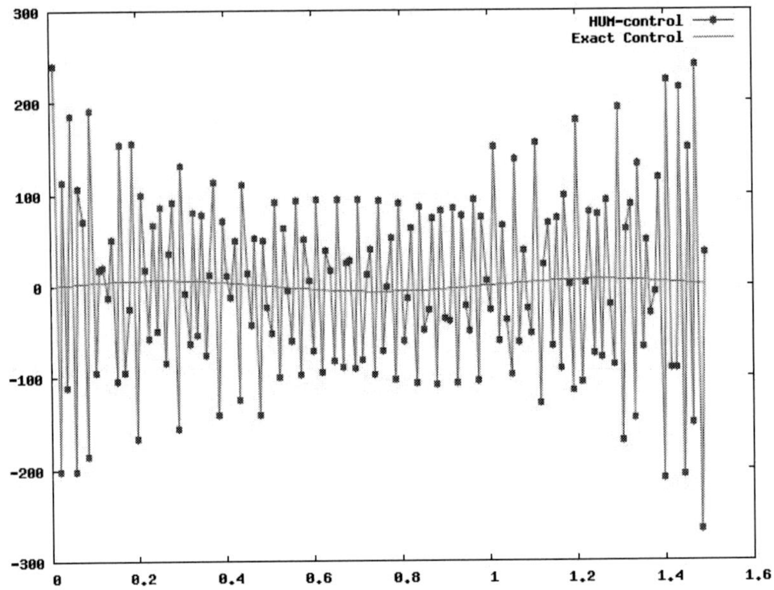

Figure 6. Example 3: Discontinuous target velocity. $T = 3/2,\ h = 1/100,\ \tau/h = 15/16,$ noise=1%,

exact control= u_{*0}, DHUM-control= $\overset{\square}{u}_{\diamond 0}$, DHUM-error= $\dfrac{\|\overset{\square}{u}_{\diamond} - u_{*}\|_{H}}{\|u_{*}\|_{H}} = 2267\%.$

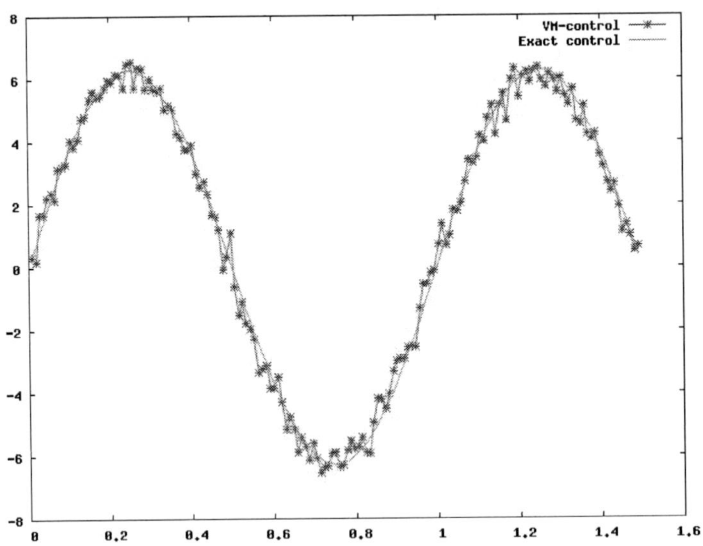

Figure 7. Example 3: Discontinuous target velocity. $T = 3/2,\ h = 1/100,\ \tau/h = 15/16,$ noise=5%,

exact control= u_{*0}, VM-control= $\overset{\square}{u}_{0}$, $r = 5$, VM-error= $\dfrac{\|\overset{\square}{u} - u_{*}\|_{H}}{\|u_{*}\|_{H}} = 8.4\%.$

Table 9. Example 3. Results of DHUM and VM for $T = 3/2, h = 1/200$, and $\tau/h = 15/16$.

Method	r	$\frac{\|\tilde{f} - f\|_F}{\|f\|_F}$	$\frac{\|u - u_*\|_H}{\|u_*\|_H}$	$\frac{\|A\tilde{u} - f\|_F}{\|f\|_F}$	# of iters
DHUM		0	469.167	0.00014	
VM	5	0	0.01580	0.00017	1
VM	15	0	0.01580	0.00017	1
DHUM		0.00541	12174	0.01429	
VM	5	0.00541	0.02029	0.00565	11
VM	15	0.00541	0.02651	0.00529	17
DHUM		0.05082	114049	0.13558	
VM	5	0.05082	0.08494	0.05141	9
VM	15	0.05082	0.11412	0.04884	15

In this Example DHUM's results became worse on the more dense grids even for exact data, while VM-error remained comparable to the noise level in the initial data and to the density of the difference grid.

7. Conclusion

In this chapter we didn't compare computational abilities of our VM with other existing numerical approaches described in [1]--[8]. It is possible that some of them might be more accurate or faster than VM under specific conditions. However in our opinion VM is noteworthy because of its noise-resistant properties and natural structure which can be easily adapted to any of the standard finite-dimensional methods used for approximation of differential equations. An additional point to emphasize is that convergence of VM is mathematically proved in Theorems 1 and 2. The only complementary information VM really needs is the value of radius r, which can be obtained from the continuous observability inequality as we showed in Remark 2 above.

References

[1] Glowinski, R.; Li, C.H.; Lions, J.L. A numerical approach to the exact boundary controllability of the wave equation (I). Dirichlet controls: Description of the numerical methods. *Japan J. Appl. Math.* 1990, 7, 1--76.

[2] Glowinski, R.; Lions, J.L. *Exact and approximate controllability of distributed parameter systems*: Part II. Acta Numerica. 1995, Cambridge University Press: Cambridge, UK, 269--378.

[3] Glowinski, R.; He, J.W.; Lions, J.L. On the controllability of wave models with variable coefficients: a numerical investigation. *Computational and Applied Mathematics*. 2002, 21(1), 191--225.

[4] Negreanu, M.; Zuazua, E. *Convergence of a multi-grid method for the controllability of a 1-d wave equation*. C.R. Acad. Sci. Paris, Série I. 2004, 338(5), 413--418.

[5] Zuazua, E. Propagation, observation, and control of waves approximated by finite difference methods. *SIAM Rev*. 2005, 47(2), 197--243.

[6] Münch, A. A uniformly controllable and implicit scheme for the 1-D wave equation. *Mathematical Modelling and Numerical Analysis*. 2005, 39(2), 377--418.

[7] Castro, C.; Micu, S.; Münch, A. Numerical approximation of the boundary control for the wave equation with mixed finite elements in a square. *IMA Journal of Numerical Analysis*. 2008, 28(1), 186--214.

[8] Glowinski, R.; Lions, J.L.; He, J.W. Exact and Approximate Controllability for Distributed Parameter Systems: a Numerical Approach; *Encyclopedia of Mathematics and its Applications,* 117; Cambridge University Press: Cambridge, UK, 2008.

[9] Lions, J.L. Exact controllability, stabilization and perturbations for distributed systems. *SIAM Rev.* 1988, 30(1), 1--68.

[10] Potapov, M.M. A stable method for solving linear equation with nonuniformly perturbed operators. *Doklady Mathematics*. 1999, 59(2), 286--288.

[11] Potapov, M.M. Strong convergence of difference approximations for problems of boundary control and observation for the wave equation. *Comput. Math. Math. Phys.* 1998, 38(3), 373--383.

[12] Potapov, M.M. Approximate solution to boundary control and observation problems for the equation describing transverse vibrations of a bar. Comput. *Math. Math. Phys.* 2005, 45(6), 978--994.

[13] Potapov, M.M. Approximation of the Dirichlet control problem and the dual problem with irregular Neumann observations for the wave equation. *Doklady Mathematics.* 2006, 73(3), 412--416.

[14] Potapov, M.M. Approximate solutions to Dirichlet control problems for the wave equation in Sobolev classes and dual observation problems. *Comput. Math. Math. Phys.* 2006, 46(12), 2092--2109.

[15] Potapov, M.M. Finite-difference approximations of Dirichlet observation problems for weak solutions to the wave equation subject to Robin boundary conditions. *Comput. Math. Math. Phys*. 2007, 47(8), 1268--1284.

[16] Tikhonov, A.N.; Leonov, A.S.; Yagola, A.G. Nonlinear *Ill-Posed Problems*; Chapman and Hall: London, 1998.

[17] Bakushinski, A.B.; Goncharsky, A.V. *Ill-posed Problems*: Theory and Application; Kluwer: Dordrecht, 1994.

[18] Komornik, V. *Exact Controllability and Stabilazation.* The Multiplier Method; Masson: Paris, John Wiley: Chichester, UK, 1994.

[19] Lasiecka, I.; Lions, J.L.; Triggiani, R. Nonhomogeneous boundary value problems for second order hyperbolic operators. *J. Math. Pures Appl*. 1986, 65, 149--192.

[20] Lasiecka, I.; Triggiani, R. Control Theory for Partial Differential Equations: Continuous and Approximation Theories. II: Abstract Hyperbolic-like Systems over a

Finite Time Horizon; *Encyclopedia of Mathematics and its Applications*, 75; Cambridge University Press: Cambridge, UK, 2000.

[21] Ho, L.F. Exact controllability of the one-dimensional wave equation with locally distributed control. *SIAM J. Control and Optimizat*. 1990, 28(3), 733--748.

[22] Dunford, N.; Schwartz, J.T. *Linear Operators. Part I:* General Theory; Interscience Publishers: New York, London, 1958.

[23] Yosida, K. *Functional Analysis*; Springer-Verlag: Berlin, Göttingen, Heidelberg, 1965.

[24] Il'in, V.A.; Moiseev, E.I. Optimization of boundary controls of string vibrations. Russ. *Math. Surv*. 2005, 60(6), 1093--1119.

In: Eye Research Developments
Editor: Alan N. Westerhouse
ISBN: 978-1-60741-177-2

Chapter VIII

Deep Anterior Lamellar Keratoplasty (DALK) in Post-Infective Corneal Scars

Antonio Leccisotti*
Visiting Professor, School of Biomedical Sciences, University of Ulster, Coleraine, UK
Director, Dept. of Ophthalmology, Casa di Cura Rugani, Siena, Italy,

Abstract

BACKGROUND: In the last years, Deep Anterior Lamellar Keratoplasty (DALK) has emerged as the standard surgical technique for the treatment of advanced keratoconus and anterior corneal dystrophies. DALK has several advantages over penetrating keratoplasty (PKP): it preserves the recipient endothelium, it is an external procedure, it has an extremely low rejection rate, and the rejection is only directed toward the stroma and is therefore well controllable.

The most popular method for DALK is the Big-Bubble technique, by which air, forcefully injected into the stroma, separates the Descemet's membrane from the recipient stromal tissue, creating a smooth interface for the donor stroma.

In post-infective corneal leukoma, DALK is less commonly performed because injected air is often unable to penetrate a severely scarred stroma. In these cases, PKP carries an increased risk of rejection because of neovascularization and, in post-herpetic scars, because of the strong immunologic stimulus and the possible recurrence of herpetic keratitis. In addition, cataract may occur after herpetic kerato-uveitis, and subsequent phacoemulsification can affect the PKP endothelium.

STUDY DESIGN: Consecutive, non-comparative, single-surgeon retrospective study.

METHODS: in post-infective stromal scars the following pre-Descemetic DALK technique is used: the cornea is trephined for approximately 450 micron by a 8 mm Hessburg-Barron disposable trephine, air is delicately injected into the stroma without achieving a big bubble, an anterior keratectomy is performed, and subsequently a deeper manual dissection with a bevel-up rounded blade is carried out, following the stromal planes, and leaving a thin stromal layer of approximately 50 microns. The donor button is cut by a Hessburg-Barron 8.25 mm punch and the Descemet's membrane with the overlying endothelium is peeled off. The donor button is then secured to the recipient stromal bed by 16 interrupted 10-0 nylon sutures.

This pre-Descemetic technique has a very low perforation risk and allows a safe dissection of severely scarred corneas, using air not to cleave the Descemet's membrane but rather to facilitate manual stromal dissection.

---

* Address: Piazza 5 Bersaglieri 2; 53100 Siena, Italy; leccisotti@libero.it

RESULTS: pre-Descemetic DALK was performed in 25 cases of post-infective corneal leukoma (12 herpetic, 9 bacterial, 4 of unknown origin). In all cases, surgery was uneventful and no perforation occurred. A transitory hazy donor-recipient interface was observed in 9 cases, but it fully resolved in 2 to 6 months. No cases of rejection were observed. In 2 cases, cataract surgery by phacoemulsification was successfully performed. At 12 months, after complete suture removal, mean post-operative best corrected visual acuity was 0.73. Mean post-operative astigmatism was 2.41 dioptres (D). In the 14 cases in which pre-operative refraction was known, DALK induced a mean -2.20 D change in spherical equivalent.

In all post-herpetic scars, prophylaxis with oral acyclovir was instituted as follows: 400 mg 3 times daily for 6 months, then twice daily for 6 months. No herpetic recurrence was observed; in 2 cases, a subtle peripheral neovascularization of the interface occurred, with no consequences.

CONCLUSION: Pre-Descemetic DALK was safely and successfully carried out in all cases of post-infective leukoma. The thin stromal layer left on the recipient bed did not affect long term visual acuity.

Introduction

In the recent years, the concept of selective tissue transplantation has considerably changed the approach to corneal grafting. Until the recent past, penetrating keratoplasty (PKP) has been the golden standard of corneal transplantation, due to easy surgical technique and to good prognosis [1]. Unfortunately, PKP in post-infective corneal scars is characterised by a less favourable prognosis, especially in post-herpetic leukoma, in which pre-existent neovascularisation and herpetic reactivation increase the risk for rejection [2, 3], in spite of antiviral prophylaxis [4, 5].

In the last years, Deep Anterior Lamellar Keratoplasty (DALK) has emerged as the standard surgical technique for the treatment of advanced keratoconus and anterior corneal dystrophies [6-9]. DALK is the most rational approach to corneal stromal diseases and has several advantages over penetrating keratoplasty (PKP): it preserves the recipient endothelium, it is an external procedure, it has an extremely low rejection rate, and the rejection is only directed toward the stroma and is therefore well controllable. In addition, tissue for lamellar keratoplasty does not require the endothelial standards needed for PKP, and is therefore more readily available. The most popular method for DALK is the Big-Bubble technique, by which air, forcefully injected into the stroma, separates the Descemet's membrane from the recipient stromal tissue, creating a smooth interface for the donor stroma [10, 11]. In post-infective corneal leukoma DALK is less commonly performed because injected air is often unable to penetrate a severely scarred stroma.

The authors of big-bubble DALK have proposed a near-Descemetic (or pre-Descemetic) approach in cases of increased risk of intraoperative perforation, such as thin or scarred corneas [12]. In near-Descemetic DALK, a gentle intrastromal air injection is followed by manual layer-to-layer dissection, leaving a stromal bed of approximately 50 micron. This technique has not been assessed in post-infective stromal scars.

In the present study, the technique, visual results and complications of pre-Descemetic DALK in post-infective corneal scars.

Surgical Technique

The instruments needed for pre-Descemetic DALK are simple and inexpensive, and can be used for PKP as well (figure 1):

- a straight Vannas scissor with blunt tip
- 2 curved scissors for corneal transplantation (1 right, 1 left), with lower blade internal and upper blade external (in case of PKP, the lower blade will only damage the endothelium that is removed) (e.g. Sir, Italy, C928)
- disposable Hessburg-Barron trephine (Altomed, Tyne & Wear, England), 8 mm diameter
- disposable Barron punch (Altomed, Tyne & Wear, England), 8 or 8.25 mm diameter
- a Barraquer solid blade eyelid speculum (Sir, Italy, E-10011)
- 10-0 nylon suture with curved needle
- a 0.5 mm gauge (PMS, Germany, E15-225)
- a bevel-up crescent knife (Alcon)
- a 15° blade for possible paracentesis
- a needle-holder with curved head for 10-0 sutures
- 2 tying forceps (1 straight, 1 curved)
- a smaller and a larger straight forceps
- a 8 mm round corneal marker with central cross
- a violet gentian felt tip pen
- a 5 cc syringe with luer-lock connection, and a 30-gauge needle
- an air filter
- ophthalmic cohesive viscoelastic (such as Pro-Visc, Alcon), only needed for PKP
- a guarded diamond blade, only needed in case of shallow trephination
- Maloney surgical keratometer
- Merocell sponges
- balanced salt solution (BSS) for irrigation and anterior chamber reformation in case of perforation
- an anterior chamber cannula.

The procedure is particularly delicate and lasts approximately 1 hour; general anaesthesia is therefore normally preferred, especially in younger patients. However, in selected cases a peribulbar block with intravenous sedation can be effectively used. The periocular skin and conjunctival sac are prepared with povidone iodine (10% on the skin and 5% in the conjunctiva). The presence of stromal neovascularisation should be carefully assessed, and major vessels invading the cornea should be cauterized at the limbus, avoiding the damage of the corneal tissue. An 8 mm circular marker tinted with gentian violet is centred on the geometrical centre of the cornea.

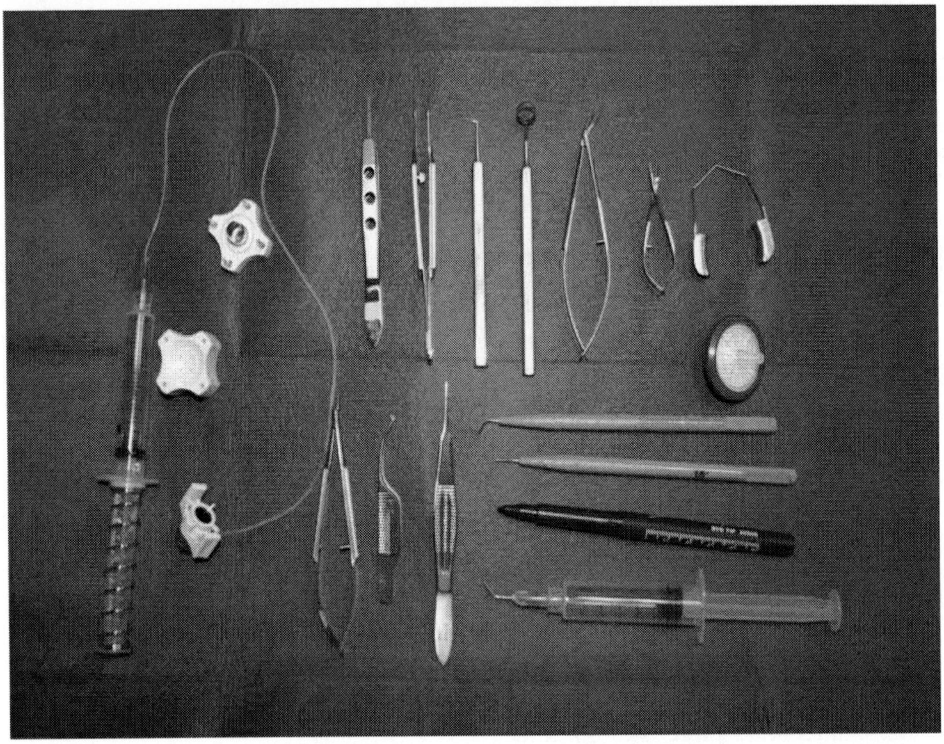

Figure 1. Surgical instrumentation for pre-Descemetic deep anterior lamellar keratoplasty (DALK).

A partial trephination is carried out with the Hessburg-Barron suction trephine (figure 2 and 3). With a peripheral thickness of 500 micron, a full turn and a half (approximately 400 micron) are advised. The depth of trephination is checked by a 0.5 mm gauge. If the cut is too shallow (because of bad suction or wrong calculation of trephination), it should be deepened by a guarded diamond blade, set at 400 micron (or less, in case of thinner cornea), to allow subsequent needle insertion and anterior dissection. A 5 cc syringe filled with sterile air is locked to a 30 gauge needle, which is bent at a 100° angle at 8 mm from the tip, with the bevel down. The 30 gauge needle is larger than usual needles for DALK, with the purpose of an easier penetration and a more efficient air penetration in the stroma. The needle is inserted at half thickness in the stroma, at 10 o'clock, holding the central corneal button with a forceps. The needle is advanced slowly but firmly, following the same corneal plane until the corneal geometrical centre (figure 4). Resistance may be encountered in particularly scarred corneas, but usually penetration is easily achieved, and the needle can be constantly checked despite corneal opacity. The syringe plunger is pushed with a constant pressure to inject intrastromal air, but excess pressure is avoided. The central area will only whiten if it is not excessively scarred, but full stromal emphysema is not necessary, let alone a big bubble. The purpose of stromal emphysema is to facilitate subsequent stromal manual dissection, so even a semi-peripheral emphysema will equally serve the purpose (figure 5). It is best to stop air injection if the limbus starts to whiten, otherwise air will reach the anterior chamber through the trabecular meshwork in the form of small bubbles, which may impair the vision of the last corneal layers in the ultimate phases of stromal dissection. The needle is retracted, and the excision of a thick part of the anterior stroma is performed with a bevel up crescent blade.

The blade is inserted superiorly at approximately ¾ of the stromal depth and maintained at the same level all over, sliding safely within a same stromal plane (figure 6). The blade does not usually encounter any particular resistance when cutting through the scarred stroma; because of its poor visualization, the blade should be in a horizontal position. When reaching the trephination cut, the blade should undermine for 1-2 mm its external edge, to allow good external apposition of the sutured margins despite their different thickness. The button is peripherally excised by corneal round scissors (figure 7). A more delicate excision of one or two additional thin stromal layers is performed, reaching a stromal bed thickness of approximately 50 microns (figure 8). In most cases, the stroma is clear at this level (figure 9), but occasionally a slight opacity is still visible. This opacity will only marginally affect final visual acuity; it is therefore advisable not to insist in total stromal removal, increasing the risk of perforation. The donor button is cut by a Barron punch, its endothelial side is gently dried with a Merocell sponge, and the endothelium marked with small dots of the felt tip pen, to assist its full removal. The central Descemet's membrane is pinched with delicate forceps and peeled off (figure 10). The prepared donor button is secured to the stromal bed by sixteen 10-0 nylon interrupted sutures (figure 11).

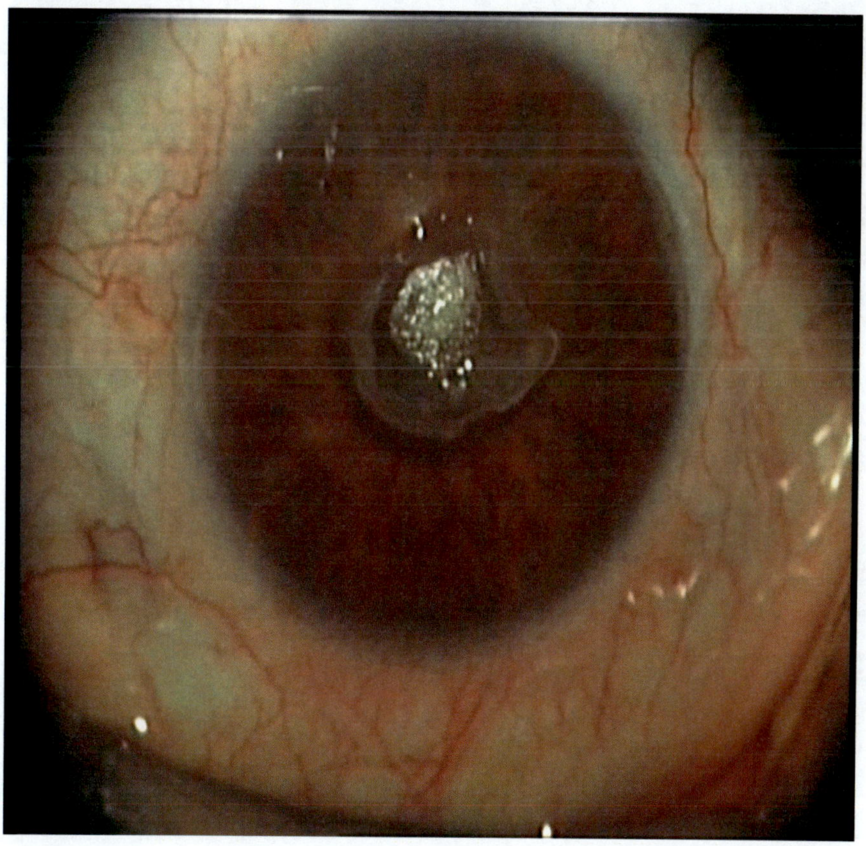

Figure 2. Pre-operative aspect of a post-herpetic stromal scar.

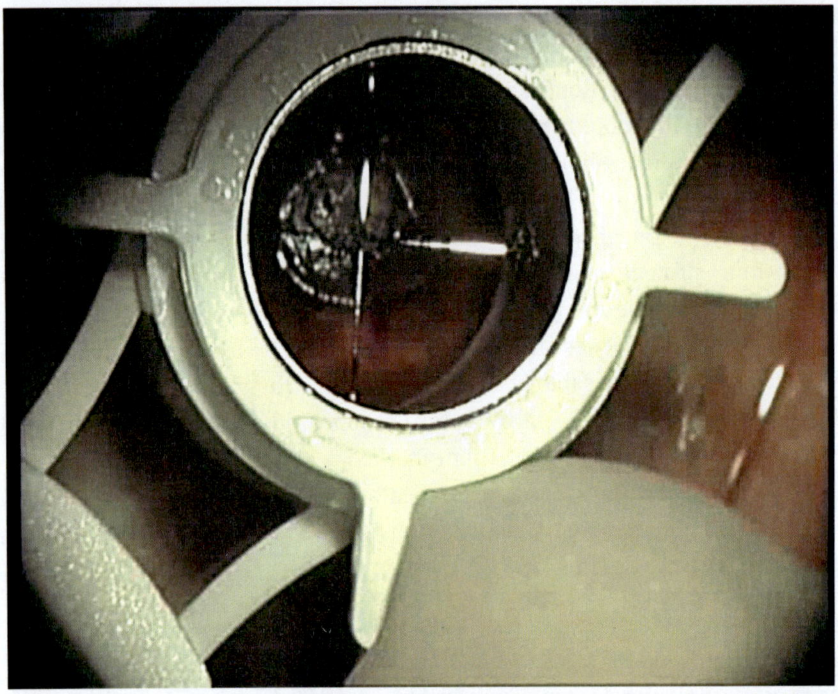

Figure 3. Partial trephination with Hessburg-Barron trephine.

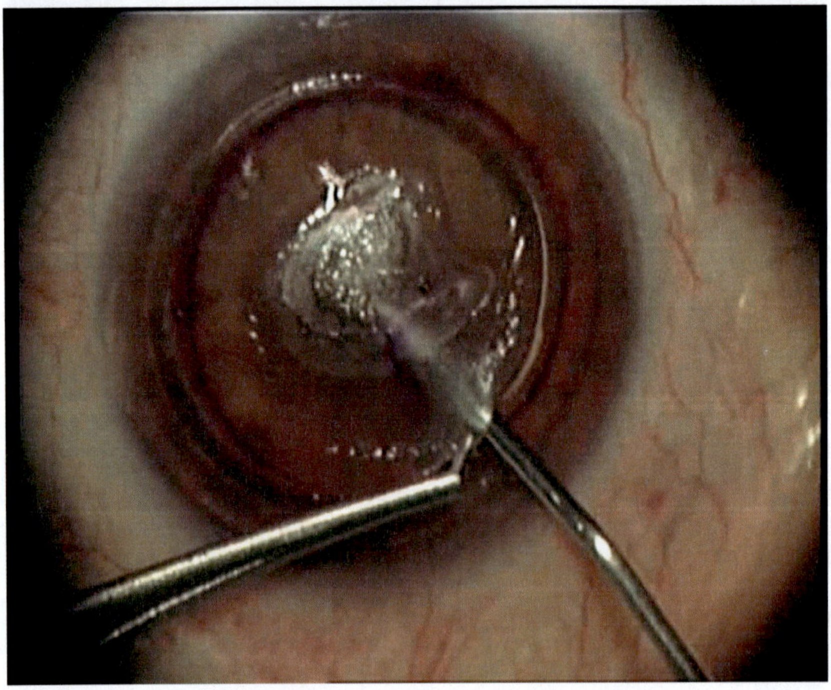

Figure 4. Needle insertion in mid stroma.

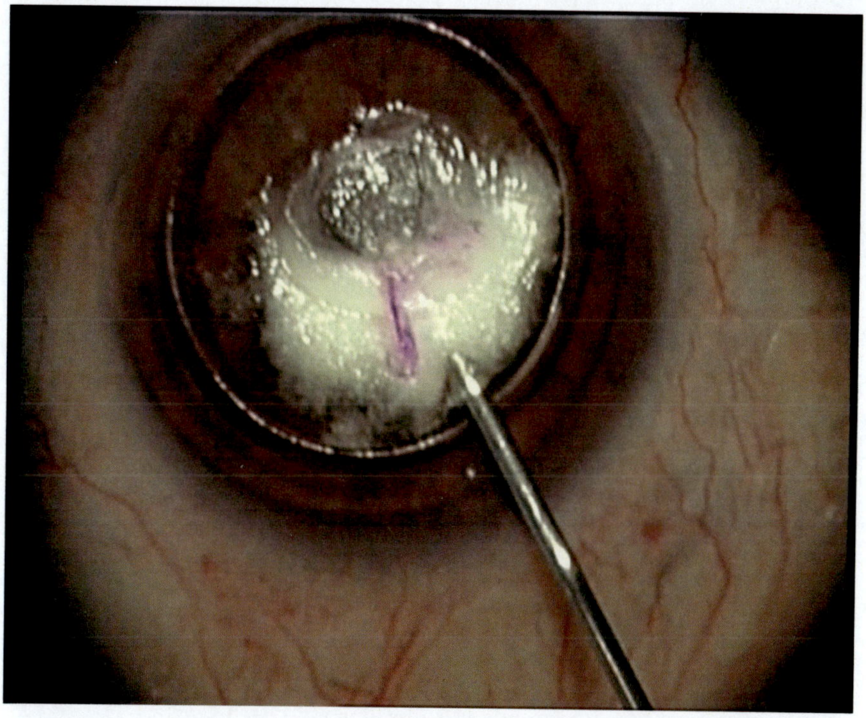

Figure 5. Intrastromal air injection. The small bubbles do not access the central scarred area.

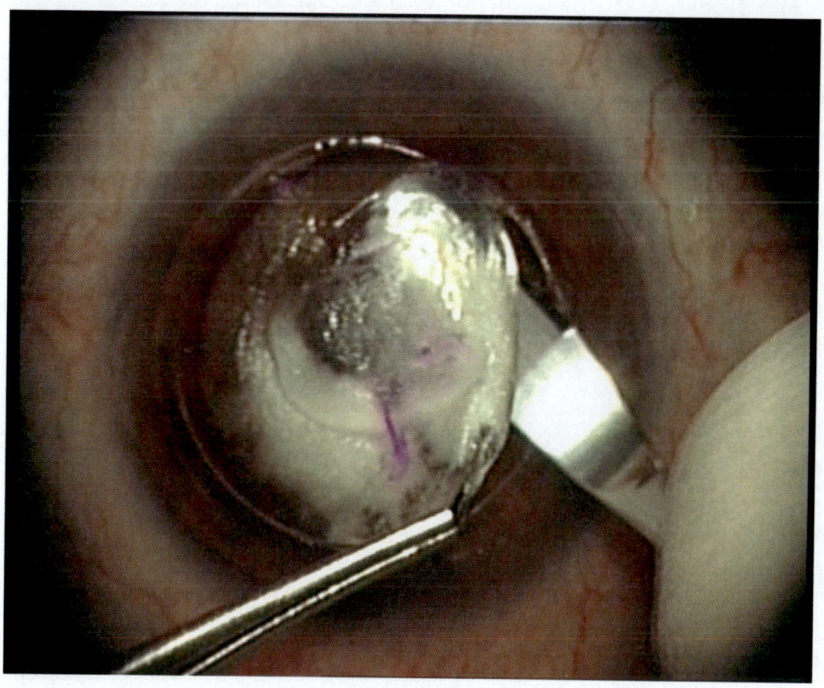

Figure 6. Anterior keratectomy with crescent blade.

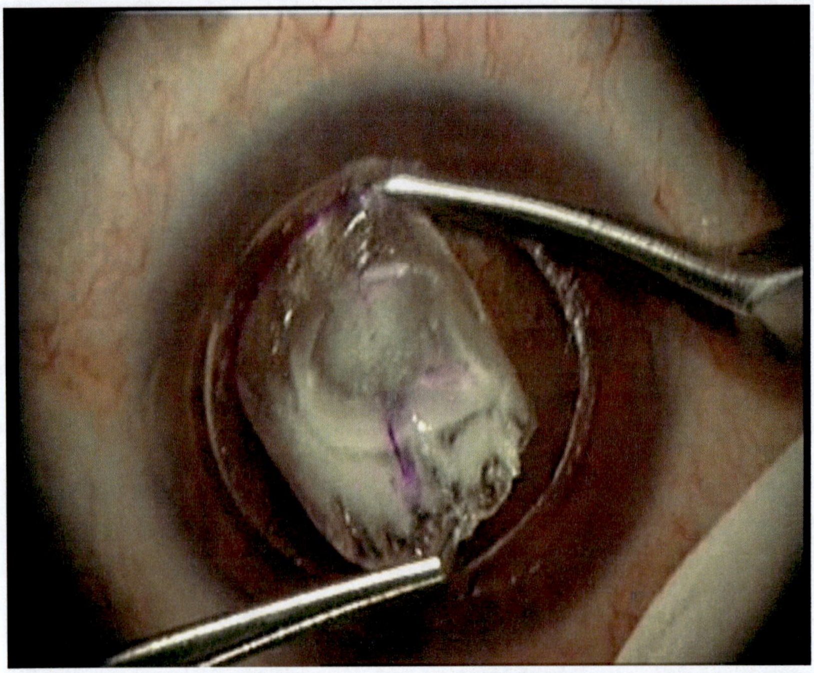

Figure 7. Excision of anterior stroma is completed by scissors.

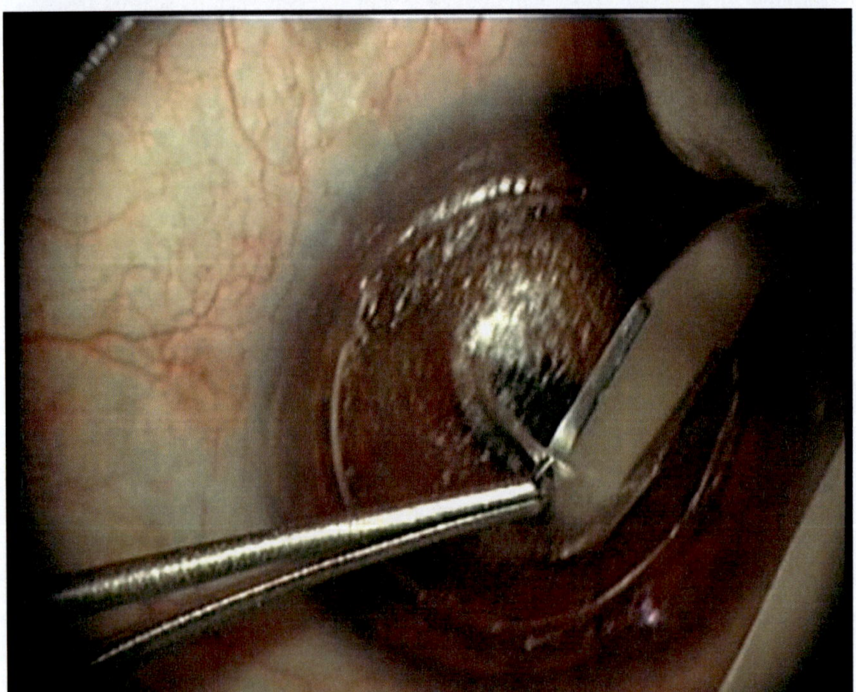

Figure 8. Deep stromal dissection with crescent blade.

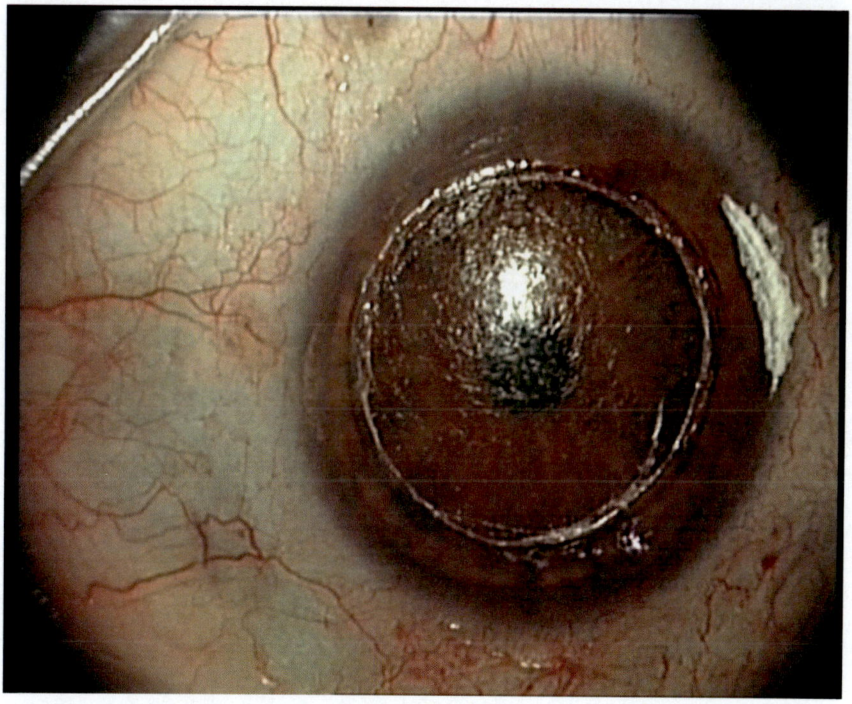

Figure 9. Stromal bed after deep dissection.

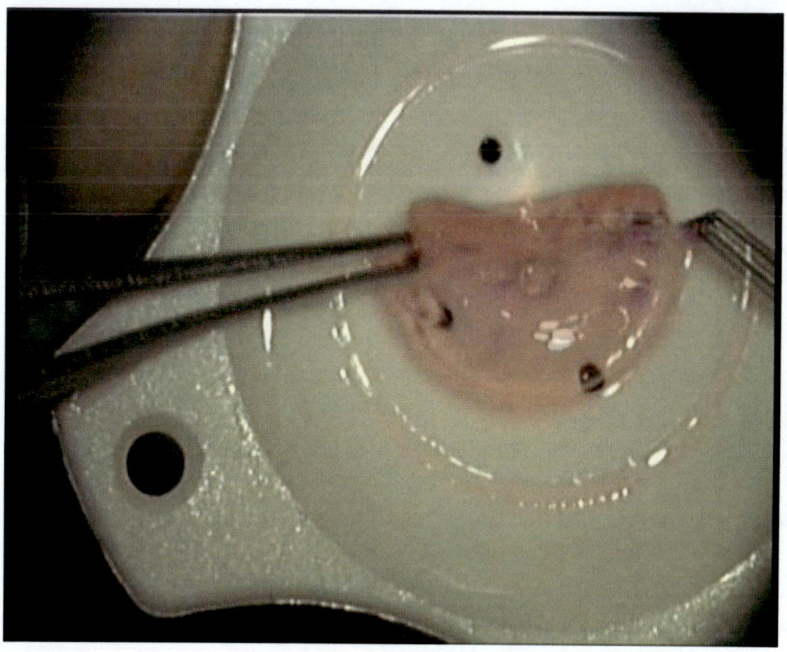

Figure 10. Peeling of Descemet's membrane from the donor button.

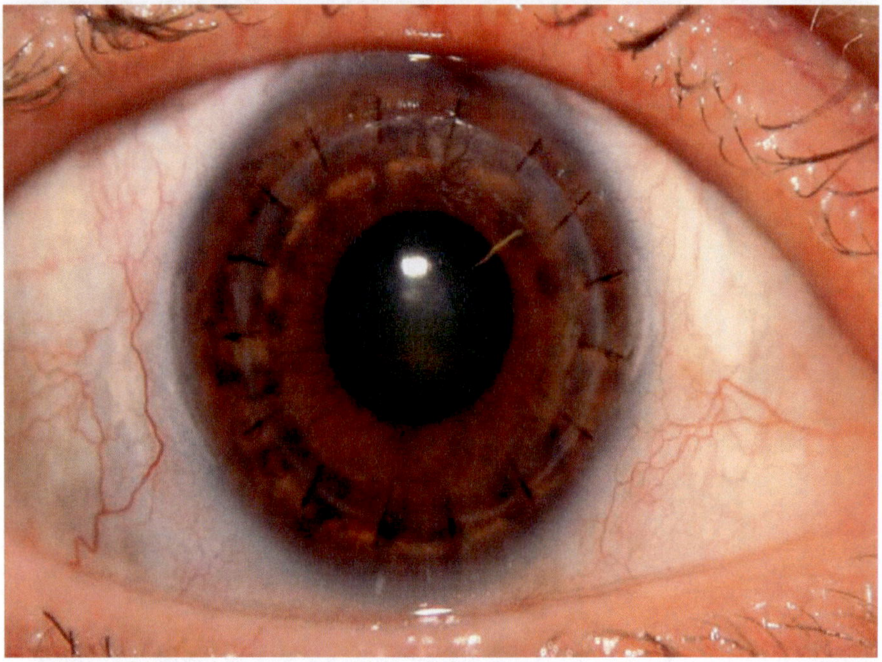

Figure 11. Two weeks after DALK, fully transparent cornea.

Intra-Operative Complications

The most feared intraoperative complication is Descemet's membrane perforation, which may occur at different stages. Perforation during trephination can be caused by errors in pachymetry or in calculation of trephination depth. This occurrence can be managed by temporarily suturing the perforation with radial sutures, continuing DALK and finally tightly suturing the button in the area of perforation.

Perforation during dissection is much more common, and is caused by the attempt of removing the deepest stromal layers. Microperforations usually allow completion of DALK if most of the stroma has been excised, but continuing dissection after perforation is often impossible because of globe softening. At the moment of perforation the surgeon should decide whether the residual stroma will compromise visual function: in such case, conversion to PKP may be required. Otherwise, if needed, the anterior chamber can be reformed by air through a paracentesis and the donor button is sutured. Larger perforations may lead to the formation of a fluid interface between the recipient Descemet and the donor stroma; if this fluid does not reabsorb, the stroma will become oedematous. An attempt to tampon the perforation with air in the anterior chamber can be done, but intraocular pressure (IOP) should be constantly monitored, because a large bubble in the anterior chamber may cause an acute IOP rise, similar to pupillary block glaucoma, with fixed dilated pupil and subcapsular cataract [13].

Post-Operative Management

During the first post-operative week the donor epithelium is gradually replaced by the overriding recipient epithelium, but sometimes, when the donor epithelium has a weak adhesion, large epithelial defects are slowly covered by the advancing recipient epithelium. This process is normally easy and uneventful, but it must be frequently checked and facilitated by frequent (every 2 hours when awake) lubrication with a preservative-free gel and topical preservative-free antibiotics and steroids. After full epithelialisation, topical dexamethasone or betamethasone should be used 4 times daily for 2 to 3 months, then treatment can be switched to loteprednol, 4 times daily until the 9th-10th month.

In all post-herpetic scars, prophylaxis with oral acyclovir must be continued as follows: 400 mg 3 times daily for 6 months, then twice daily for 6 months. Suture management is of paramount importance: all loose sutures must be removed, to avoid inflammation, neovascularisation and stromal melting. Beginning from the 3rd month, excessively tight sutures (recognized at corneal topography by localized steepening) can be removed to reduce astigmatism. Contrarily to DALK in keratoconus, in which donor adhesion is slow, post-keratitis DALK has a fast healing, so that early suture removal is safe. All sutures must be removed before the 12th month, to avoid their degradation and a difficult late removal. Stromal rejection is exceedingly rare, and should be managed by increasing topical steroid administration.

Post-DALK refractive errors can be surgically managed by excimer laser (contraindicated in post-herpetic scars, because ultraviolet light may reactivate the virus), by refractive lens exchange (for large spherical errors in presbyopic age), by phakic intraocular lenses (for large spherical errors in younger patients), and by astigmatic keratotomy (especially for mixed astigmatism).

Results

Pre-Descemetic DALK was performed in 25 cases of post-infective corneal leukoma (12 herpetic, 9 bacterial, 4 of unknown origin). In all cases, surgery was uneventful and no perforation occurred. A transitory hazy donor-recipient interface was observed in 9 cases, but it fully resolved in 2 to 6 months. In one case, due to extensive peripheral neovascularization, blood remained in the interface for several weeks; in the same case, scar involved the deepest stroma, but did not affect the final visual recovery (figure 12). No cases of rejection were observed. In 2 cases, in which a cataract was present before DALK, phacoemulsification and in-the-bag implantation of an intraocular lens (IOL) was successfully performed, respectively 4 and 7 months after DALK. Mean post-operative astigmatism was 2.41 dioptres (D). In the 14 cases in which pre-operative refraction was known, DALK induced a mean -2.20 D change in spherical equivalent. Pre-operative mean best-spectacle corrected visual acuity (BSCVA) was 0.23; at 12 months, after complete suture removal, mean post-operative BSCVA was 0.73.

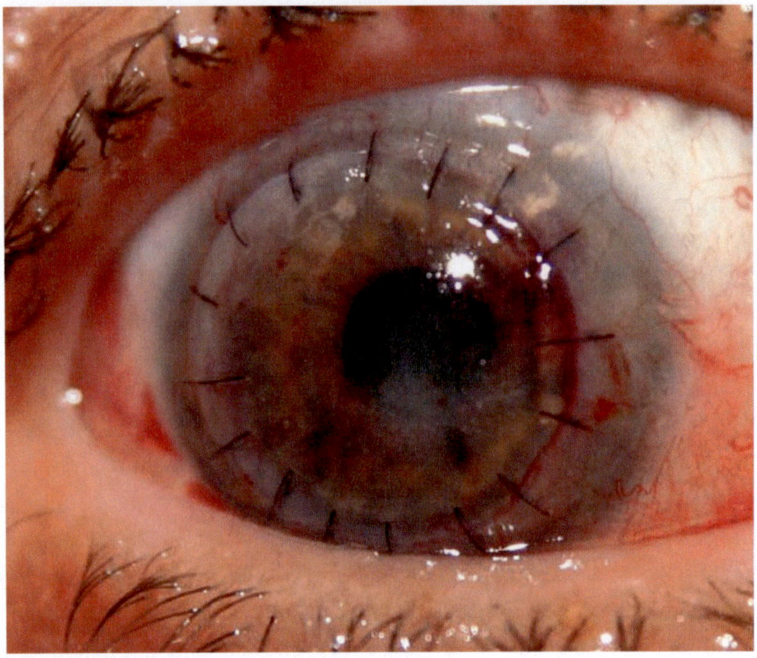

Figure 12. In a case with extensive neovascularisation and deep stromal scar, blood in the interface and paracentral opacity of the stromal bed, 1 day after DALK.

Conclusion

Pre-Descemetic DALK is the most logical approach to stromal scars, because it only replaces the diseased tissue and preserves the healthy endothelium. This is even more important in post-herpetic leukoma, where viral recurrence may require repeat DALK and where neovascularization increases the risk of rejection. In such cases, replacement of a DALK button is simple and safe, contrarily to repeat PKP. In addition, early removal of suture can be safely be accomplished in DALK, contributing to a faster visual rehabilitation and to a faster elimination of a stimulus to inflammation and rejection.

In the present series no cases of intraoperative perforation occurred, due to the prudent pre-Descemetic approach, deliberately avoiding the formation of a big-bubble and the exposure of the Descemet's membrane. In rare cases, stromal scar may extend to deeper levels and cannot be fully excised by pre-Descemetic DALK, but we must remember that most of the visual impairment in stromal scars is caused by the superficial irregularity and by the overall corneal opacification. As shown by one of our cases, a thin residual stromal opacity does not considerably affect the final visual acuity.

Surgical difficulties of DALK in scarred corneas include the impossibility of complete stromal emphysema when air is injected, and the impaired visualization of the blade during the first anterior keratectomy. However, complete emphysema is not necessary, provided that air is at least in the peripheral stroma, especially in its superior aspects, where manual dissection is started. The blade is safely advanced between the stromal planes, and its perfect visualization is not necessary.

The risk of herpetic recurrence is well controlled by prolonged systemic antiviral prophylaxis with acyclovir; with this approach, we had no cases of stromal re-infections.

DALK with Descemet's membrane baring techniques has been reported in post-infectious corneal opacities, but the risk of intraoperative perforation and conversion to PKP has been evidenced by most series [14-17]. A 10-eye series of DALK with no perforations included only one case of presumed post-infectious scar [18]. In all these reports, despite successful Descemet's membrane exposure, visual results are comparable to the present study; we feel therefore that pursuing Descemet's membrane exposure in post-infectious stromal opacity is unnecessarily risky.

Recently, the use of femtosecond laser for DALK has been reported [19-20]. Unfortunately, femtosecond laser requires an almost perfectly clear tissue for penetration; its use is therefore limited to keratoconic corneas with no apical scarring, and cannot be extended to corneal leukomas, in which manual dissection has no current alternatives.

In conclusion, the pre-Descemetic approach to DALK allows low-risk surgery in post-infective corneal opacity. Visual rehabilitation can be slower than that achieved by PKP, but the preservation of a healthy endothelium, the completely external surgery, the low risk of rejection in such difficult eyes, and the use of more readily available donor tissue make pre-Descemetic DALK the most logical approach to disabling stromal scars.

References

[1] Dorrepaal SJ, Cao KY, Slomovic AR. Indications for penetrating keratoplasty in a tertiary referral centre in Canada, 1996-2004. *Can. J. Ophthalmol.* 2007;42:244-250

[2] Sterk CC, Jager MJ, Swart-vd Berg M. Recurrent herpetic keratitis in penetrating keratoplasty. *Doc. Ophthalmol.* 1995;90:29-33

[3] Tuppin P, Poinard C, Loty B, Delbosc B. Risk factors for corneal regraft in patients on the French waiting list. *Cornea.* 2004;23:704-711

[4] van Rooij J, Rijneveld WJ, Remeijer L, et al. Effect of oral acyclovir after penetrating keratoplasty for herpetic keratitis: a placebo-controlled multicenter trial. *Ophthalmology.* 2003;110:1916-1919

[5] Ghosh S, Jhanji V, Lamoureux E, Taylor HR, Vajpayee RB. Acyclovir therapy in prevention of recurrent herpetic keratitis following penetrating keratoplasty. *Am. J. Ophthalmol.* 2008;145:198-202

[6] Archila EA. Deep lamellar keratoplasty dissection of host tissue with intrastromal air injection. *Cornea.* 1984/85;3:217-218

[7] Sugita J, Kondo J. Deep lamellar keratoplasty with complete removal of pathological stroma for vision improvement. *Br. J. Ophthalmol.* 1997;81:184-188

[8] Melles GRJ, Lander F, Rietveld FJR, Remeijer L, Beekhuis WH, Binder PS. A new surgical technique for deep stromal, anterior lamellar keratoplasty. *Br. J. Ophthalmol.* 1999;83:327-333

[9] Duong MH, Thimel S, Hoang Xuan T. Kératoplastie lamellaire avec aero-visco dissection. *J. Fr. Ophthalmol.* 2001;24:930-936

[10] Anwar M, Teichmann KD. Big-bubble technique to bare Descemet's membrane in anterior lamellar keratoplasty. *J. Cataract. Refract. Surg.* 2002;28:398-403

[11] Anwar M, Teichmann KD. Deep lamellar keratoplasty. Surgical techniques for anterior lamellar keratoplasty with and without baring of Descemet's membrane. *Cornea.* 2002;21:374-383

[12] Anwar M, Teichmann KD. Planned near-Descemet's dissection in deep lamellar keratoplasty, using air or fluid. In John T (ed) Surgical Techniques in Anterior and Posterior Lamellar Corneal Surgery. New Delhi: Jaypee, 2006;125-139

[13] Leccisotti A. Descemet's membrane perforation during deep anterior lamellar keratoplasty: Prognosis. *J. Cataract. Refract. Surg.* 2007;33:825-829

[14] Noble BA, Agrawal A, Collins C, Saldana M, Brogden PR, Zuberbuhler B. Deep Anterior Lamellar Keratoplasty (DALK): visual outcome and complications for a heterogeneous group of corneal pathologies. *Cornea.* 2007;26:59-64

[15] Wylegała E, Wróblewska EM, Tarnawska D, Mierzwa M. [Applying deep lamellar keratoplasty in corneal disorders without endothelial abnormalities] [Article in Polish] *Klin. Oczna.* 2003;105:263-6

[16] Bodenmueller M, Goldblum D, Frueh BE. [Retrospective analysis of deep lamellar keratoplasties] [Article in German] *Klin. Monatsbl. Augenheilkd.* 2004;221:307-10

[17] Wylegała E, Tarnawska D, Dobrowolski D. Deep lamellar keratoplasty for various corneal lesions. *Eur. J. Ophthalmol.* 2004;14:467-72

[18] Vajpayee RB, Tyagi J, Sharma N, Kumar N, Jhanji V, Titiyal JS. Deep anterior lamellar keratoplasty by big-bubble technique for treatment corneal stromal opacities. *Am. J. Ophthalmol.* 2007;143:954-957

[19] Hoffart L, Proust H, Matonti F, Catanèse M, Conrath J, Ridings B. Kératoplastie lamellaire antérieure assistée par laser femtoseconde *J. Fr. Ophtalmol.* 2007;30:689-694

[20] Yoo SH, Kymionis GD, Koreishi A, et al. Femtosecond laser-assisted sutureless anterior lamellar keratoplasty. *Ophthalmology.* 2008;115:1303-1307

In: Eye Research Developments: ...
Editor: Alan N. Westerhouse

ISBN: 978-1-60741-177-2

Chapter IX

Eales' Disease

Sandeep Saxena*
CSM Medical University
(Erstwhile King George's Medical University), Lucknow, India.

Abstract

Eales' disease is an idiopathic retinal periphlebitis that primarily affects the peripheral retina in young adults. Eales' disease is characterized by retinal periphlebitis, peripheral retinal ischemia, and neovascularization. Visual loss is characteristically caused by recurrent vitreous haemorrhage. Eales' disease appears to be an immunologic reaction that may be triggered by an exogenous exposure. Eales' disease is distinctively characterized both by stage of inflammation as well as stage of proliferation. Hypoxia-induced expression of vascular endothelial growth factor is only one aspect of the complicated processes in intraocular neovascularization. The increased expression of VEGF, when compared to other conditions inducing neovascularization, might explain the severity of neovascular growth and the propensity of repeated vitreous hemorrhage in Eales' disease. Photocoagulation is the mainstay of therapy in proliferative stage of the disease. Chemokines have also been found to play a role in the intraocular neovascularization. Anti-cytokine therapeutic agents may prove to be beneficial.

Introduction

Eales' disease is an idiopathic retinal periphlebitis that primarily affects the peripheral retina in young adults. Eales' disease was first described by Henry Eales, a British ophthalmologist, in 1880 and 1882.[1,2] He found it in seven young, male patients ranging in age from 14 to 29 years with recurrent vitreous hemorrhage. In addition, these patients had history of headache, variation in peripheral circulation, chronic constipation and epistaxis. In the next century, the disease was redefined by several investigators. [3-6] Elliot first recognized the inflammation of retinal vein and described it as periphlebitis retinae. [4] Subsequently several investigators documented both venular and arteriolar inflammation.[5,7]

* e-mail: sandeepsaxena2020@yahoo.com, cell: +91- 9415160528

Eales' disease most commonly affects healthy young adult males and is an important cause of preventable blindness in young adults. The predominant age of onset of symptoms is 20-30 years. The disease is more commonly seen in the Indian subcontinent. However, it has been reported from United Kingdom, U.S.A., Canada, Germany, Greece and Turkey.

Eales' disease is characterized by retinal periphlebitis (Fig. 1), peripheral retinal ischemia (Fig. 2), and neovascularization (Fig.3). Visual loss is characteristically caused by recurrent vitreous haemorrhage. [8] Vascular involvement in Eales' disease may be peripheral or central. Central Eales' disease is markedly uncommon (Fig. 4). [9-11]

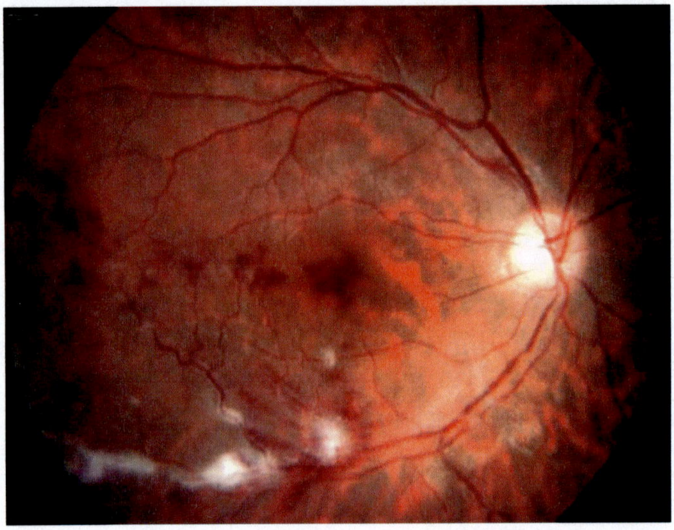

Figure 1. Color fundus photograph shows retinal periphelbitis along with superficial retinal hemorrhages.

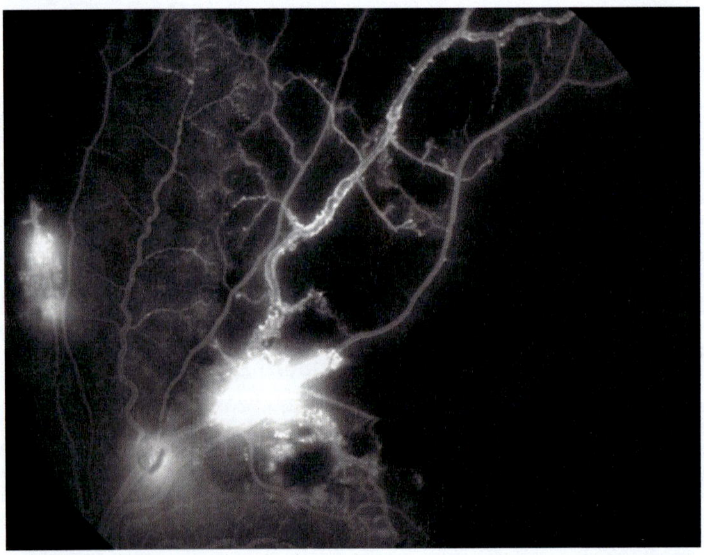

Figure 2. Fundus fluorescein angiography shows capillary non perfusion, microaneurysms and leakage of fluorescein dye from retinal neovascularization.

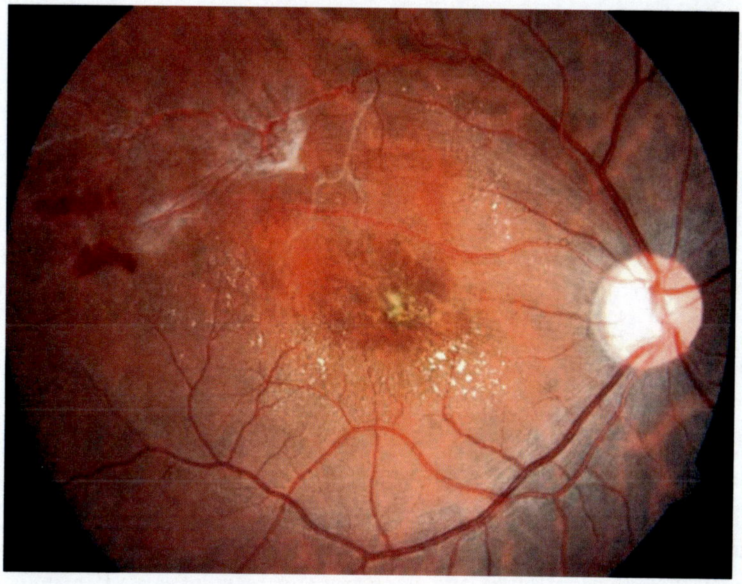

Figure 3. Color fundus photographs shows neovascularization elsewhere, sheathing of retinal vessels and hard exudates at macula.

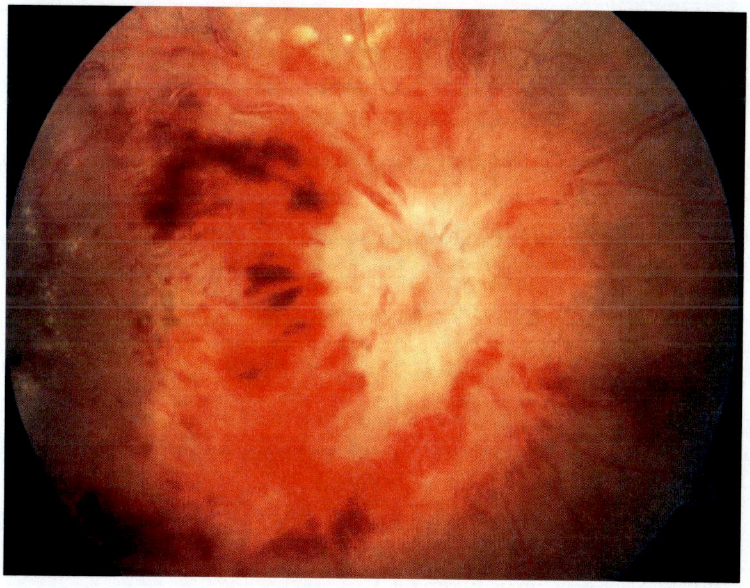

Figure 4. Central Eales' disease.

Etiopathogenesis

Eales' disease appears to be an immunologic reaction that may be triggered by an exogenous exposure. Retinal S-antigen and Interphotoreceptor Retinoid Binding Protein play a role in the etiopathogenesis of this condition. An extraneous agent results in the exposure of normally sequestered uveitopathogenic antigens of the immune system, leading to an immune response in the eye that initiates the disease process. [12]

Oxidative stress has been found to play an important role in the etiopathogenesis. [13-20] Lowered levels of antioxidant vitamins E and C and consequent accumulation of oxygen and lipid free radicals, or vice versa, could explain the inflammation, neovascularization and retinal pathology in patients with Eales' disease. Also, vitamin A deficiency could aggravate retinal illness. Elevated lipid peroxides have been found in the proliferative stage, which induce synthesis of cytokines and growth factors in retina during neovascularization. [15]

Eales' disease is distinctively characterized both by stage of inflammation as well as stage of proliferation.[7] Cytokines play an important role in intraocular inflammation.[8,9] The cascade of multiple angiogenic cytokines induced by oxidative damage, associated with tissue hypoxia, may interact to promote sustained retinal neovascularization.[10] During the inflammatory and proliferative stages of the disease statistically significant increase in IL-1β, IL-6, IL-10 and TNF-α expression was observed as compared to controls, highlighting the role of pro- and anti-inflammatory cytokines in the pathogenesis.

Markedly raised levels of IL-1β and TNF-α have been observed in the inflammatory stage which persisted in the proliferative stage (unpublished data). Raised levels of IL-1β, in the inflammatory stage, decreased significantly in the proliferative stage. Elevated TNF-α levels, observed in the inflammatory stage, increased significantly in the proliferative stage where clinically, inflammation (periphlebitis) had subsided but retinal neovascularization and vitreous hemorrhage had developed with the occurrence of retina hypoxia and ischemia. This data suggests that despite clinical absence of periphlebitis in the proliferative stage of the disease, IL-1β and TNF-α levels remain raised significantly as compared to controls. The synergism of IL-1 and TNF is a commonly reported phenomenon. IL-1 and TNF initiate the cascade of inflammatory mediators by targeting the endothelium. Although the receptors for TNF and IL-1 are clearly different, the post receptor events are similar. IL-1 often synergizes with TNF for NO induction which mediates cell death.[11] Nitrosoactive stress has been found to promote retinal vasculitis in Eales' disease.[12] Significant TNF-α expression was observed during the proliferative stage. These findings indicate that angiogenesis during the proliferative stage is induced by TNF-α. Angiogenesis induced by TNF-α, during post-ischemic inflammation, may be modulated through induction of potent angiogenic factors.[14] Hypoxia-induced expression of vascular endothelial growth factor is only one aspect of the complicated processes in intraocular neovascularization.[15] Chemokines have also been found to be involved in the recruitment of neutrophils and monocytes into the vitreous and play a role in the intraocular neovascularization.[16] Thus, the IL-1 system represents a novel target for controlling inflammatory activity and/or the associated long-term sequelae related to angiogenesis in Eales' disease. Role of TNF-α in the inflammatory as well as proliferative stage of the disease has implications for anti-TNF-α therapy in Eales' disease. Reducing the biological activities of IL-1 and TNF may be accomplished by several different, but highly specific strategies, which involve neutralizing antibodies, soluble receptors, receptor antagonist, and inhibitors of proteases that convert inactive precursors to active, mature molecules. Anti-cytokine therapeutic agents such as TNF-neutralizing antibodies, soluble TNF receptors, and IL-1 receptor antagonist may prove beneficial. Infliximab (anti-TNF-α) may prove to be beneficial in patients of Eales' disease.A close relationship between the prominent neovascular proliferation in Eales' disease and the intense expression of VEGF has been found. The increased expression of VEGF, when compared to other conditions inducing neovascularization, might explain the severity of neovascular growth and the propensity of repeated vitreous hemorrhage in Eales' disease.[21]

Retinal photoreceptors and platelets have been shown to be an easy target of oxidants because of high proportion of polyunsaturated fatty acids. The decreased membrane fluidity in platelets suggests alterations in the physiological events, which may result in alterations in functioning of retinal photoreceptors. [20]

Mycobacterium tuberculosis DNA has also been detected by polymerase chain reaction, in the vitreous of such patients. [22-24] However, the role of mycobacterium genome in the pathogenesis is yet to be ascertained.

Clinical Features

Eales' disease with a characteristic clinical picture, fluorescein angiographic findings and natural course is considered a specific disease entity. Recurrent vitreous hemorrhage is the hall mark of this disease. A new classification system has been proposed recently by the author. [25] This staging system, based on standard terminology and features, provides a simple method to categorize, according to the severity of the disease. This staging system takes into consideration the fundoscopic and fluorescein angiographic variables that have been shown to be prognostic of visual outcome (Table). Macular involvement is uncommon. Macular ischemia and traction macular detachment are associated with poor visual outcome (Fig. 5).[26]

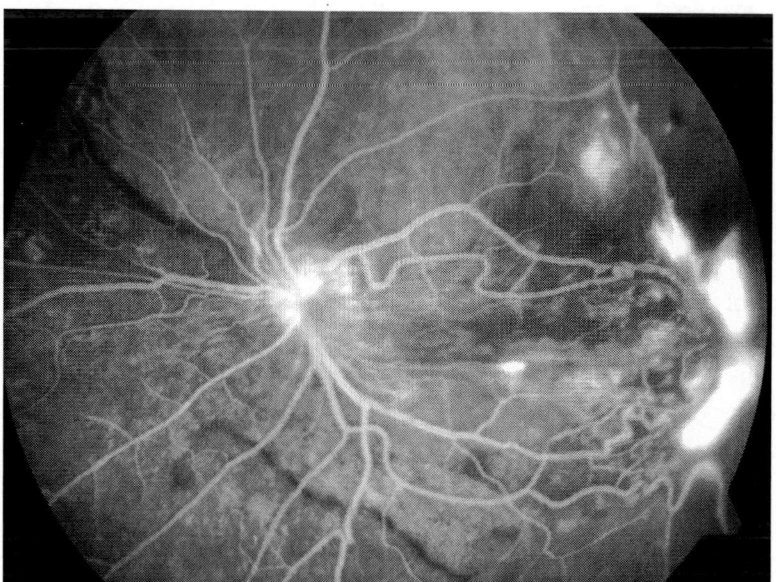

Figure 5. Fundus fluorescein angiography shows traction macular detachment, neovascularization elsewhere associated with capillary non perfusion and early neovascularization at the disc.

Table. Classification system for Eales' disease.

Stages	Features
A. Eales' disease	
Stage 1a	Periphlebitis of small caliber vessels with superficial retinal hemorrhages
Stage 1b	Periphlebitis of large caliber vessels with superficial retinal hemorrhages
Stage 2a	Peripheral capillary nonperfusion
Stage 2b	Neovascularization elsewhere / Neovascularization of the disc
Stage 3a	Fibrovascular proliferation
Stage 3b	Vitreous hemorrhage
Stage 4a	Traction / combined rhegmatogenous detachment
Stage 4b	Rubeosis iridis, neovascular glaucoma, complicated cataract, and optic atrophy
B. Central Eales' disease	

The new classification system is consistent, simple and easy to recall. It can also be used to monitor the effect of medical, laser and/or surgical treatment.

Fluorescein Angiography

In cases of active retinal periphlebitis, staining of the veins can be seen in the early venous phase with extravasation of dye in the late phase (Fig. 6). In the healed stage, only staining of the vessel wall occurs without any leak in the late venous phase. Areas of capillary non-perfusion and retinal neovascularization can be easily delineated by fluorescein angiography (Fig. 7). Capillary non-perfusion of more than 20 disc area and 60 disc area are associated with neovascularization elsewhere (NVE) and neovascularization of the disc (NVD) (Fig. 8). [27] Retinal neovascularization sites have been found to cluster around specific anatomic foci. The quadrantic distribution of the sites of NVE in Eales' disease is: superotemporal, 45.95%; inferotemporal, 24.32%; superonasal, 16.22%; and inferonasal, 13.51%.[28]

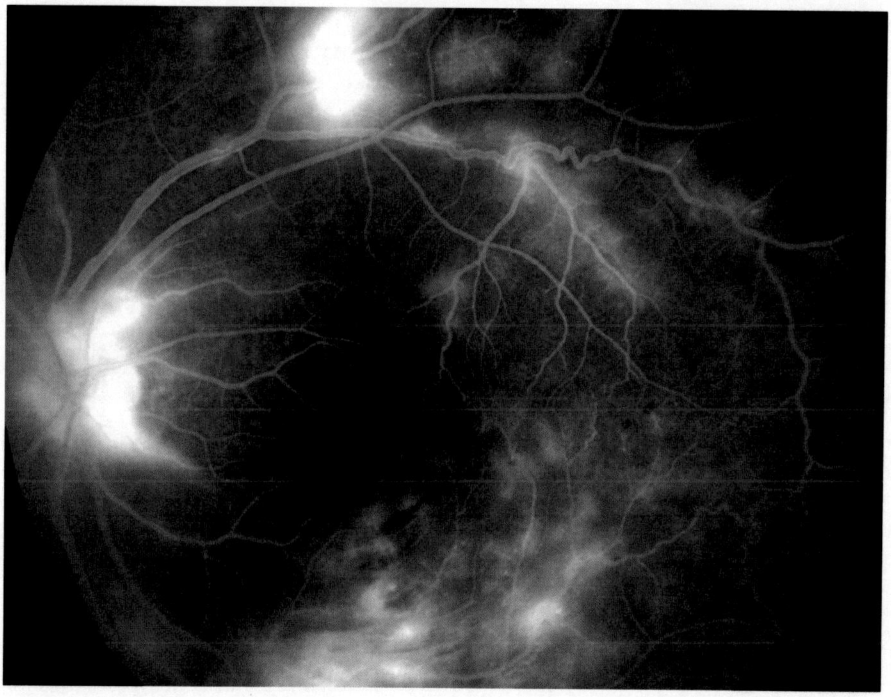

Figure 6. Fundus fluorescein angiography shows leakage of fluorescein dye from neovasculazation at the disc, neovascularization elsewhere and areas of retinal periphlebitis.

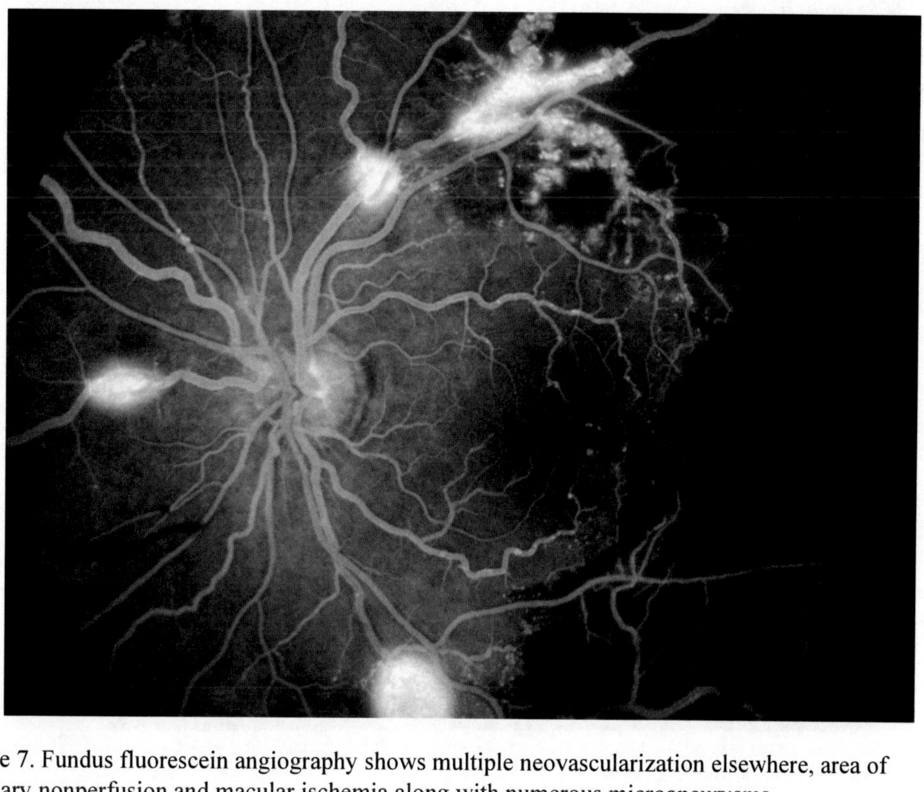

Figure 7. Fundus fluorescein angiography shows multiple neovascularization elsewhere, area of capillary nonperfusion and macular ischemia along with numerous microaneurysms.

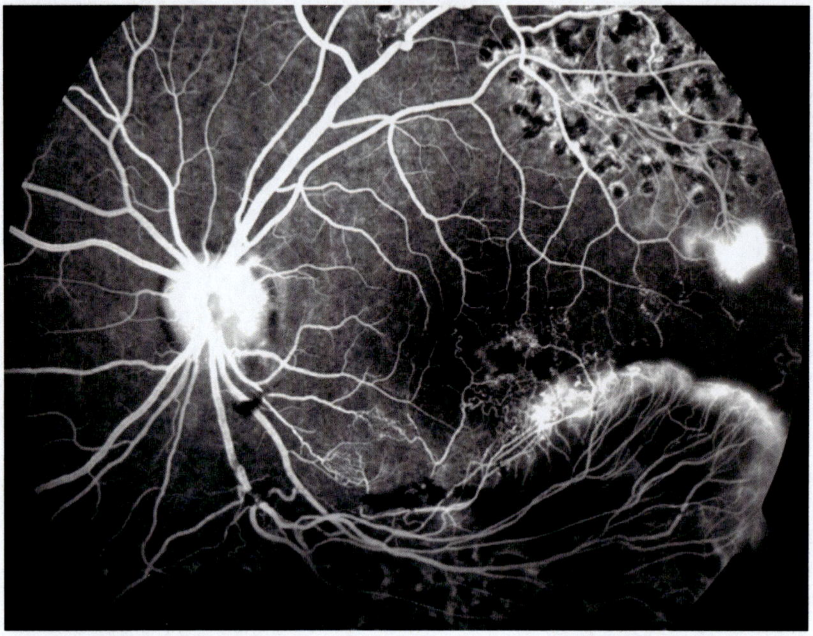

Figure 8. Fundus fluorescein angiography shows neovascularization at the disc, neovascularization elsewhere, multiple laser spots, collateral vessel formation and ischemia at macula.

Central Eales' disease is relatively uncommon. Such central retinal periphlebitis has a similar presentation as central retinal vein occlusion. Branch retinal vein occlusion with peripheral retinal periphlebitis (Fig. 9) and central Eales' disease have been found to be associated with favorable visual outcome. [29,30]

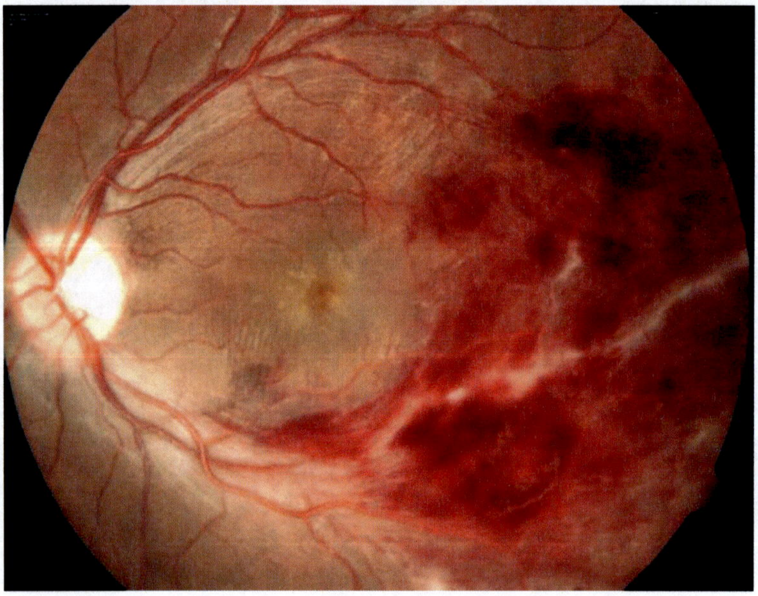

Figure 9. Color fundus photograph shows inferotemporal retinal vein occlusion, retinal periphlebitis and macular edema.

Management

The management of Eales' disease depends on the severity of the disease. Management strategies can also be defined according to the stage of the disease. Stage 1, the stage of inflammation, is amenable to medical therapy. Stage 2, the stage of ischemia and neovascularization, requires observation/laser photocoagulation. Stage 3, the stage of proliferation, requires laser / pars plana vitrectomy and laser. Stage 4, the stage of complications, requires sophisticated surgical management strategies. [25]

a. Observation

Patients with inactive retinal periphlebitis can be observed periodically at 6-month interval. Patients with fresh vitreous hemorrhage can also be observed at intervals of 4-6 weeks if underlying retina is found to be attached by indirect ophthalmoscopy or by ultrasound.

b. Medical Therapy

Corticosteroids: Anti-inflammatory corticosteroid drugs arc potent therapeutic agents for a wide range of ocular and systemic disorders and remain the mainstay of therapy in retinal periphlebitis in Eales' disease (1mg/kg/day).

Methotrexate: Predominantly T-cell involvement has been demonstrated in the lymphocytic infiltration of epiretinal and subretinal membranes in Eales' disease. Hence, treatment should be directed to the down regulation of the activated T-cells. Search for safer and more specific forms of treatment have lead to certain immunosuppressives, like methotrexate, which have found a role in patients with immunologically driven systemic diseases. As opposed to the more 'cytostatic' effects of corticosteroids, the 'cytotoxic' immunosuppressives exert their beneficial effects by actually killing the rapidly dividing clones of lymphocytes that are responsible for inflammation. Methotrexate, a folic acid antagonist, has anti-inflammatory and immunomodulatory actions. The drug reduces the synthesis of DNA by acting on the enzyme dihydrofolate reductase. Methotrexate is used as a weekly 'pulsed' therapy. A 'pulse' differs from chronic moderate dose therapy in its ability to "reset" an aberrant immune response. Inhibition of the proliferating lymphocyte clones, the temporary removal of recirculating T-lymphocytes from the blood and eye, and the profound suppression of peripheral inflammation, all occur simultaneously. Antigens exposed by viral, bacterial or autoimmune injury are normally perpetuated by the inflammatory response but in such a system a pulse may abolish the source of antigen at the same time as it suppresses the immune response. When memory T-cells recirculate, the disease falters in the absence of the antigen. [31, 32]

c. Photocoagulation

Photocoagulation is the mainstay of therapy in proliferative stage of the disease. [33] Laser photocoagulation leads to resolution of retinal neovascularization due to its anti-VEGF effect. In cases of gross capillary non-perfusion photocoagulation is suggested. For NVE and NVD, sectoral scatter photocoagulation and pan retinal photocoagulation, respectively is suggested (Figs. 10 and 11).

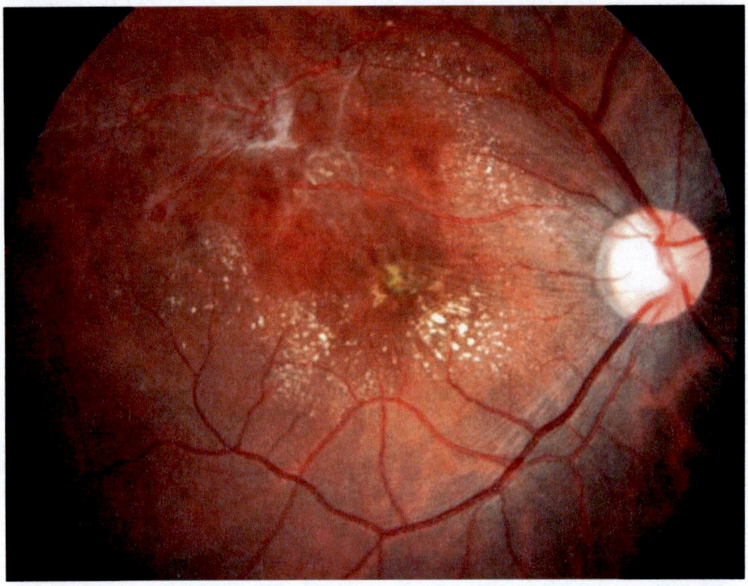

Figure 10A. Color funduis photograph shows neovascularization elsewhere.

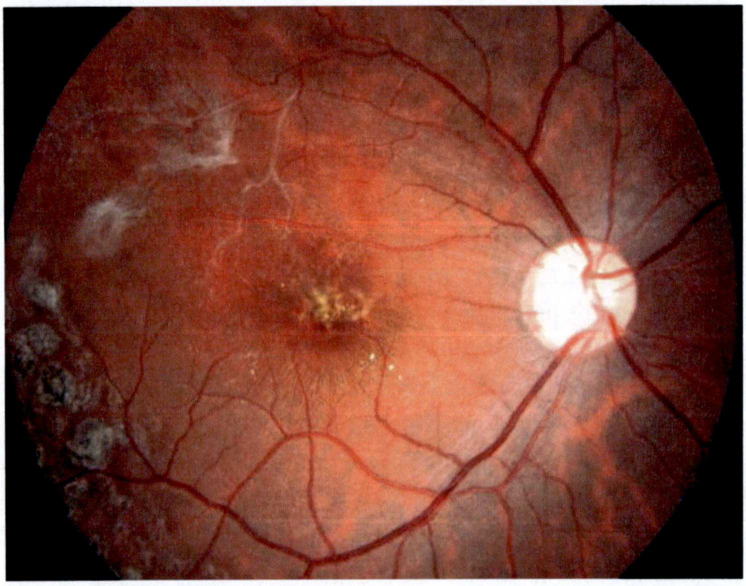

Figure 10B. Color fundus photograph shows regression of retinal neovascularization following laser photocoagulation.

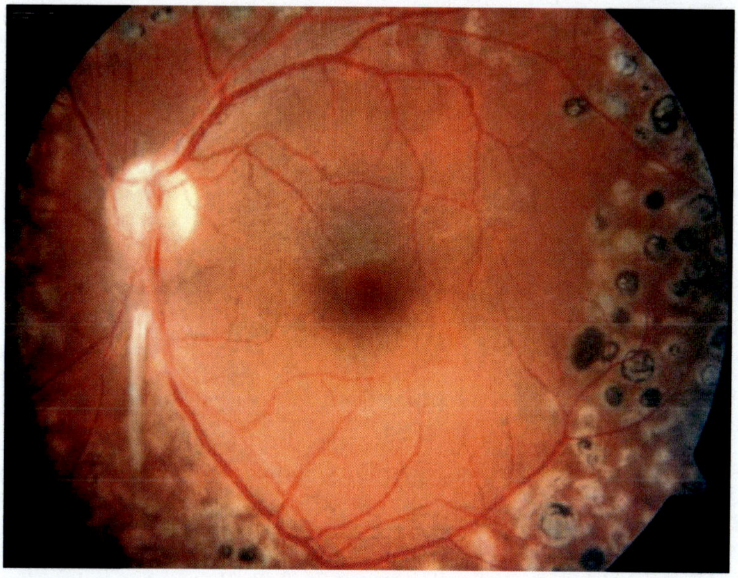

Figure 11. Color fundus photograph after laser photocoagulation shows residual fibrous proliferation from the disc following resolution of neovascularization at the disc.

d. Vitreoretinal Surgery

Vitrectomy alone or combined with other vitreoretinal surgical procedures is often required. Vitrectomy for non-resolving vitreous hemorrhage done at 3-6 months has better visual outcome than done after 6 months. Patients with fewer episodes of vitreous hemorrhage and preoperative laser have better visual prognosis. [34,35]

e. Anterior Retinal Cryo Ablation

Anterior retinal cryo ablation is usually reserved as an adjunct to photocoagulation in Eales' disease for effect in peripheral retina.

References

[1] Eales H. Retinal haemorrhage associated with epistaxis and constipation. *Brim Med Rev* 1880;9:262.

[2] Eales H. Primary retinal haemorrhage in young men. *Ophthalmic Rev* 1882;1:41.

[3] Duke-Elder S, Dobree JH. *Primary perivasculitis of the retina: Eales disease, in Duke* Elder, Perkins EJ (eds): System of Ophthalmology, Vol. X. London, Henry Kimpton, 1967, pp 222-236.

[4] Elliot AJ. 30-year observation of patients with Eales disease. *Am J Ophthalmol* 1975;80:404-408.

[5] Kimura SJ, Carriker FR, Hogen MJ. Retinal vasculitis with intraocular hemorrhage. Classification and results of special studies. *Arch Ophthalmol 1*956;56:361-365.

[6] Cross AG. Vasculitis retinae. *Trans Ophthalmol Soc UK* 1963;83:133.

[7] Keith-Lyle T, Wybark A. Retinal vasculitis. *Br J Ophthalmol* 1961;45:77-78.

[8] Gilbert TW. *Periphlebitis and endovasculitis of retinal vessels.* Klin Monatsbl Augenheilkd 1935;94:335-349.

[9] Kumar D, Saxena RC, Saxena S. Vitreous hemorrhage in Eales' disease. *Afro-Asian J Ophthalmol* 1995;13:109-112.

[10] Atmaca LS, Idil A, Gunduz K. Visualization of retinal vasculitis in Eales disease. *Ocul Immunol Inflammol* 1993;1:41-48.

[11] Das T, Biswas J, Kumar A, Namperumalsamy P, Nagpal PN, Patnaik B, Tewari HK. Eales'disease. *Ind J Ophthalmol* 1994;42:3-18.

[12] Saxena S, Rajasingh J, Biswas S, Kumar D, Shinohara T, Singh V.K. Cellular response to Retinal S-antigen and Interphotoreceptor Retinoid Binding Protein fragments in patients with Eales' disease. *Pathobiology* 1999;67:37-44.

[13] Saxena S, Khanna VK, Kumar D, Srivastava P, Seth PK. Enhanced oxidative stress in Eales' disease. *Ann Ophthalmol* 2001;33:40-42.

[14] Saxena S, Kumar D, Srivastava P, Khanna VK, Seth PK. Low levels of platelet glutathione in Eales' disease. *Med Sci Res* 1999;42:125-126.

[15] Srivastava P, Saxena S, Khanna VK, Kumar D, Nath R, Seth PK. Raised platelet thiobarbituric acid reacting substances in proliferative Eales disease. Indian *J Ophthalmol* 2000;48:307-310.

[16] Saxena S, Khanna VK, Kumar D, Srivastava P, Seth PK. Impaired antioxidant defense mechanism in central Eales' disease. *Ann Ophthalmol* 2004;36:29-31.

[17] Bhooma V, Sulochana KN, Biswas J, Ramakrishnan S. Eales' disease: accumulation of reactive oxygen intermediates and lipid peroxides and decrease of antioxidants causing inflammation, neovascularization and retinal damage. *Curr Eye Res* 1997;16:91-95.

[18] Sulochana KN, Biswas J, Ramakrishnan S. Eales' disease: increased oxidation and peroxidation products of membrane constituents chiefly lipids and antioxidant enzymes and reduced glutathione in vitreous. *Curr Eye Res* 1999;19:254-259.

[19] Swamy-Mruthinti S, Miriam KC, Kumar SK, Biswas J, Ramakrishnan S, Nagaraj RH, Sulochana KN. Immunolocalization and quantification of advanced glycation end products in retinal neovascular membranes and serum: a possible role in ocular neovascularization. *Curr Eye Res* 2002;25:139-145.

[20] Saxena S, Srivastava P, Kumar D, Khanna VK, Seth PK. Decreased platelet membrane fluidity in retinal periphlebitis in Eales' disease. *Ocul Immunol Inflamm* 2006;14:113-116.

[21] Perentes Y, Chan CC, Bovey E, Uffer S, Herbort CP. *Massive vascular endothelium growth factor (VEGF) expression in Eales' disease*. Klin Monatsbl Augenheilkd. 2002;219:311-314.

[22] Madhavan HN, Therese KL, Doraiswamy K. Further investigations on the association of Mycobacterium tuberculosis with Eales' disease. *Ind J Ophthalmol* 2002;50:35-39.

[23] Biswas J, Therese L, Madhavan HN. Use of polymerase chain reaction in detection of Mycobacterium tuberculosis complex DNA from vitreous samples of Eales' disease. *Br J Ophthalmol* 1999;83:994.

[24] Madhavan HN, Therese KL, Gunisha P, Jayanti U, Biswas J. Polymerase chain reaction for detection of Mycobacterium tuberculosis in epiretinal membrane in Eales' disease. *Invest Ophthalmol Vis Sci* 2000;41:822-825.

[25] Saxena S, Kumar D. A new staging system of idiopathic retinal periphlebitis. *Eur J Ophthalmol* 2004;14:236-239.

[26] Saxena S, Kumar D. Macular involvement in Eales' disease. *Ann Ophthalmol* 2000;32:98- 100.

[27] Saxena S, Kumar D, Maitreya A, Srivastava P, Khanna VK, Nath R, Seth PK. Ann *Ophthalmol* 2003;35:25-27.

[28] Saxena S, Kumar D. *Topographic distribution of retinal neovascularisation in Eales' disease.* 2005;37:273-275.

[29] Saxena S, Kumar D. Visual outcome in Eales' Disease with Branch Retinal Vein Occlusion. *Ann Ophthalmol* 1999;31:173-175.

[30] 30. Saxena S, Kumar D. Visual outcome in Central Eales' disease. *Ann Ophthalmol* 2001;33:300- 302.

[31] Saxena S, Kumar D, Kapoor S. The efficacy of oral methotrexate pulsed therapy in Eales' disease. *Ann Ophthalmol* 2000;32:60-62.

[32] Bali T, Saxena S, Kumar D, Nath R. Response time and efficacy of oral methotrexate pulsed therapy in idiopathic retinal periphlebitis. *Eur J Ophthalmol* 2005;15:374-378.

[33] El-Asrar AM, Al-Kharashi SA. Full panretinal photocoagulation and early vitrectomy improve prognosis of retinal vasculitis associated with tuberculoprotein hypersensitivity (Eales' disease). *Br J Ophthalmol.* 2002;86:1248-1251.

[34] Kumar A, Tiwari HK, Singh RP, Verma L, Prasad N. Comparative evaluation of early vs. deferred vitrectomy in Eales' disease. *Acta Ophthalmol Scand* 2000;78:77-78.

[35] Shanmugam MP, Badrinath SS, Gopal L, Sharma T. Long term visual results of vitrectomy for Eales disease complications. *Int Ophthalmol* 1998;22:61-64.

In: Eye Research Developments
Editor: Alan N. Westerhouse

ISBN: 978-1-60741-177-2

Chapter X

Does an Association Exist between Intraocular Pressure-Lowering Medication and Ocular Ischemic Events? A Case-Control Analysis

***Carlo E. Traverso*[1], *John G. Walt*[2], *Lee S. Stern*[*3] *and Margarita Dolgitser*[3]**

[1] Centro di Ricerca Clinica e laboratorio per il Glaucoma e la Cornea, Clinica Oculistica, Di.N.O.G., University of Genova, Genova, Italy;
[2] Outcomes Strategy and Research, Allergan, Inc., Irvine, CA;
[3] Analytica International, New York, NY

Abstract

Objective: Determine whether IOP-lowering medications reduce the risk of retinal arterial occlusions or retinal venous occlusions.

Study Design and Setting: A retrospective case-control study evaluated patients with central retinal arterial occlusion (CRAO), branch retinal arterial occlusion (BRAO), central retinal venous occlusion (CRVO), or branch retinal venous occlusion (BRVO) and their matched controls. Conditional logistic regression models (based on matched variables) predicted the likelihood of each outcome while adjusting for the following covariates: treatment with IOP-lowering medication in the year pre-index date (incrementally defined as 2 to 10 prescriptions), descriptives and comorbidities.

Results: In univariate analysis, CRVO, BRVO, and CRAO patients and matched controls had similar numbers of IOP-lowering prescriptions in the year pre-index date. After adjusting for covariates, CRVO and BRVO patients treated with IOP-lowering medications in the year pre-index date were slightly less likely to develop ocular ischemic events. As the number of prescriptions used to define the treatment cutoff increased, the likelihood of experiencing a retinal venous occlusion decreased. This trend was significant for CRVO ($P<0.0001$) and BRVO ($P=0.0110$) patients, but not observed in CRAO and BRAO patients.

Conclusion: Prolonged treatment with IOP-lowering medication may be protective against retinal venous occlusions.

---

[*] Please address correspondence and reprint requests to: Lee S. Stern, MS; Vice President, Global Health Economics and Pricing; Analytica International; 450 Park Avenue South, 12th Floor; New York, NY 10016; Phone: (212) 686-4100; Fax: (212) 686-8601; Email: lstern@analyticaintl.com

Keywords: case-control, glaucoma, IOP-lowering medication, ocular ischemic events, retinal occlusions, retrospective claims database.

What is New?

- Prolonged treatment with IOP-lowering medications may reduce the risk of retinal venous occlusions
- This study takes the first step in confirming the hypothesis that an association exists between IOP-lowering medications and retinal venous occlusions
- To our knowledge, this is the first study using a large sample of real-world data to assess the association between IOP-lowering medications and retinal venous occlusions
- Future research is necessary in order to confirm the association observed in our study
- If this protective effect can be confirmed in future studies, IOP-lowering medications may provide a new therapeutic approach to patients at risk for retinal venous occlusions

Introduction

During the last decade there has been increasing interest in the study of hemodynamics in ocular tissues as linked to disturbances in blood supply and disease progression. While elevated intraocular pressure (IOP) is recognized as a major risk factor in glaucoma, growing evidence indicates that the disease is multifactorial [1-7], and that ocular ischemia plays a major role in disease pathogenesis. Several studies have demonstrated a positive association between elevated intraocular pressure (IOP) and ocular ischemic events [8-10].

Vascular factors leading to tissue ischemia either through vasospasm or capillary underperfusion impact the initiation and progression of glaucoma in certain patients [11, 12]. Reduced blood flow to the optic nerve may occur due to deficient autoregulation of optic nerve head circulation, ocular or generalized vasospastic disorder or generalized vascular disease [13]. Glaucoma patients reportedly have a reduced optic nerve blood flow that correlates with the degree of glaucomatous damage [14].

Acute retinal vascular disorders collectively constitute one of the major causes of blindness or seriously impaired vision [9]. There is controversy with regard to their pathogenesis, clinical features and management; this has been attributed to multiple misconceptions - addressed elsewhere [9]. Retinal vascular occlusions are serious conditions that often lead to blindness. The importance of simultaneous disease management of IOP and blood flow to target both mechanical and vascular factors (recognizing that both play important and interacting roles in disease onset and progression) has been demonstrated [4].

This retrospective case-control study was designed to determine whether treatment with IOP-lowering medications reduces the risk of the following ocular ischemic events: retinal arterial occlusions [including central (CRAO) and branch (BRAO)], or retinal venous occlusions [including central (CRVO) or branch (BRVO)].

Materials and Methods

Patient Selection

The patient population was drawn from the PharMetrics Anonymous Patient-Centric database; a source-linked claims database containing medical and pharmacy information on over 50 million covered patients belonging to 64 national and regional managed care organizations in the United States. The records are representative of the national managed care population on a variety of demographic measures, including age, gender, and product type (i.e., type of provider organization).

Patients were identified as either cases or controls based on specified criteria (table 1).

Table 1. Study Design

	Inclusion Criteria	Exclusion Criteria
Cases	≥1 International Classification of Diseases, Ninth Revision (ICD-9) diagnosis code for one of the following conditions of interest: Central retinal artery occlusion (CRAO, 362.31) Branch retinal artery occlusion (BRAO, 362.32) Central retinal vein occlusion (CRVO, 362.35) Branch retinal vein occlusion (BRVO, 362.36)	No diagnosis for an ocular ischemic event of interest in PharMetrics database
	≥1 year of follow-up prior to index date	≤19 years of age at time of first diagnosis (defined as index date)
Controls	≥1 diagnosis of any other ophthalmic condition	Diagnosis of any of the case defining conditions
	≥1 year of follow-up prior to index date	≤19 years of age at time of last claim in database (defined as index date)

Inclusion criteria for the case study population were as follows: at least one International Classification of Diseases, Ninth Revision (ICD-9) [15] diagnosis of a retinal arterial occlusion (CRAO or BRAO) or a retinal venous occlusion (CRVO or BRVO) from 1996 through 2004; at least one year of follow-up prior to first diagnosis; and at least 19 years of age at the time of first diagnosis (so they would have been at least 18 in the year of follow-up prior to index date). A pool of eligible controls was identified according to the following inclusion criteria: no ICD-9 codes for any ocular ischemic event and at least one diagnosis of any other ophthalmic condition from 1996 through 2004 (to ensure that they were selected from the same underlying population from which the cases arose); at least one year of follow-up prior to last claim date available; and at least 19 years of age at the time of the last claim. Patients with non-arteritic anterior ischemic optic neuropathy (NAION) were not included in this analysis due to clinical and physiopathological differences between NAION and the included conditions.

Controls were randomly selected from the pool of eligible patients in a 1:1 matching ratio based on the following descriptive criteria: age (matched within 5 year increments, with 19 year-olds being grouped with 20-24 year-olds); index year (matched on exact index year with the exception of the grouping of 1996 and 1997); gender; and Charlson Comorbidity Index

(CCI; a continuous measure of overall health status) [16]. One BRAO case, 2 cases each of CRVO and BRVO, and 3 CRAO cases did not have a match from the pool of eligible controls that fit all four of the above criteria; controls were therefore hand-selected for these cases based on the closest index year available.

Each eligible patient was selected as a case for only the first ocular ischemic event with which he/she was diagnosed. Provided they met the appropriate matching criteria, eligible patients had the potential to be selected as controls for more than one condition. Index date was defined as the date of first ischemic event diagnosis (CRAO, BRAO, CRVO, or BRVO) for cases and last claim date in the PharMetrics database for controls.

Statistical Analyses

For cases and controls of each outcome, frequencies (numbers and proportions) and distributions (mean, standard deviation, median, and range) of descriptive statistics were evaluated for categorical and continuous measures, respectively. The mean number of IOP-lowering prescriptions in the year prior to index date were calculated and compared for treated cases and controls using a student t-test.

Conditional multivariate logistic regression models (based on matched variables) were used to predict the likelihood of each ocular ischemic event based on treatment with IOP-lowering medication in the year prior to index date. Treatment was defined using cutoffs from >=2 to >=10 prescriptions, with each of the cutoffs used separately in 9 individual models (for each condition). The trend of the model odds ratio (OR) with the increase in number of prescriptions used as a cutoff was assessed using regression. Each model controlled for covariates of interest, including descriptives (region, payer type, product type, years of follow-up in PharMetrics); presence of ocular hypertension (OHT), pre-glaucoma, or primary open-angle glaucoma (POAG) in the year prior to index date (defined as >=1 ICD-9 diagnosis code for one of the three conditions or treatment with IOP-lowering medication); presence of comorbidities (diabetes, systemic hypertension, cardiovascular disease, or hyperlipidemia; >=2 diagnoses) any time prior to index date; number of ophthalmologist visits and number of IOP measurements taken in the year prior to index date; and presence of trabeculectomy and/or trabeculoplasty any time prior to index date. An interaction term, number of IOP measurements by treatment with IOP-lowering medication, was also tested. All variables were initially included; a backwards selection procedure removed covariates from the final models whose p-values exceeded 0.2. All statistical analyses were conducted using SAS version 9.1 [17].

Results

The final case study population for each ocular ischemic event was as follows: CRAO, N = 734; BRAO, N = 1336; CRVO, N = 1930; and BRVO, N = 3511. The BRVO study population was majority female (56%); the remaining study populations had approximately equal gender distribution (table 2). BRVO cases and controls had the highest mean age (61 ±

13 years) while BRAO cases and controls had the lowest (58 ± 14 years). Age for all study populations ranged from 19 to 98 years (table 2). Most patients were from the Midwest (ranging from 36% CRAO to 40% BRAO cases), followed by the Northeast (ranging from 29% BRAO to 34% CRAO cases). Approximately one third of the patients in all cohorts were from the South and West (table 3).

Table 2. Descriptive Statistics: Matched Variables – All Conditions

		CRAO (N=1468)	BRAO (N=2672)	CRVO (N=3680)	BRVO (N=7022)
Age (years)		60.7+15.3	57.9+13.6	60.7+15.4	61.4+13.1
Gender	Male (%)	51	51	51	44
	Female(%)	49	49	49	56
Index Year	1996-1997	1	1	1	0
	1998	3	3	2	2
	1999	8	7	8	7
	2000	9	9	10	10
	2001	20	17	18	19
	2002	26	29	29	27
	2003	24	25	23	24
	2004	9	9	9	11
CCI		4.5+3.1	3.7+2.8	4.1+2.9	3.9+2.6

Table 3. Descriptive Statistics for Cases of Retinal Arterial and Vein Occlusions

		CRAO N=734	BRAO N=1336	CRVO N=1930	BRVO N=3511
Payer Type (%)	Commercial	47	57	51	53
	Medicare Risk	33	23	33	30
	Self-Insured	6	5	5	5
	Medicaid	2	1	1	1
	Unknown	12	14	10	11
Product Type (%)	HMO	61	52	60	56
	PPO	19	26	21	23
	POS	11	14	11	13
	Indemnity	4	4	3	4
	Unknown	5	4	5	4
Region (%)	Midwest	36	40	38	39
	Northeast	34	29	31	32
	South	18	19	19	17
	West	12	12	12	12
Years of Follow-Up		2.2+1.0	2.3+1.3	2.1+1.0	2.2+1.1

The most common index year for all four ocular ischemic events was 2002 (table 2). Within all outcome groups, controls had a significantly longer duration of follow-up than cases ($p<.0001$ for all conditions). Mean Charlson score ranged from 3.7 ± 2.8 among BRAO cases and controls to 4.5 ± 3.1 among CRAO cases and controls (table 2).

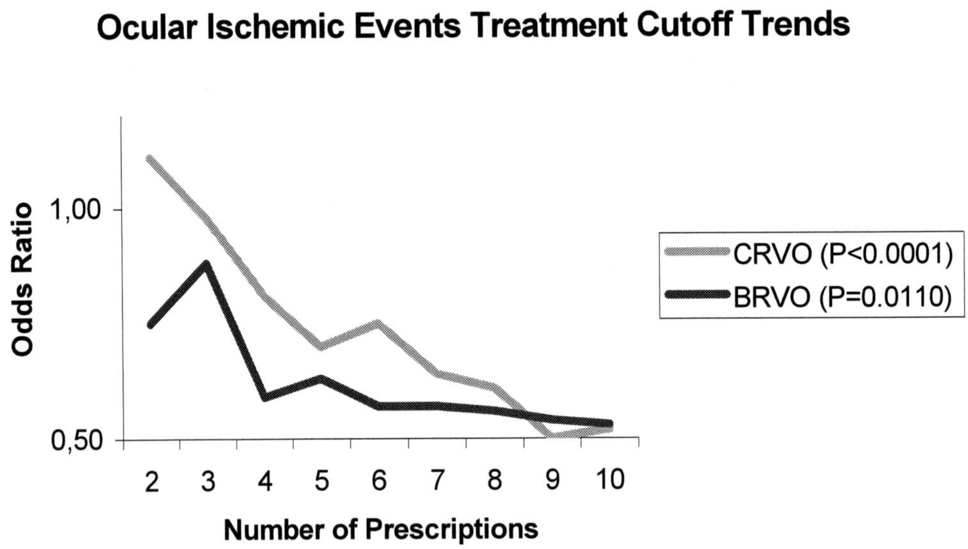

Figure 1. Multivariate Trend Analysis: Odds of cases versus controls being treated with IOP lowering medication (treatment definition varies with prescription cutoff) during year prior to index date

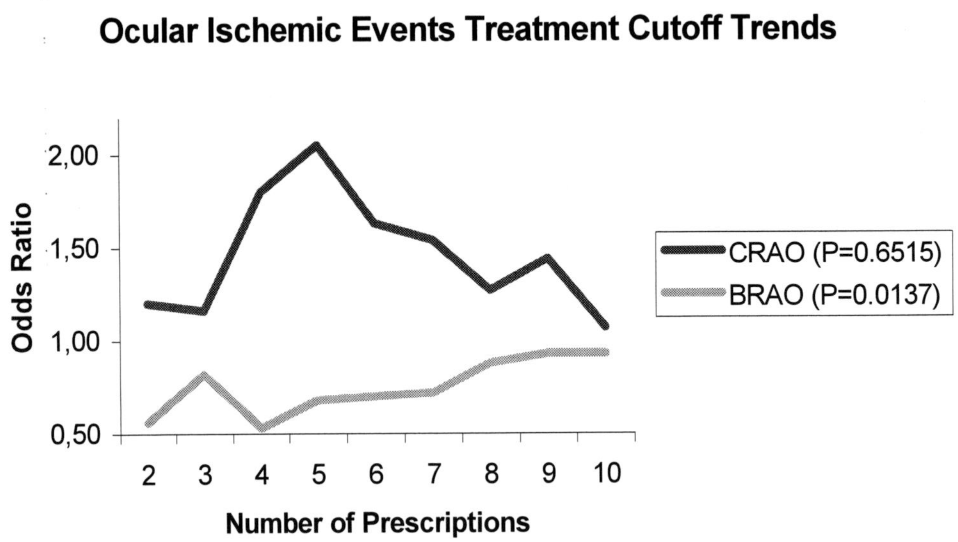

Figure 2. Multivariate Trend Analysis: Odds of cases versus controls being treated with IOP lowering medication (treatment definition varies with prescription cutoff) during year prior to index date.

In unadjusted analyses of treated patients (those with at least one prescription for an IOP-lowering medication in the year prior to index date), there were no significant differences in the number of IOP-lowering prescriptions for cases and controls of all four subtypes (table 4).

When adjusted for covariates, CRVO and BRVO patients treated with IOP-lowering medications in the year prior to index date were less slightly likely to develop ocular ischemic events. As the number of prescriptions used to define the treatment cutoff increased, so did the protective effects of the OR (table 5). In other words, the more IOP-lowering prescriptions a patient received, the less likely he was to experience a retinal venous occlusion. This trend was significant for both CRVO (P=0.0002) and BRVO (P=0.0192) patients (figure 1). However, a similar trend was not observed in the CRAO and BRAO patients (table 5 and figure 2).

Table 4. Univariate Analysis: Mean number of IOP-lowering prescriptions during year prior to index date for treated cases versus treated controls

Cohort	N	Mean	Std	T-value	P-values
CRAO					
Cases	53	6.68	5.21	0.11	0.9095
Controls	38	6.87	9.31		
BRAO					
Cases	79	6.56	6.08	-1.20	0.2328
Controls	76	5.46	5.27		
CRVO					
Cases	280	6.01	6.22	1.59	0.1140
Controls	144	7.22	7.98		
BRVO					
Cases	291	6.99	6.99	0.78	0.4367
Controls	209	7.47	6.76		

Table 5. Multivariate Trend Analysis: Odds of cases versus controls being treated with IOP lowering medication (treatment definition varies with prescription cutoff) during year prior to index date

Condition	Prescription Cutoff	Odds Ratio	Confidence Interval	Trend P-Value
CRVO	2	1.11	0.83 – 1.50	<0.0001
	3	0.98	0.88 – 1.09	
	4	0.81	0.57 – 1.15	
	5	0.70	0.47 – 1.04	
	6	0.75	0.48 – 1.15	
	7	0.64	0.40 – 1.00	
	8	0.61	0.37 – 1.00	
	9	0.50	0.30 – 0.84	
	10	0.52	0.30 – 0.89	
BRVO	2	0.75	0.59 – 0.97	0.0110
	3	0.88	0.80 – 0.96	
	4	0.59	0.44 – 0.79	
	5	0.63	0.46 – 0.86	
	6	0.57	0.41 – 0.80	
	7	0.57	0.40 – 0.82	
	8	0.56	0.38 – 0.81	
	9	0.54	0.36 – 0.81	
	10	0.53	0.34 – 0.81	

Table 5. (Continued)

CRAO	2	1.20	0.69 – 2.06	0.6515
	3	1.16	0.94 – 1.41	
	4	1.80	0.90 – 3.61	
	5	2.05	0.96 – 4.38	
	6	1.63	0.72 – 3.66	
	7	1.54	0.65 – 3.61	
	8	1.27	0.54 – 3.00	
	9	1.44	0.53 – 3.91	
	10	1.07	0.37 – 3.07	
BRAO	2	0.56	0.35 – 0.88	0.0137
	3	0.82	0.69 – 0.97	
	4	0.53	0.31 – 0.91	
	5	0.68	0.38 – 1.22	
	6	0.70	0.37 – 1.33	
	7	0.72	0.37 – 1.43	
	8	0.88	0.43 – 1.81	
	9	0.93	0.41 – 2.10	
	10	0.93	0.39 – 2.21	

Discussion

To the best of our knowledge, this retrospective cohort study is the first large-scale study designed to examine the association between use of IOP-lowering medication and risk of ocular ischemic events.

The importance of simultaneous disease management of IOP and ocular ischemia in glaucoma has been documented [4]. Based on our analysis, after controlling for covariates in multivariate models, patients with retinal venous occlusions were less likely to have received IOP-lowering medication in the year prior to index date than controls. As the number of prescriptions for IOP-lowering medications increased, the odds of a retinal venous occlusion decreased. The strongest protective effect of treatment with IOP-lowering medications was seen in CRVO; this result is consistent with literature reporting that elevated IOP is a risk factor for CRVO [8, 10]. This may be due to the fact that veins have very thin walls that contain smooth muscle, which can cause changes in the diameter of the venous vessel. Due to these properties, veins are quite distensible and their diameters can change passively in response to minor changes in transmural distending pressure [18].

While use of a comprehensive patient-centric database has several advantages in terms of large sample size, varied patient population, and access to 'real world' data representing true practice patterns outside of a clinical trial, there are limitations with this approach. Since this study used a retrospective claims database, only information collected and recorded at the time of the healthcare service or procedure was available for analysis. As determination of severity of ophthalmic illness was not possible, number of ophthalmic visits and number of IOP measurements were used as a proxy for disease severity. Furthermore, due to limitations of the data, intra-ocular pressures were unavailable, thus limiting our ability to assess and control for the association between intra-ocular pressure and ocular ischemic events. It is important to consider the possibility that the lower pressure, brought about by the presence of prescriptions, has a protective effect on risk of ischemia. Nonetheless, IOP-lowering prescriptions are still a necessary antecedent in this relationship.

Another recognized limitation is the potential for selection bias; the rare occurrence of ocular ischemic events required us to design this study to identify an event and then look back at the period prior to the event in order to determine treatment. Our study inclusion criteria specified that patients have at least one year of continuous enrollment in the health plan—these patients may be those that tend to seek out medical coverage more often. In the multivariate model, patients with longer enrollment were less likely to experience ocular ischemic events.

As is the case with retrospective reviews and analyses, our findings are suggestive of trends and data may not be generalizable to the overall US population. Managed care patients are generally younger and healthier than the population most at risk for an ocular ischemic event (i.e., the elderly). Additional research is needed to assess the effects of treatment on ocular ischemic events in order to determine whether there is a causal relationship between use of IOP-lowering medication and decreased ocular ischemic events.

Results of our study suggest that prolonged treatment with IOP-lowering medication may be protective against retinal venous occlusions. If this protective effect can be confirmed in future studies, it could provide a new therapeutic approach to patients at risk.

Acknowledgments

The authors would like to thank Paul P. Lee, MD, JD and Leonard A. Levin, MD, PhD for their assistance in reviewing this manuscript.

References

[1] European Glaucoma Prevention Study Group. Results of the European Glaucoma Prevention Study. *Ophthalmology*. 2005; 112:366-375.

[2] Bengtsson B. Aspects of the epidemiology of chronic glaucoma. *Acta Ophthalmol.* 1981; 146 Suppl:1-48.

[3] Gordon MO, Beiser JA, Brandt JD, et al. The ocular hypertension treatment study: Baseline factors that predict the onset of primary open-angle glaucoma. *Arch. Ophthalmol.* 2002; 120:714-720.

[4] Siris ES, Harris ST, Rosen CJ, et al. Adherence to bisphosphonate therapy and fracture rates in osteoporotic women: relationship to vertebral and nonvertebral fractures from 2 US claims databases. *Mayo Clin. Proc. Aug.* 2006; 81:1013-1022.

[5] Hollows FC, Graham PA. Intra-ocular pressure, glaucoma, and glaucoma suspects in a defined population. *Br. J. Ophthalmol.* 1966; 50:570-586.

[6] Nemesure B, Honkanen R, Hennis A, et al. Barbados Eye Studies Group. Incident open-angle glaucoma and intraocular pressure. *Ophthalmology.* 2007; 144:1810-1815

[7] Quigley HA, Nickells RW, Kerrigan LA, et al. Retinal ganglion cell death in experimental glaucoma and after axotomy occurs by apoptosis. *Invest. Ophthalmol. Vis. Sci.* 1995; 36:774-786.

[8] Beaumont PE, Kang HK. Clinical characteristics of retinal venous occlusions occurring at different sites. *Br. J. Ophthalmol.* 2002; 86:572-580.

[9] Hayreh SS. Prevalent misconceptions about acute retinal vascular occlusive disorders. *Prog. Retin. Eye Res. Jul.* 2005; 24:493-519.

[10] Hayreh SS, Zimmerman MB, Beri M, et al. Intraocular pressure abnormalities associated with central and hemicentral retinal vein occlusion. *Ophthalmology.* Jan. 2004; 111:133-141.

[11] Michelson G, Langhans MJ, Harazny J, et al. Visual field defect and perfusion of the juxtapapillary retina and the neuroretinal rim area in primary open-angle glaucoma. *Graefes Arch. Clin. Exp. Ophthalmol.* 1998; 236:80-85.

[12] Stroman GA, Stewart WC, Golnik KC, et al. Magnetic resonance imaging in patients with low-tension glaucoma. *Arch. Ophthalmol.* 1995; 113:168-172.

[13] Pillunat LE, Bohm AG, Koller AU, et al. Effect of topical dorzolamide on optic nerve head blood flow. *Graefes Arch. Clin. Exp. Ophthalmol.* Jun 1999; 237:495-500.

[14] Grunwald JE, Piltz J, Hariprasad SM, et al. Optic nerve blood flow in glaucoma: effect of systemic hypertension.[see comment]. *Am. J. Ophthalmol.* May 1999; 127:516-522.

[15] ICD-9-CM. International Classification of Diseases, 9th Revision, *Clinical Modification.* 5th ed: Medicode Publications; 1999.

[16] Charlson ME, Pompei P, Ales KL, et al. A new method of classifying prognostic comorbidity in longitudinal studies: development and validation. *J. Chron. Dis.* 1987; 40:373-383.

[17] SAS Version 9.1 [computer program]. Version: SAS Institute; 2002-2004.

[18] Mohrman DE HL. Cardiovascular physiology. In: Lange physiology series. 5th ed. New York: Lange Medical Books/McGraw-Hill. 2003:13-15.

In: Eye Research Developments: ...
Editor: Alan N. Westerhouse

ISBN: 978-1-60741-177-2

Chapter XI

Clinical Outcomes and Results of Microbiological Contamination After IOL Implantation – A Comparative Study*

Nada Jiráskova*†, *Pavel Rozsíval, Jana Pozlerova, Marie Ludvíkova, Eugenie Pozlerova, Jana Nekolova
University Hospital, Hradec Králové, Czech Republic

Abstract

Purpose: To compare the incidence of perioperative complications, microbiological contamination of the anterior chamber and postoperative outcomes after two standard methods of implantation of the hydrophilic acrylic intraocular lens (IOL)

Setting: Departments of Ophthalmology and Clinical Microbiology, University Hospital, Hradec Králové, Czech Republic

Methods: In this prospective randomized clinical study 60 eyes were implanted with the IOL CORNEAL ACR6D SE after uncomplicated phacoemulsification under topical anesthesia. Injector was used in 30 eyes and folding and insertion forceps in 30 eyes. After delivery of the IOL in the capsular bag, viscoelastic material was removed and an anterior chamber aspirate for microbiological examination was collected. The anterior chamber was reformed with balanced salt solution, intracameral injection of antiobiotic was used and the stroma alongside the primary incision and the side port incisions were lightly irrigated.

Results: No perioperative complications occurred in this series. The incidence of anterior chamber contamination after IOL implantation was 0 %, as all aspirates proved culture negative. Only threetimes sporadic colonies of *Staphylococcus plasmacoagulase-negative* were isolated from the liquid medium after reincubation, that were described by the microbiologist as almost certain contamination of the

* Presented in part at the ASCRS Symposium on Cataract, IOL and Refractive Surgery, Chicago, Il, USA, April 2008 and XXVI Congress of the ESCRS, Berlin, Germany, September 2008

Supported in part by research project MZO 00179906 from the Ministry of Health, Prague, Czech Republic
None of the authors has a financial or proprietary interest in any product mentioned.

† Department of Ophthalmology, University Hospital, Sokolska 581, 500 05 Hradec Králové, Czech Republic, e-mail: jirasnad@fnhk.cz, telephone: 420 495 833 392

sample (sampling and laboratory errors). In two of these three cases forceps were used for implantation, once injector. Anaerobic and mycologic examinations of all samples were negative. There was no evidence of postoperative inflammation or wound related complications in any case. Visual acuity was excellent immediately after surgery.

Conclusions: Both methods of the IOL implantation are safe and effective for small-incision cataract surgery.

Synopsis: Both implantation techniques (injector or folding and insertion forceps) proved to be safe and effective, with no significant differences comparing the microbiological contamination of the anterior chamber after implantation, perioperative findings and postoperative outcome.

Key words: intraocular lens; implantation; injector; forceps

Introduction

As a result of small-incision cataract surgery, the use of foldable intraocular lenses (IOLs) in cataract surgical interventions has increased worldwide. There were 1548 intraocular implants produced by 33 manufacturers available for use by surgeons as of January 2004[1]. The foldable IOLs are made of silicone elastomers or acrylate-methacrylate polymers. Acrylic IOLs offer advantages over lenses made of other materials such as controlled unfolding movement, lower aqueous flare intensity, and clear postoperative capsules[2, 3]. Moreover, acrylic polymers allow larger optics and permit less distortion and better distension of the capsular bag, that results in better stability and centration after implantation [4, 5].

Although no major breakthroughs have emerged in the area of lens insertion techniques and technology, small incremental advancements continue to take place for the delivery of foldable IOLs through small incisions. Ophthalmic surgeons and instrument manufacturers continue to strive to improve the methods and instrumentation for insertion of IOLs[6].

There are two standard methods of IOL folding and implantation: with a folding forceps or with an injector (folder). Injector systems have become more popular in many surgeons for their ability to fold lenses effectively and to allow insertion through smaller incisions. Folders have a further advantage in the possibility of greater sterility by the passage of the IOL from the outside nonsterile environment into the anterior chamber. On the other hand some surgeons still use folding and insertion forceps for implantation for reasons of more controlled unfolding movement, poor quality of some single-use cartridges and injectors that may cause damage of the IOL, and last but not least the price of the disposable devices that makes implantation using injector systems more expensive than using forceps.

In vitro results showed that a significantly higher number of bacteria adhered to forceps-folded hydrophobic acrylic IOLs than to nonfolded or injector-folded IOLs [7]. A retrospective survey has suggested, but not proven, that use of foldable IOLs inserted via a sterile injector lowers the incidence of postoperative endophthalmitis [8]. In another retrospective study, Kumar et al.[9] found significantly more wound-related complications after incision enlargement for IOL implantation. Our prospective clinical study was therefore designed to assess the results of microbiological contamination of the aqueous humor, operative complications and postoperative results after implantation of hydrophilic acrylic IOL CORNEAL ACR6D SE using single-use injector or folding and insertion forceps.

Materials and Methods

This prospective clinical study included 60 eyes (56 patients) with lens opacification scheduled for cataract surgery at the Department of Ophthalmology, University Hospital, Hradec Králové. The mean age of the 32 women (57 %) and 24 men (43 %) was 71.4 years (range 51 to 87 years). Patients with ocular surface diseases, endothelial or stromal corneal dystrophies, other anterior segment diseases, as well as with congenital or traumatic cataract were excluded. Exclusion criteria also included a secondary procedure that might affect wound stability such as trabeculectomy, a limbal relaxing incision, astigmatic keratotomy, and other major surgical procedures such as pars plana vitrectomy. The study purpose, procedures, and responsibilities were explained to all potential participants, and informed consent was obtained from all selected patients. Before surgery, a complete eye examination was performed.

Surgeries were performed under topical anesthesia by two surgeons (PR, NJ).

A 10 % benzododecinii bromati solution was used for peri-orbital skin antisepsis (eyelids, nose, cheek, eyebrow, and forehead). Povidone-iodine 5 % solution was then applied liberally to the conjunctiva, eyelids, eyelashes, and eyebrow. The eyelashes were kept out of the surgical field with a sterile plastic tape and the eyelids were retracted with a Lieberman stainless steel speculum. A 2.8 limbal tunnel incision was created by diamond knife (Storz Instruments, Bausch&Lomb) for phacoemulsification and 2 side-port incisions using a single use, 30-degree ophthalmic knife (Alcon). Anterior continuous circular capsulorhexis was done under viscoelastic device. Modified quick-chop phacoemulsification was performed in routine manner after hydrodissection and bimanual irrigation/aspiration (I/A) was used to remove the cortical material and clean the capsule. Viscoelastic material was injected to fill the anterior chamber and the capsular bag and posterior chamber (PC) IOL CORNEAL ACR6D SE was implanted in all cases. It is a single-piece hydrophilic acrylic IOL with a 26 % water content in equilibrium and refractive index of 1.465. It is purchased either as a unit consisting of a single-use injector containing the IOL (model PREMIER) or without any insertion devices (model STANDARD). In 30 eyes STANDARD model was implanted using folding and insertion forceps (2-778 and 4-718, Storz Instruments, Bausch&Lomb) and in 30 eyes injector system (model PREMIER) was used.

Forceps Folding

The incision was enlarged to 3.4 mm. IOL was removed from its package and positioned in the folding forceps following the manufacturer´s instructions. The forceps was gradually and carefully tightened until the IOL was correctly folded on the 6 o´clock to12 o´clock axis. Then it was grasped with the insertion forceps and inserted through the incision inside the anterior chamber. After the leading haptic had been delivered under the distal capsulorhexis, the forceps were slowly opened allowing the lens to unfold. Aided by a spatula, the lens optic and the second haptic was dialed into the capsular bag.

Injector Folding

The wound was not enlarged. According to the manufacturer´s instructions, the container with injector was partially opened and saline solution poured out. Than the container was opened completely and some viscoelastic material was added in order to lubricate IOL. The lever was closed onto the body of the injector and the folded IOL was checked. The piston was gently pressed to move the IOL fully in the cannula. The end of the cannula was introduced into the 2.8 mm incision and the IOL was inserted in the bag by pushing the central cylinder. Proper position of both haptics and centration of the implant in the bag was completed by spatula.

After implantation, viscoelastic material was carefully removed using bimanual I/A and the anterior chamber aspirate (0.2-0.3 mL) was drowned with a sterile cannula attached to a 1 mL syringe. The anterior chamber was reformed with balanced salt solution, intracameral antiobiotic solution (cefuroximum natricum 1mg/ 0.1 mL) was injected and the stroma alongside the primary wound and the side-port incisions were lightly irrigated. The stability of all incisions were tested by applying light external pressure with the cannula. At the conclusion of the operation, tobramycin 3.0 mg /mL and dexamethasonum 1.0 mg/mL (Tobradex®) and timolol (Timolol-POS 0.5%) were applied topically and the eye dressed in the usual manner.

All patients received topical tobramycin 3.0 mg /mL and dexamethasonum 1.0 mg/mL (Tobradex®) five times daily for 2 weeks postoperatively, followed by dexamethasonum 1.0 mg/mL (Dexamethason®) three times daily for 2 weeks.

On the first postoperative day uncorrected and best corrected Snellen visual acuity at distance were measured and a complete eye examination was performed with intent on wound stability, corneal clarity, anterior chamber flare and position and centration of the IOL. All patients were routinely followed-up for the next three months.

The anterior chamber aspirates were labeled in a coded manner for the laboratory staff and sent for microbiological examination. Each specimen was plated on chocolate blood agar incubated in carbon dioxide 5%, sheep blood agar, MacConkey agar, Sabouraud agar and anaerobe blood agar with brainheart infusion incubated within 2 hours of collection. All plates were held at 37 °C for 3 days. Then colonies were isolated and identified using current bacteriological techniques, for example BBL™ Crystal™ Identification Systems (Becton Dickinson), Vitek® 2 Compact (BioMerieux).

Results

No intraoperative complications occurred in this series. Folding and implantation of the IOL were in all eyes done smoothly and easily and there was no case of torn or other damage of the IOL after implantation. No patient reported pain during IOL insertion or enlargement of the wound in eyes where forceps were used. None of the eyes required a suture for unstable wound or insufficient watertightness at the end of surgery. Best corrected visual acuity was 1.0 -0.8 on the first postoperative day in all patients. No eye had a incision leak or other wound related complication. There was no evidence of postoperative inflammation in any case during the whole follow-up period.

All anterior chamber samples proved culture negative. Only threetimes were sporadic colonies of *Staphylococcus plasmacoagulase-negative* isolated from the liquid medium after reincubation, that were described by the microbiologist as almost certain contamination of the sample (sampling and laboratory errors). At two from these three cases forceps were used for implantation, once injector. Anaerobic and mycologic examinations of all samples were negative.

Discussion

Modern cataract surgery has a high success rates. Very fast visual rehabilitation, nearly no surgically induced astigmatism, reduced postoperative intraocular inflammation, possibility of topical anesthesia and outpatient cataract surgery are the advantages of small-incision surgery. Incision sizes of 2.0-3.5 mm are recommended today to insert foldable IOLs. There are two standard methods for implantation of these lenses: using specially manufactured folding and insertion forceps or injector systems.

In general, there appears to be more of a trend away from folding and insertion forceps toward cartridge injector systems. New cartridge injectors are inreasing in popularity because of their ease of use, ability to pass lenses effectively through smaller incisions, and the possibility of greater sterility [6]. The large variety of injector systems reflects the diversity of IOLs. Familiarity with the various devices used for insertion of foldable lenses takes on increasing importance. Most of them need the manipulation of the IOL: with forceps the IOL has to be taken out of the package and positioned into the cartridge or into the folding chamber. A certain amount of viscoelastic material protects the IOL during injection. Advancing of the IOL is done by pushing or by rotating the central cylinder. The IOL CORNEAL ACR6D SE (model PREMIER) is purchased as a unit consisting of a single-use injector containing single-piece hydrophilic acrylic IOL. The lens is placed directly in the injector cartrige (container) filled with the preserving saline solution and does not need manipulation with forceps. The insertion of this type of IOL is straight from the sterile environment of the container and injector to the anterior chamber. The same IOL CORNEAL ACR6D SE (model STANDARD) is purchased without any insertion devices and in our study folding and insertion forceps were used for implanation. Folding and implatation of the IOL were in all eyes done smoothly and easily and there was no case of torn or other damage of the IOL after implatation. No patient reported pain during IOL insertion or widening of the incision.

Theoretically, any additional step involving a knife in the eye, in particular for procedure in topical anesthesia, can be associated with increased complication rates [9]. In our study 30 eyes recieved an IOL CORNEAL PREMIER through 2.8 mm incision and 30 eyes were implanted with IOL CORNEAL STANDARD after enlargement of the incision to 3.4 mm. We found no clinical difference in wound statibility or possible complications between both techniques for the IOL implantation. None of the eyes required a suture for unstable wound or insufficient watertightness at the end of surgery. There was no case of incision leak or other evidence of wound complications during the whole follow-up period. Visual acuity was excellent in all eyes immediately after surgery.

Infections are potentially serious complications of cataract surgery. Although the incidence is relatively low, infections represent a serious clinical concern because of morbidity, increased medical costs, and prolongation of the the treatment [10, 11]. The occurrence, severity and clinical course of endophthalmitis depend on the route of infection, the virulence and number of inoculated pathogens as well as the patient´s immune state and the time of examination. There is a range of technical factors relating to the surgery that influence the risk of endophthalmitis [12]. Cataract extraction and IOL implantation require an incision be made in the anterior chamber, exposing it to the microorganisms that colonize the adjacent ocular surface and adnexa [13]. It has been shown that bacteria routinely enter the anterior chamber during cataract extraction and remain there at the end of surgery in a significant proportion of patients [13, 14, 15]. To reduce the risk of postoperative infectious endophthalmitis, a primary objective is to minimize the entry of the organisms into the anterior chamber during the whole procedure and to close carefully all incisions at the end of surgery. In our study we did not find any difference between either method – nor in the wound stability and watertightness, nor in the microbiological contamination of the anterior chamber after implantation. All anterior chamber aspirates proved culture negative and there was no evidence of postoperative inflammation in any case during the whole follow-up period.

In conclusion, both implantation techniques (injector or folding and insertion forceps) proved to be safe and effective, with no significant differences comparing the microbiological contamination of the anterior chamber after implantation, perioperative findings and postoperative outcome.

References

[1] Holladay JT. International Intraocular Lens & Implant Registry 2004. *J Cataract Refract Surg* 2004; 30:207-229

[2] Apple DJ, Kincald MC, Mamalis N, Olson RJ. *Intraocular Lenses; Evolution, Designs, Complications, and Pathology*. Baltimore, MD, Wiliams & Wilkins, 1989

[3] Omar O, Mamalis N, Veiga J, et al. Scanning electron microscopic characteristics of small-incision intraocular lenses. *Ophthalmology* 1996; 103:1124-1129

[4] Mamalis N. Explantation of intraocular lenses. *Curr Opin Ophthalmol* 2000; 11:289-295

[5] Subramaniam S, Tuft SJ. Early decentration of plate-haptic silicone intraocular lenses. *J Cataract Refract Surg* 2001; 27:330-332

[6] Hoffman RS, Fine IH. New Techniques and instruments for lens implantation. *Curr Opin Ophthalmol* 1999; 10:16-21

[7] Mencucci R, Dei R, Danielli D, et al. Folding procedure for acrylic intraocular lenses Effect on optic surfaces and bacterial adhesion. *J Cataract Refract Surg* 2004; 30:457-463

[8] Mayer E, Cadman D, Ewings P. A 10 year retrospective study of cataract surgery and endophthalmitis in a single eye unit: injectable lenses lower the incidence of endophthalmitis. *Br J Ophthalmol* 2003; 87:867-869

[9] Kumar R, Reeves DL, Olson RJ. Wound complications associated with incision enlargement for foldable intraocular lens implantation during cataract surgery. J *Cataract Refract Surg* 2001; 27:224-226

[10] Somani S, Grinbaum A, Slomovic AR. Potoperative endophthalmitis: incidence, predisposing surgery, clinical course and outcome. *Can J Ophthalmol* 1997; 32:303-310

[11] Mamalis N, Kearsley L, Brinton E. Post-operative endophthalmitis. *Curr Opin Ophthalmol* 2002; 13:14-18

[12] Masket S. Preventing, diagnosing, and treating endophthalmitis. *J Cataract Refract Surg* 1998; 24:725-726

[13] Sherwood DR, Rich WJ, Jacob JS, et al. Bacterial contamination of intraocular and extraocular fluids during extracapsular cataract extraction. *Eye* 1989; 3:308-312

[14] Dickey JB, Thompson KD, Jay WM. Anterior chamber aspirate cultures after uncomplicated cataract surgery. *Am J Ophthalmol* 1991; 112:278-282

[15] Mistlberger A, Ruckhofer J, Raithel E, et al. Anterior chamber contamination during cataract surgery with intraocular lens implantation. *J Cataract Refract Surg* 1997; 23:1064-1069

In: Eye Research Developments
Editor: Alan N. Westerhouse
ISBN: 978-1-60741-177-2

Chapter XII

Role of RGM, an Axon Guidance Protein, in the Degeneration and Regeneration of the Optic Nerve – Implication for the Treatment of Glaucoma

Sylvie Julien [*] ***and Sven Schnichels***
Section for experimental Vitreoretinal Surgery, Centre for Ophthalmology, Institute for Ophthalmic Research, Schleichstr. 12/1, 72076 Tübingen, Germany

Glaucoma

Glaucoma refers to a specific pattern of optic nerve damage and visual field loss caused by a number of different eye pathologies that affect the optic nerve, the retina and the vascular network. It is the second leading cause of blindness worldwide. About 60 millions people will be affected by this disease in the year 2010 [1]. Most, but not all, of these conditions are characterized by elevated intraocular pressure (IOP), which is not the disease itself, but the most important risk factor for the development of glaucoma. It has been suggested that high values of IOP produce direct mechanical damage to the axons of the optic nerve by interfering with the axonal cytoplasm flow and create gradual ischemia of the retina by mechanical compression of the vascular network of the retina. These processes can generate a chain of metabolic events that lead to slow axonal degeneration of retinal ganglion cells (RGC) and ultimately to apoptotic death of these cells [2].

Optic nerve damage in glaucomatous patients remains a challenge. Although many factors have recently been recognized to mediate RGC degeneration in glaucoma, the molecular mediators that participate in this process are largely unknown.

[*] E-Mail: sylvie.julien@med.uni-tuebingen.de

Axotomy of the Optic Nerve

Following optic nerve axotomy in adult rats, initial reduction of the original population of RGC is observed 5-7 days after injury. A rapid process of cell death takes place, and >80% of the RGCs die within 2 weeks after the injury [3]. Because a relatively long interval precedes this massive death, it can be speculated that a time window exists, in which protective intervention can be employed with modulators that attenuate or prevent cell death. Indeed, partial and temporal rescue of RGC from axotomy-induced apoptosis was obtained by several approaches. These included early treatment with microglial inhibitors [4, 5], glial or brain-derived neurotrophic factors [6], caspase inhibitors [5, 7], implantation of stimulated macrophages [8], overexpression of Bcl-2 [9] and intravitreal injection of β- or γ-crystallins [10] or an endonuclease inhibitor [11].

Moreover, in a study from Shirvan *et al.*, the authors observed that complete axotomy of optic nerve in rats, with minimal damage to the vascular supply and meningeal structure, led to the induction of the axon guidance protein semaphorin 3A in the retina 48-72 h following injury [12]. Morphological evaluation of the retina indicated that axotomy-induced death was indeed apoptotic and that rescue of RGCs from axotomy-induced degeneration could be achieved by treatment of the injured retina by intraocular administration of anti-Sema3A function-blocking antibodies. Nevertheless functional studies of the surviving neurons, and further studies of their ability to receive and integrate synaptic inputs are still necessary. Furthermore, future studies should also examine whether longer-term survival can be obtained using this strategy [12].

The Concept of Guidance by Repulsion

A common feature of all optic neuropathies is the loss of axons. Since axonal damage is involved in both axotomy and glaucoma, Shirvan *et al.* [12] hypothesize that similar molecular mediators are involved in RGC death in both neuropathies. A similar neuronal population is lost following total optic nerve axotomy and in glaucoma. In the former condition the cell bodies of the ganglion cells die typically within a month [13], while the death process in glaucoma is more prolonged and often takes years or decades. The injured ganglion cells have the genetic program to grow new axons toward their target cells, but are prevented from doing so probably by the presence of extracellular molecules that inhibit the growth process and/or by non-neuronal surrounding cells, which are non permissive to axonal growth. The discovery of several gene families containing members that can function as axon repellents has defined the concept of "guidance by repulsion" at the molecular level [14]. As has been shown for growth-promoting or attractive guidance cues, repulsive cues can either be short-range, surface-bound (i.e. contact repellents), or long-range, diffusible (i.e. chemorepellents) in nature. Recently characterized chemorepellents include ephrins, netrins, slits, and semaphorins [15, 16]. Some of these chemorepulsive axon guidance cues continue to be expressed in the mature rodent and human nervous system [17, 18]. This sustained expression of chemorepulsive proteins during adulthood, as well as injury-induced recapitulation of their expression, may significantly influence the course of axonal regeneration [19].

RGM, the Repulsive Guidance Molecule

Evidence is now emerging that the proteins governing developmental axon guidance may contribute to the failure of injured central neurons to regenerate [19-21]. The expression of chemorepulsive netrin-1, semaphorins and ephrins has been shown to relate to the success or failure of injured axons to regenerate [19, 22, 23] through damaged CNS (optic nerve and spinal cord). The Repulsive Guidance Molecule (RGM), an axon guidance protein of 33 kDa, has been cloned and functionally characterized as a molecular determinant for retinotectal map formation [24-26]. It is a membrane-associated glycoprotein which shares no sequence homology with any other known guidance cues. RGM is attached to membranes *via* a glycosylphosphatidylinositol (GPI) anchor.

To date, three RGM genes have been isolated in the mouse genome [27]: RGMA, RGMB and RGMC. Furthermore, neogenin, which was known to be a netrin-1 receptor, was also demonstrated to function as an RGMA receptor [28]. In the human genome the three RGMs and neogenin are highly conserved, whereas in the rat genome only RGMA, RGMC and neogenin could be identified yet. The expression patterns of the three homologues were identified in the mouse embryo by in-situ hybridization [27, 29]. RGMA and RGMB are predominantly expressed in the developing and adult central nervous system (CNS) in complementary patterns with little overlap. RGMC expression is restricted to all striated muscles and the myocardium. It has been demonstrated that recombinant chick RGMA induces collapse of temporal but not nasal growth cones of RGCs and guides temporal retinal axons *in vitro*, demonstrating a repulsive and axon-specific guiding activity [24]. As a step toward elucidation of the role of chemorepulsive molecules in axonal regeneration, we have studied the effects of spinal cord injury (SCI) on the expression of RGMA [30]. The presence of RGMA in a glial barrier and its inhibitory activity *in vitro* made it plausible that it might exert inhibitory effects on regenerating axons in the glial scar. Indeed, it was recently shown in rats after SCI that inhibition of RGMA enhanced growth of injured axons, promoted functional recovery [31] and induced synaptic rearrangements of spared axonal projections [32]. Thus, reexpression of embryonic repulsive cues in adult tissues contributes to failure of axon regeneration in the central nervous system [33].

Expression Patterns of RGM and Its Receptor Neogenin in the Mouse Visual System: C57BL/6J vs. the Glaucoma Model DBA/2J

Recently, we analyzed the expression patterns of RGMA, its receptor neogenin, RGMB and RGMC in the developing and mature mouse visual system [34] of a genetically determined murine pigmentary glaucoma strain, the DBA/2J mouse [35], versus the wild-type

C57BL/6J strain. In the DBA/2J mouse, glaucoma results in a slowly progressing decrease in the population of RGCs. The period of elevated IOP extends from six months to 16 months. An important transition to high IOP for many mice is with eight to nine months of age [36]. The majority of mice aged 10.5 months and older (>75%) showed moderate to severe ganglion cell loss [37]. Optic nerve degeneration follows IOP elevation, with the majority of optic nerves being severely damaged by twelve months of age [36].

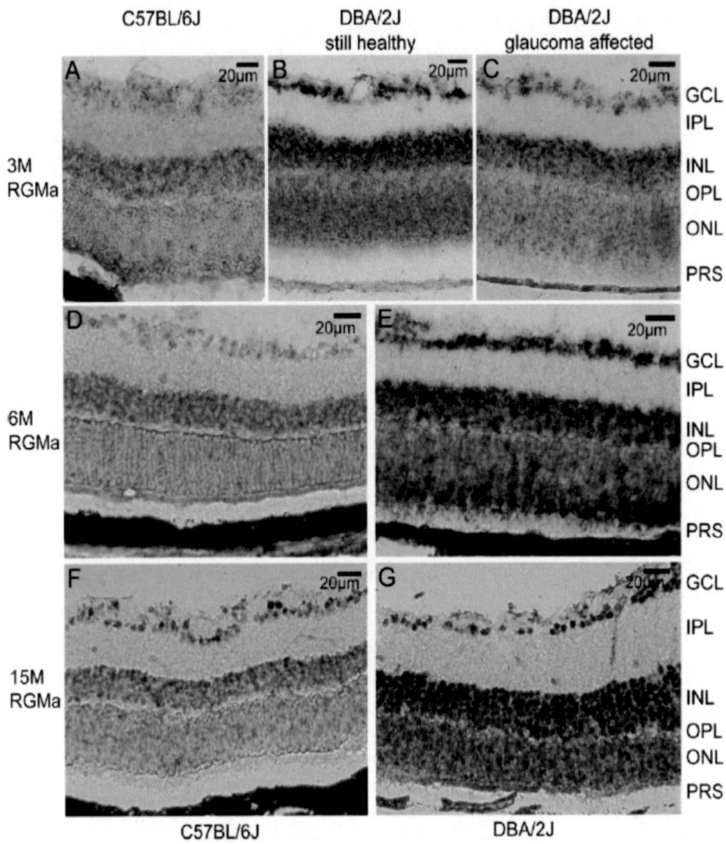

Figure 1. Differences in the expression of RGMa in mature C57BL/6 and DBA/2J retinas: In 3-month-old mice, the level of RGMA-expression in glaucoma affected DBA/2J mice was 2.3 times higher in the GCL and between 1.1 and 1.3 times higher in the ONL and INL than in the C57BL/6J mice, respectively. With increasing age, the expression of RGMA in C57BL/6J decreased in both the INL and the ONL (figure 1A, D and F), in contrast to DBA/2J mice, where the expression did not decrease at all with age (figure 1B, C, E and G). We observed the highest RGMA expression in the retina sections of 6-month-old DBA/2J mice, the onset of glaucoma in most of the mice. Quantification of the signal intensity revealed a 3.0 times higher expression in the GCL, a 1.9 higher expression in the INL and a 2.4 higher expression in the ONL of 6-month-old mice, respectively. In 15- month-old mice, the difference was not so striking (this might be due to the ongoing RGC death in the DBA/2J glaucoma strain). We observed a 1.9 times higher expression in the GCL and ONL, and a 1.4-fold higher expression in the INL. [34] Reprinted from Gene Expression Patterns, Vol. 8, Issue 1, Sven Schnichels, Sabine Conrad, Katrin Warstat, Sigrid Henke-Fahle, Thomas Skutella, Ulrich Schraermeyer and Sylvie Julien, Gene expression of the repulsive guidance molecules/neogenin in the developing and mature mouse visual system: C57BL/6J vs. the glaucoma model DBA/2J, Pages No. 1-11, 2007, with permission from Elsevier.

Therefore, these mice provide a powerful model system for determining mechanisms that insult RGCs in glaucoma and for characterizing specific damaging pathways. Indeed, the RGC loss in DBA/2J inbred mice is natural, age related, variable, with an asynchronous progressive course that in this way resembles the human glaucoma [36]. The progression of the disease is asymmetric [37]. Both eyes can therefore be treated as independent [36]. In order to understand the role of RGMs and neogenin in glaucoma, we characterized their expression patterns in the developing and mature mouse retina and in the optic nerve by *in-situ* hybridization. RGMA, RGMB and neogenin expression was detected in the ganglion cell layer (GCL) at all investigated stages from post-natal day (P) 0 to 15 months (M). From P10 to 15M, we found RGMA, RGMB and neogenin expression in the inner nuclear layer (INL) and the outer nuclear layer (ONL). In P10- and older mice, the expression patterns of RGMA and its receptor neogenin were similar, while that of RGMB differed from both. As expected, no specific retinal expression of RGMC was detected in any of the age groups investigated. C57BL/6J mice and DBA/2J mice displayed no differences in the expression pattern of RGMA, RGMB, RGMC and neogenin in the developing retina (embryonic age 14.5 days (E14.5), P0 & P10). Interestingly, we found a higher expression of RGMA (figure 1), RGMB and neogenin in the retinas of all glaucoma-affected mice than in the age-matched control strain. Furthermore, we detected a higher RGMA and RGMB expression in the optic nerves of glaucoma-affected DBA/2J-mice older than 11M than in C57BL/6J mice of the same age, whereas the expression of neogenin did not change (figures 2-4).

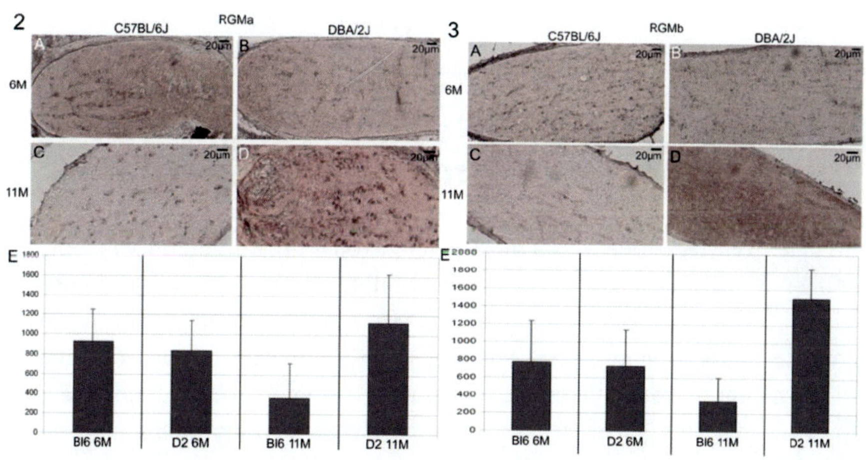

Figures 2 and 3. Differences in RGMA and RGMB expression in the optic nerves of aging C57BL/6J and DBA/2J mice. No significant difference in the expression of RGMA and RGMB was observed in the optic nerves of 6-month-old C57BL/6J mice (respectively 2A, 3A) and DBA/2J (respectively 2B, 3B). C57BL/6J mice older than 11 months (2C and 3C) showed a lower expression than mice younger than 11 months, whereas the expression increased in DBA/2J mice aged 11 months (2D and 3D). Quantitative analysis of the optic nerve sections (2E and 3E). The RGMA and RGMB signals were equal in 6-month-old mice, whereas the expressions in 11-month-old mice were respectively 3 times and 5 times higher in DBA/2J (D2) mice [34]. Reprinted from Gene Expression Patterns, Vol. 8, Issue 1, Sven Schnichels, Sabine Conrad, Katrin Warstat, Sigrid Henke-Fahle, Thomas Skutella, Ulrich Schraermeyer and Sylvie Julien, Gene expression of the repulsive guidance molecules/neogenin in the developing and mature mouse visual system: C57BL/6J vs. the glaucoma model DBA/2J, Pages No. 1-11, 2007, with permission from Elsevier.

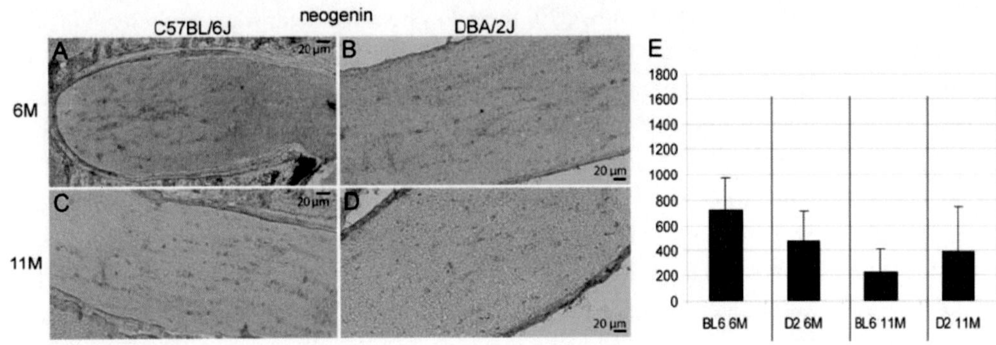

Figure 4. Differences in neogenin expression in the optic nerves of aging C57BL/6J and DBA/2J mice. In mice younger than 10M, the expression of neogenin in the optic nerve was slightly higher in C57BL/6J (A) mice than in DBA/2J mice (B). The expression in 11M-old DBA/2J mice (D) did not rise higher than with 6M of age. In contrast to RGMA and RGMB, expression of neogenin in the two strains did not invert with age. Quantitative analysis of the optic nerve sections (E): The neogenin signals of the C57BL/6J (BL6) mice decreased with age, whereas the expression of neogenin in the DBA/2J (D2) stayed at approximately the same level. (Schnichels et al., unpublished data).

Although several lines of evidence indicate that RGMA and its receptor neogenin may belong to the factors that determine whether axonal regeneration will succeed or fail, probably mediated by the Rho pathway [38], further studies will be necessary to establish a causal relationship between RGMA function and the failure of regeneration in the optic nerve.

Possible Rescue of Retinal Ganglion Cells with RGMA Function-Blocking Antibody

Since to date, RGMA is one of the most potent axonal growth inhibitors identified [30], we suggest that RGMA is a key protein that modulates the cell fate of axotomized or glaucoma damaged RGC. Neutralization of RGMA repulsive function by injection of a function-blocking antibody may serve, but not necessary exhaustive, as a promising new approach for treatment of traumatic injury in the adult mammalian central nervous system or of ophthalmologic diseases such as glaucoma and ischemic optic neuropathy that induce apoptotic RGC death. In previous studies in primates, we demonstrated that a full-length intravitreally injected antibody (bevacizumab/Avastin®) was able to penetrate the retina as easily as an antibody fragment [39] and that this antibody penetrated quickly into the macula, the retinal veins and the optic nerve [40].

References

[1] Quigley HA, Broman AT. The number of people with glaucoma worldwide in 2010 and 2020. *Br. J. Ophthalmol.* 2006 Mar;90(3):262-7.

[2] Quigley HA. Neuronal death in glaucoma. *Prog. Retin. Eye Res.* 1999 Jan;18(1):39-57.

[3] Berkelaar M, Clarke DB, Wang YC, Bray GM, Aguayo AJ. Axotomy results in delayed death and apoptosis of retinal ganglion cells in adult rats. *J. Neurosci.* 1994 Jul;14(7):4368-74.

[4] Thanos S, Mey J. Type-specific stabilization and target-dependent survival of regenerating ganglion cells in the retina of adult rats. *J. Neurosci.* 1995 Feb;15(2):1057-79.

[5] Heiduschka P, Fischer D, Thanos S. [Neuroprotection and regeneration after traumatic lesion of the optic nerve]. *Klin. Monatsbl. Augenheilkd.* 2004 Aug;221(8):684-701.

[6] Isenmann S, Klocker N, Gravel C, Bahr M. Short communication: protection of axotomized retinal ganglion cells by adenovirally delivered BDNF in vivo. *Eur. J. Neurosci.* 1998 Aug;10(8):2751-6.

[7] Kermer P, Klocker N, Labes M, Bahr M. Insulin-like growth factor-I protects axotomized rat retinal ganglion cells from secondary death via PI3-K-dependent Akt phosphorylation and inhibition of caspase-3 In vivo. *J. Neurosci.* 2000 Jan 15;20(2):2-8.

[8] Lazarov-Spiegler O, Solomon AS, Schwartz M. Link between optic nerve regrowth failure and macrophage stimulation in mammals. Vision Res. 1999 Jan;39(1):169-75.

[9] Chierzi S, Cenni MC, Maffei L, Pizzorusso T, Porciatti V, Ratto GM, et al. Protection of retinal ganglion cells and preservation of function after optic nerve lesion in bcl-2 transgenic mice. *Vision Res.* 1998 May;38(10):1537-43.

[10] Fischer D, Hauk TG, Muller A, Thanos S. Crystallins of the beta/gamma-superfamily mimic the effects of lens injury and promote axon regeneration. *Mol. Cell Neurosci.* 2008 Mar;37(3):471-9.

[11] Heiduschka P, Thanos S. Aurintricarboxylic acid promotes survival and regeneration of axotomised retinal ganglion cells in vivo. *Neuropharmacology.* 2000 Mar 3;39(5):889-902.

[12] Shirvan A, Kimron M, Holdengreber V, Ziv I, Ben-Shaul Y, Melamed S, et al. Anti-semaphorin 3A antibodies rescue retinal ganglion cells from cell death following optic nerve axotomy. *J. Biol. Chem.* 2002 Dec 20;277(51):49799-807.

[13] Quigley HA, Davis EB, Anderson DR. Descending optic nerve degeneration in primates. *Invest. Ophthalmol. Vis. Sci.* 1977 Sep;16(9):841-9.

[14] Tessier-Lavigne M, Goodman CS. The molecular biology of axon guidance. *Science.* 1996 Nov 15;274(5290):1123-33.

[15] Mueller BK. Growth cone guidance: first steps towards a deeper understanding. *Annu. Rev. Neurosci.* 1999;22:351-88.

[16] Song HJ, Poo MM. Signal transduction underlying growth cone guidance by diffusible factors. *Curr. Opin. Neurobiol.* 1999 Jun;9(3):355-63.

[17] Livesey FJ, Hunt SP. Netrin and netrin receptor expression in the embryonic mammalian nervous system suggests roles in retinal, striatal, nigral, and cerebellar development. *Mol. Cell Neurosci.* 1997;8(6):417-29.

[18] Mark MD, Lohrum M, Puschel AW. Patterning neuronal connections by chemorepulsion: the semaphorins. *Cell Tissue Res.* 1997 Nov;290(2):299-306.

[19] Low K, Culbertson M, Bradke F, Tessier-Lavigne M, Tuszynski MH. Netrin-1 is a novel myelin-associated inhibitor to axon growth. *J. Neurosci.* 2008 Jan 30;28(5):1099-108.

[20] Cramer SC, Chopp M. Recovery recapitulates ontogeny. *Trends Neurosci.* 2000 Jun;23(6):265-71.

[21] Wizenmann A, Thies E, Klostermann S, Bonhoeffer F, Bahr M. Appearance of target-specific guidance information for regenerating axons after CNS lesions. *Neuron.* 1993 Nov;11(5):975-83.

[22] Knoll B, Drescher U. Ephrin-As as receptors in topographic projections. *Trends Neurosci.* 2002 Mar;25(3):145-9.

[23] Pasterkamp RJ, Verhaagen J. Emerging roles for semaphorins in neural regeneration. *Brain Res. Brain Res. Rev.* 2001 Mar;35(1):36-54.

[24] Monnier PP, Sierra A, Macchi P, Deitinghoff L, Andersen JS, Mann M, et al. RGM is a repulsive guidance molecule for retinal axons. *Nature.* 2002 Sep 26;419(6905):392-5.

[25] Muller BK, Jay DG, Bonhoeffer F. Chromophore-assisted laser inactivation of a repulsive axonal guidance molecule. *Curr. Biol.* 1996 Nov 1;6(11):1497-502.

[26] Stahl B, Muller B, von Boxberg Y, Cox EC, Bonhoeffer F. Biochemical characterization of a putative axonal guidance molecule of the chick visual system. *Neuron.* 1990 Nov;5(5):735-43.

[27] Schmidtmer J, Engelkamp D. Isolation and expression pattern of three mouse homologues of chick Rgm. *Gene Expr. Patterns.* 2004 Jan;4(1):105-10.

[28] Rajagopalan S, Deitinghoff L, Davis D, Conrad S, Skutella T, Chedotal A, et al. Neogenin mediates the action of repulsive guidance molecule. *Nat. Cell Biol.* 2004 Aug;6(8):756-62.

[29] Oldekamp J, Kramer N, Alvarez-Bolado G, Skutella T. Expression pattern of the repulsive guidance molecules RGM A, B and C during mouse development. *Gene Expr. Patterns*. 2004 May;4(3):283-8.

[30] Schwab JM, Conrad S, Monnier PP, Julien S, Mueller BK, Schluesener HJ. Spinal cord injury-induced lesional expression of the repulsive guidance molecule (RGM). *Eur. J. Neurosci*. 2005 Mar;21(6):1569-76.

[31] Hata K, Fujitani M, Yasuda Y, Doya H, Saito T, Yamagishi S, et al. RGMa inhibition promotes axonal growth and recovery after spinal cord injury. *J. Cell Biol.* 2006 Apr 10;173(1):47-58.

[32] Kyoto A, Hata K, Yamashita T. Synapse formation of the cortico-spinal axons is enhanced by RGMa inhibition after spinal cord injury. *Brain Res.* 2007 Dec;1186:74-86.

[33] Yamashita T, Mueller BK, Hata K. Neogenin and repulsive guidance molecule signaling in the central nervous system. *Curr. Opin. Neurobiol.* 2007 Feb;17(1):29-34.

[34] Schnichels S, Conrad S, Warstat K, Henke-Fahle S, Skutella T, Schraermeyer U, et al. Gene expression of the repulsive guidance molecules/neogenin in the developing and mature mouse visual system: C57BL/6J vs. the glaucoma model DBA/2J. *Gene Expr. Patterns.* 2007 Dec;8(1):1-11.

[35] John SW, Smith RS, Savinova OV, Hawes NL, Chang B, Turnbull D, et al. Essential iris atrophy, pigment dispersion, and glaucoma in DBA/2J mice. Invest. *Ophthalmol. Vis. Sci.* 1998 May;39(6):951-62.

[36] Libby RT, Anderson MG, Pang IH, Robinson ZH, Savinova OV, Cosma IM, et al. Inherited glaucoma in DBA/2J mice: pertinent disease features for studying the neurodegeneration. *Vis. Neurosci.* 2005 Sep-Oct;22(5):637-48.

[37] Schlamp CL, Li Y, Dietz JA, Janssen KT, Nickells RW. Progressive ganglion cell loss and optic nerve degeneration in DBA/2J mice is variable and asymmetric. *BMC Neurosci.* 2006;7:66.

[38] Kubo T, Hata K, Yamaguchi A, Yamashita T. Rho-ROCK inhibitors as emerging strategies to promote nerve regeneration. *Curr. Pharm. Des.* 2007;13(24):2493-9.

[39] Heiduschka P, Fietz H, Hofmeister S, Schultheiss S, Mack AF, Peters S, et al. Penetration of bevacizumab through the retina after intravitreal injection in the monkey. *Invest. Ophthalmol. Vis. Sci.* 2007 Jun;48(6):2814-23.

[40] Julien S, Heiduschka P, Hofmeister S, Schraermeyer U. Immunohistochemical localisation of intravitreally injected bevacizumab at the posterior pole of the primate eye: implication for the treatment of retinal vein occlusion. *Br. J. Ophthalmol.* 2008 Oct;92(10):1424-8.

In: Eye Research Developments
Editor: Alan N. Westerhouse
ISBN: 978-1-60741-177-2

Chapter XIII

The Impact of Ischemia in Glaucoma

Antonio Martinez
Instituto Galego de Oftalmoloxia, Santiago de Compostela, Spain

Abstract

Whereas intraocular pressure (IOP) is considered a major risk factor in glaucoma, growing evidence now indicates that it is not the only one.

There is increasing evidence that ocular ischemia plays a major role not only in the pathogenesis but also in the progression of the glaucomatous damage.

By virtue of this and because many existing techniques are able to evaluate the blood supply in the different vascular beds, it is essential that current and future investigations for glaucoma evaluate the role of ischemia on the progression of the glaucomatous optic neuropathy.

During the last decade, the study of haemodynamics in ocular tissues has been increasing interest and we observed exceptional advances in the development of new devices.

Furthermore, the eye offers a unique opportunity for non-invasive measurements of blood flow in humans.

Many different blood flow measurement techniques are used to visualized and measure directly or calculate indirectly in vivo ocular blood flow (OBF). However, there is still no a single method that can provide all the relevant information in one reading.

On the other hand, the fact that the different measurement techniques available also measure different aspects of ocular haemodynamics and targeting to different tissue layers makes direct comparisons between techniques all but easy.

The fact that altered blood flow can be observed not only in the ocular and retrobulbar vessels, but even in the naildfold-capillaries, indicates that the OBF reduction may be not only secondary either due to IOP increase or due to glaucomatous optic neuropathy.

Disturbances of the blood supply to the ocular tissue are believed to be linked to disease progression and we witness new perspectives beyond glaucoma therapy for IOP reduction.

1. Introduction

The term glaucoma covers a wide range of diseases, traditionally including any and all conditions associated with increased intraocular pressure (IOP) and visual field loss.

The European Glaucoma Society defines primary open-angle glaucoma (POAG) as chronic and progressive optic neuropathies, which have in common characteristics morphological changes at the optic nerve head and retinal nerve fiber layer (RNFL) in the absence of other ocular diseases or congenital anomalies [1].

Elevated IOP has long been associated with glaucoma in retrospective studies [2]. Recent prospective studies in ocular hypertensive patients have suggested the relationship between IOP and the onset of POAG [3] and shown that topical ocular hypotensive medication can prevent or delay the onset of glaucoma in patients with ocular hypertension (OHT) [4].

Further more we have evidence suggesting that decreasing intraocular pressure actually helps to slow the progression of the glaucomatous damage not only in high pressure POAG [5-7] but also in glaucoma patients with statistically normal IOP [8].

Nevertheless, the assumption that IOP is the only relevant risk factor is changing. There is sufficient evidence to suggest that elevated IOPs are not responsible for the development of all glaucoma cases and that reducing IOP is not effective in avoiding the deterioration of visual function of each and every glaucoma patient.

The Ocular Hypertension treatment Study (OHTS) [4] reported that the conversion rate of ocular hypertensive patients to glaucoma is low (at 60 months, the cumulative probability of developing POAG was 9.5% in the observation group).

The Early Manifest Glaucoma Trial (EMGT) [7] was a multicenter study designed to compare the effect of immediately lowering the intraocular pressure (IOP), vs. no treatment or later treatment, on the progression of newly detected open-angle glaucoma (OAG). Although the risk of visual field progression was significantly lower for the treated group, compared to the control group, 59% of the patients in this group were estimated to progress after 8 years.

The Advanced Glaucoma Intervention Study (AGIS) [5], suggested that in the eyes with 100% of IOP measurements (through out 6 years of follow-up) below 18 mm Hg (mean IOP 12.3 mm Hg) a worsening of four or more units of visual field defect score from baseline was experienced by 13.1% of eyes at 2 years, 13.9% at 5 years, and 14.4% at 7 years. In summary, it seems clear that maintaining intraocular pressure less than 18 mm Hg does not ensure the preservation of the visual field.

There is increasing evidence that ocular blood flow changes are involved in both the pathogenesis of glaucoma [9-11] and in progression of glaucomatous damage [12-15].

In a prospective study, published by our group [14], designed to assess the value of color Doppler imaging (CDI) of the ophthalmic artery (OA) and short-posterior ciliary arteries (SPCA) in the prognosis of disease progression in POAG patients, the authors prospectively follow a cohort of newly diagnosed untreated POAG patients. According to results of this study, the only independent predictors of progression were the resistivity indices (RI) of the OA and SPCA.

The eyes with RI above the optimal points (i.e. the points that provide best discrimination for both sensitivity and specificity) in the OA and SPCA showed a significantly greater rate of progression even when the curves were adjusted for other factors. In summary, ischemia is a primary and independent factor for progression in eyes with POAG and elevated IOP.

Based on the body of evidences suggesting the role of ocular blood flow (OBF) disturbances in the pathogenesis of glaucoma, much effort has been made to investigate the ocular circulation in detail.

This chapter aims to give an overview over:

1. To briefly review the different techniques available for the assessment of ocular blood flow in humans.
2. To review the current data regarding the role of ocular blood flow in patients with glaucoma.
3. To evaluate the relationship between ocular blood flow disturbances and glaucoma progression.

2. Techniques for Assessing Ocular Blood Flow

Although there have been many advances in techniques over the past 30 years, unfortunately there is not a single method that can provide all the relevant information in one reading. The measurement of the ocular blood flow is complicated by the fact that the posterior pole of the eye receives the blood supply by two different vascular beds, the retina and the choroid (table 1).

Table 1. Arterial Blood Supply of the Anterior Optic Nerve Head

Optic Nerve Head Regions	Vessels	Blood Supply
Superficial nerve fiber layer	Central retinal artery (CRA)	1. Recurrent retinal arterioles 2. ONH Centripetal branches from recurrent arteries 3. Temporal region may have contribution from the cilioretinal artery, when it is present.
Prelaminar region	Short-posterior ciliary artery (SPCA)	1. Direct branches from SPCA 2. Branches from circle of Zinn-Haler, when it is present 3. Small centripetal arteries or arterioles branches from the larger vessels from the choroidal vasculature
Laminar region	SPCA	1. Direct branches from SPCA 2. Branches from circle of Zinn-Haler, when it is present 3. Occasionally branches from pial arteries 4. Small centripetal arteries or arterioles branches from the larger vessels from the choroidal vasculature
Retrolaminar region	CRA;SPCA	1. Branches from SPCA 2. Pial artery branches coursing adjacent to the retrolaminar region. 3. Pial arteries originate from the CRA and from branches of the SPCA

In addition, the interpretation of the results is hampered by the fact that it is difficult to decide whether an increase in blood flow velocity is caused by an increase of blood flow, or by vasoconstriction within the measured vascular bed.

The fact that the different devices available also measures different aspects of ocular hemodynamics and at different locations (for instance retrobulbar blood flow or choroidal blood flow) in the eye makes direct comparisons between techniques all but easy (table 2).

Table 2. Summary of ocular blood flow measurement techniques and the parameters used. Adapted from Flammer et al [11]

Method	Vascular bed	Parameter measured	Interpretation
Doppler Ultrasound	Retrobulbar vessels	Blood flow velocity	Retrobulbar blood flow velocity Resistivity Index
Langham`s pneumotonometer	Choroid	Intraocular pressure (IOP)	Pulsatile choroidal blood flow
Laser Interferometry	Choroid, optic disc	Varying distance between cornea and retina	Ocular fundus pulsation
Laser Doppler flowmetry	Choroid, optic disc	Effect of capillary blood flow on laser light	Capillary blood flow in the choroid or optic disc
Laser Doppler velocimetry	Retina	Blood flow velocity in retinal vessels	Blood flow velocity in large retinal vessels
Confocal scanning laser Doppler flowmetry	Optic disc, retina	Effect of capillary blood flow on retinal surface as well as on laser light	Capillary blood flow in the innermost layers of the retina or the optic disk
Fluorescein angiography	Retina	Velocity of small intravascular substances	Velocity of retinal blood flow
Indocyanine green	Choroid	Velocity of intravascular proteins	Velocity of choroidal blood flow
Retinal vessels diameter analyzer	Retina	Retinal vessels diameter variation over time	Vascular diameter of the retinal vessels
Canon laser Doppler blood flowmetry	Retina	Retinal vessels diameter and blood flow velocity	Retinal blood flow
Laser speckle phenomenon	Retina, optic disc	Effect of varying surface irregularities on laser light	Capillary blood flow in the innermost layers of the retina or the optic disk
Blue field entoptic technique	Foveal retina	Entoptic phenomenon produced by leukocytes	Capillary blood flow of the retina in immediate proximity of the fovea
Color Doppler optical coherence tomography	Retina	Blood flow velocity in retinal vessels	Blood flow velocity in large retinal vessels
Retinal oximetry	Retina	Retinal oxygen levels	Oxygen saturation
Nailfold capillary microscopy	Nailfold capillaries	Blood flow velocity	Capillary blood flow velocity
Method	Vascular bed	Parameter measured	Interpretation
Corneal temperature	Integrative measure of ocular blood flow with overwhelming influence of the choroid	Corneal temperature	Uveal blood flow
Smart lens	Retina	Intraocular pressure	Allows to assess the effect of IOP on retinal blood flow
Peripheral laser Doppler flowmetry	Peripheral vessels precapillaries, capillaries and shunt-vessels of the skin	Effect of capillary blood flow on laser light	Capillary blood flow in the skin

2.1. Doppler Ultrasound

Doppler ultrasound combines B-scan images from tissue structures with velocity information obtained from the Doppler shift of the moving blood cells. A Doppler ultrasound test uses reflected sound waves to evaluate blood as it flows through a blood vessel.

This method has been widely used in many different field of medicine. In ophthalmology is used to measure blood flow velocities in the retrobulbar vessels.

During Doppler ultrasound, a handheld instrument (transducer) is passed lightly over the skin above a blood vessel. The transducer sends and receives sound waves that are amplified through a microphone. The sound waves bounce off solid objects, including blood cells. The movement of blood cells causes a change in pitch of the reflected sound waves (called the Doppler Effect).

There are four types of Doppler Ultrasound:

- "B"Bedside" or continuous wave Doppler. This type uses the change in pitch of the sound waves to provide information about blood flow through a blood vessel.
- Duplex Doppler. Duplex Doppler ultrasound uses standard ultrasound methods to produce a picture of a blood vessel and the surrounding organs. In addition, a computer converts the Doppler sounds into a graph that provides information about the speed and direction of blood flow through the blood vessel being evaluated.
- Color Doppler. Color Doppler uses standard ultrasound methods to produce a picture of a blood vessel. In addition, a computer converts the Doppler sounds into colors that are overlaid on the image of the blood vessel and that represent the speed and direction of blood flow through the vessel.
- Power Doppler. Power Doppler is a newer ultrasound technique that is up to 5 times more sensitive in detecting blood flow than color Doppler. Power Doppler can obtain some images that are difficult or impossible to obtain using standard color Doppler. However, power Doppler is most commonly used to evaluate blood flow through vessels within solid organs.

The most commonly used in Ophthalmology is the Color Doppler Imaging (figure 1). The CDI is a variation in the technology of pulse Doppler processing. The frequency shift information contained in the radiofrequency pulses returning to the transducer along one line is decoded at a given depth along this line, depending on the corresponding time delay. A mean value of the frequency shift is extracted for each point along this line. This is then done for multiple lines as defined as a color box [16-19].

The resistivity index (RI), calculated as [RI= PSV-EDV/PSV], varies from 0 to 1 with higher values supposedly indicating higher vascular distal resistance. However, it is unclear whether the RI represents an adequate measure of retinal vascular resistance [22]. Measurements of the OA and CRA can be obtained relatively easy, whereas obtaining data from the short posterior ciliary arteries requires some experience.

The reproducibility of CDI measurements has been studied using test/retest analysis and also depends on the experience of the observer [23-25].

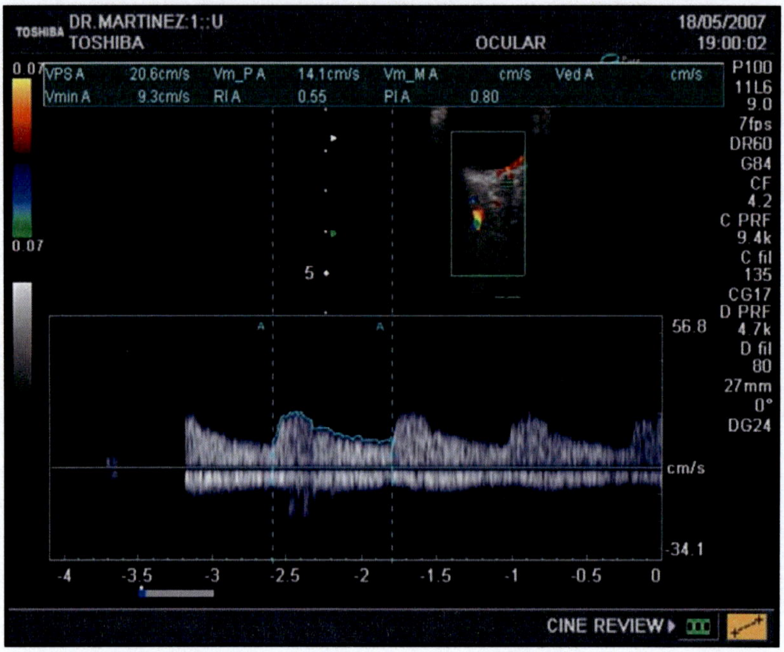

Figure 1. Color Doppler imaging of the central retinal artery and vein taken with a 7.5 MHz linear probe (Toshiba Aplio). The Doppler shifted spectrum (time velocity curve) is displayed at the bottom of the image of the image. Red and blue pixels represent blood movement toward and away from the transducer, respectively.

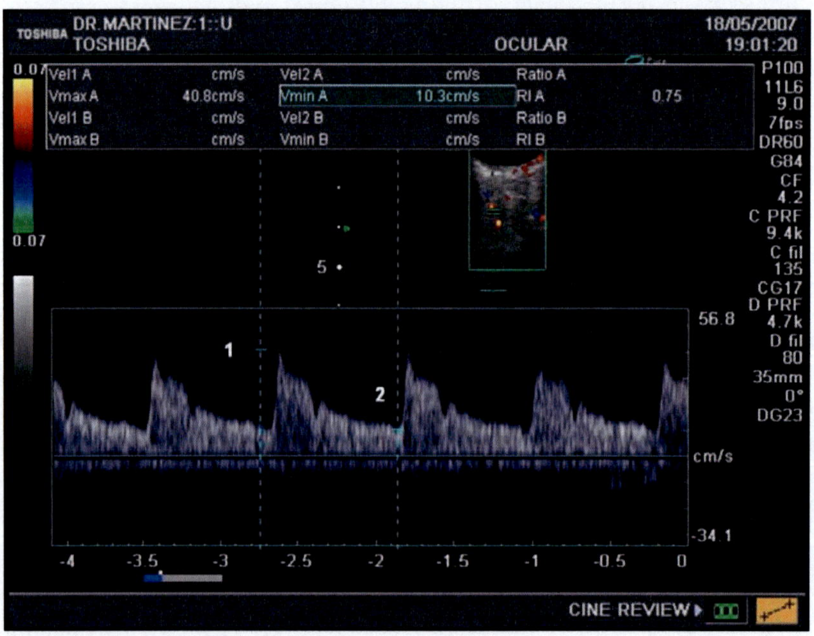

Figure 2. Color Doppler imaging of the ophthalmic artery taken with a 7.5 MHz linear probe (Toshiba Aplio). 1. represents the peak systolic velocity (PSV) (the highest velocity at systole); 2. represents the end-diastolic velocity EDV) (the lowest velocity at diastole). Pourcelot`s Resistivity Index (RI) can be calculated according with the following formula: RI= PSV – EDV / PSV.

One important limitation of this technique is that no quantitative information of vessels diameter is obtained. Therefore, calculation of blood flow is not possible with this method.

The operator identifies the peak systolic velocity (PSV) (Highest velocity at systole) and the end-diastolic velocity (EDV) (lowest velocity at diastole), from these points both velocities are measured (figure 2). In addition, the pulsatility and resistivity indices can be calculated [20, 21].

2.2. Pulsatile Ocular Blood Flow

The pulsatile ocular blood flow (POBF) device is a modified pneumotonometer interface with a microcomputer that records IOP and IOP pulse amplitudes, which are then converted to a calculation of total blood flow [26, 27].

This technique estimates the changes in IOP during the cardiac cycle; blood surges into the blood vessels during systole and continues to flow in more gradually during diastole.

The Langham ocular blood flow system measures the pulse wave of the rhythmic change in IOP during the cardiac cycle (figure 3). Using this principle, it has been proposed that real time measurements of IOP can be used to calculate the pulsatile component of blood flow [28, 29].

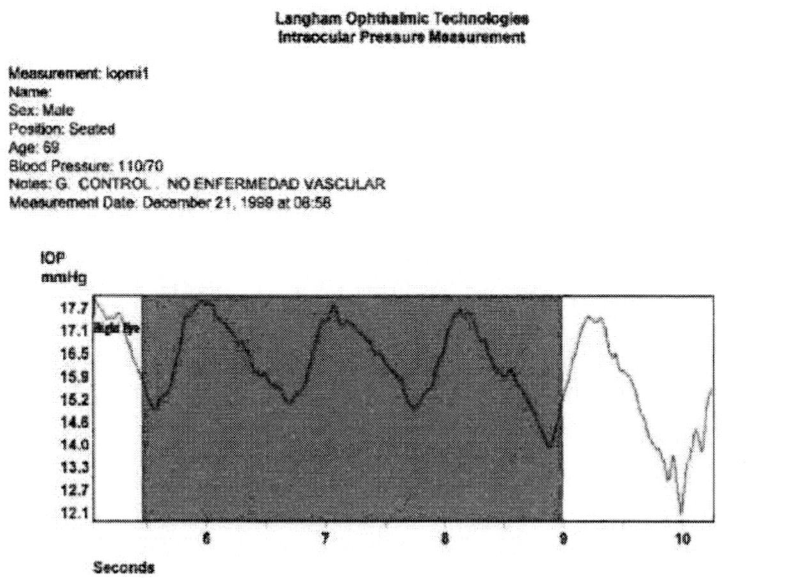

Pulse	Start Time (sec)	IOPmin (mmHg)	IOPmax (mmHg)	Amplitude (mmHg)	Volume (microlit)	POBF (microlit/min)
1	6.57	15.25	18.24	2.99	6.62	806.33
2	6.66	15.42	18.07	2.65	5.86	759.26
3	7.75	15.28	17.87	2.59	5.79	710.11
Avg		15.32	18.06	2.74	6.09	758.57

Figure 3. Langham`s pneumotonometry image. This image corresponds to a 69 years-old female, in sitting position. Three different measurements are obtained in each sitting. The data obtained are: Column 3: Minimum intraocular pressure (IOP); Column 4: Maximum IOP; Column 5: Amplitude of IOP; Column 6: Volume; Column 7: Pulsatile ocular blood flow. Image courtesy of Javier Benitez Del Castillo, MD.

Another approach to the measurement of the POBF is measuring distance changes between cornea and retina during the cardiac cycle [30, 31]. This phenomenon is called fundus pulsation amplitude (FPA).

Both approaches (pneumotonometer and interferometry [32]) are convenient for intra-individual studies rather than comparing different groups.

Although the exact proportion of the total ocular blood flow that is pulsatile is currently unknown, estimates indicate it to be between 50 and 80% [26].

Nonetheless, the physiological interpretation of POBF recording remains uncertain. Because most of the blood flow into the eye is within the choroidal circulation, it is presumed that POBF primarily measures the pulsatile component of choroidal perfusion, independent from the retinal circulation [26].

It seems clear that the main limitation of these techniques is related to the lack of information on the non-pulsatile component of ocular blood flow.

2.3. Laser Doppler Techniques

According to the Doppler Effect, the change in wavelength of the reflected radiation is a function of the targeted object's relative velocity. Thus, the velocity of the object can be obtained by measuring the change in wavelength of the reflected laser light, which is done by forming an interference fringe pattern.

Measurement of red cell blood velocities using this technique was first described in 1972 by Riva and co-workers [33, 34]. The laser Doppler principle can be used in different ways.

2.3.1. Laser Doppler Flowmetry

Laser Doppler flowmetry (LDF) is an established technique for the real-time measurement of microvascular red blood cell perfusion in tissue. Perfusion is sometimes also referred to as microvascular blood flow or red blood cell flux.

Based on the scattering theory for light in tissue formulated by Bonner and Nossal [35] that assumes a complete randomization of light directions impinging on the erythrocytes, relative measures of the mean velocity of the red cells can be obtained [36, 37].

This technique measures the blood flow in capillary beds, with the laser directed to areas between larger vessels [35, 38].

Probably, the most important issue of this technique is the depth of penetration by the light used, in order to know which component of the tissue are being studied [39]. Two wavelengths have been used, the first one uses a visible light wavelength to measure the blood flow in the optic nerve head and retina, while the second one uses a longer wavelength that penetrates the tissue further and measures choroidal blood flow underneath the macula [37, 40].

These methods provide information on capillary blood flow at a select location over a fixed period of time in Blood Perfusion Units (BPU) which is a relative unit scale defined using a carefully controlled motility standard comprising a suspension of latex spheres undergoing Brownian motion.

This technique does not allow easy comparison between individuals because of a considerable variation in scattering properties between subjects. This variation is thought to be related to variations in vascular density and vessels orientation within the relatively small volume of tissue sample by LDF.

Ergo, interindividual comparisons of baseline values are generally not useful in LDF techniques. Nevertheless, given the relatively high intraindividual reproducibility [41], which may even be improved by introducing correction factors [42], LDF has considerable potential in investigation reactivity of the ocular vasculature to different physiological and pharmacological stimuli [19].

One important limitation of this technique is the difficulty for interpreting the LDF data, as the source of measured Doppler shifts may be both the retinal and choroidal vasculature [43]. LDF is now, consequently, more often used to measure choroidal blood flow in the foveal avascular zone [29, 44].

2.3.2. Laser Doppler Velocimetry

Laser Doppler Velocimetry (LDV) is a non-intrusive technique that measures three directional components and can virtually access any flow region with the aid of fiber optics.

LDV makes use of the coherent wave nature of laser light. The crossing of two laser beams of the same wavelength produces areas of constructive and destructive interference patterns. Velocity measurements are made when particles 'seeded' in the flow pass through the fringe pattern created by the intersection of a pair of laser beams. These particles scatter light in all directions when going through the beam crossing. The frequency of the scattered light is Doppler shifted and referred to as the Doppler frequency of the flow.

This method provides fast, direct, and quantitative measurements of absolute blood velocity [45, 46]. From concomitant measurement of retinal vessels diameter, cross-sectional area total retinal blood flow in one single vessel can be calculated [47]. However, this method provides only data on a single vessel and not information about the perfusion in the rest of the eye [11].

2.3.3. Confocal Scanning Laser Doppler Flowmetry

The confocal scanning laser Doppler flowmetry or Heidelberg Retinal Flowmeter (HRF) technique combines the principles of laser Doppler flowmetry with confocal scanning laser tomography [48, 49].

Using an infrared laser, the retina or optic disc is scanned two-dimensionally. Light reflected or scattered at moving objects is frequency shifted due to the optical Doppler Effect. It interferes with unchanged light reflected at surrounding tissue. The interference causes characteristic temporal intensity variations of the measurable reflected light intensity. The HRF measures this temporal intensity variation at each point in the two-dimensional scan field by multiple scanning. The Doppler frequency shift of the reflected light is computed from the acquired data and used to quantify the local velocity of moving particles. This device obtains images of 2560 μm x 640μm x 400μm deep region of the retina or optic nerve head with a measure accuracy of 10μm. Upon completion of the scan, the HRF computer performs a fast Fourier transformation to extract the point-by-point Doppler frequency shift or reflected light.

On its default setting, the HRF analyzes a 10 pixel x 10 pixel (100μm x 100μm region of tissue [48-50].

This is a non-invasive method and results are rapidly obtained. However, it requires clear optic media and good fixation [11].

The reproducibility of the small sampling boxes (10 pixel x 10 pixel) has been demonstrated to be time dependent, with the coefficients of variation of measurements taken each week for 4-weeks averaging 30% of the mean [29, 51].

Application of improved and sophisticated software may provide better results [52, 53].

Measures in the retina are, however, hindered by the fact that a contribution from the underlying choriocapillaris cannot be excluded and information very high and very low speeds could be lost due to the narrow frequency band used [19, 54].

2.4. Angiography

Angiography visualizes the passage of fluorescent dye through ocular vessels. Most approaches are based on the measurement of the time required for the dye to pass through the retinal circulation. The arterio-venous passage time, defined as the time between the first appearance of the dye in a retinal artery and in the corresponding vein [55], has been used to assess retinal blood velocities.

Fluorescein makes it possible to study the retinal circulation in great detail and the optic nerve head with some extent, while indocyanine green is used for better visualization of choroidal circulation [56, 57].

These approaches have been adapted employing videoangiography [55, 58] and scanning laser ophtalmoscopy [59, 60].

Scanning laser ophthalmoscope (SLO) was first introduced by Robert Webb and colleagues [61]. The fundus is illuminated with a narrow laser beam that is scanned over surface of retina and a detector captures the reflected light.

In SLO the laser beam is scanned horizontally and vertically and the timing is designated to synchronize with a wide range of computer and video equipment. The image of the fundus is viewed in real time on a monitor, typically with frame rate ranging 20-30 frames per second.

Typical image pixilation numbers are 512 x 512 or 1024 x 1024 pixel per image. Recently, a new scanning laser ophthalmoscope has been introduced that has a pixilation 2000 x 2000 for a single frame and a field view oa120 degrees.

SLO increases the capability of quantitative angiography by enhancing image contrast and temporal resolution. The SLO can be used for fluorescein or indocyanine green angiography [62-64].

Several caveats should be considered when interpreting data from this technique [19]. The foremost limitation of SLO is that the technique is based on the assumption that all the blood flow of an area supplied by one specific artery is drained by the corresponding vein, which may not hold true in all cases [57, 60]. In addition, SLO imaging is required used of highly invasive techniques, including pupil dilation and dye injections. Furthermore, indocyanine green dye-dilution techniques are not widely used and therefore have limited comparison.

Although SLO techniques are highly accuracies methods for assessing retinal and choroidal circulation, their invasive used and difficult interpretation make difficult to justify their used for many patients.

2.5. Retinal Vessels Diameter Analyzers

The technique mentioned so far are limited by the fact that only information about blood velocity is available but not blood flow per se.

Thus, to determine blood flow, we need to know the exact diameter of the vessels.

2.5.1. Retinal Vessels Analyzer

The Retinal Vessel Analyzer (RVA) is a measuring device for online measurement of the diameter of retinal vessels in relation to time and locations along the vessel. An essential part of the RVA is the fundus camera (FF450, Zeiss Jena, Germany). This optical instrument enables the examination of the background area of the eye. It incorporates two optical pathways, the illumination pathway and the observation pathway. Both of them use the (dilated) pupil as an entrance to the patient's eye. The illumination light reflected by the different layers of the retina is delivered to an observation ocular and the measuring CCD-camera simultaneously [65].

Continuous recording of the vessel diameter during a measurement session results in a measuring data basis, available for further analysis after the end of the measurement.

Reproducibility, of this technique, strongly depends on measuring conditions. Influencing factors are variation of measuring location inside image field and on the vessel, measuring time (vasomotoric waves), eye movements in vessel direction and others [66].

For research in microcirculation the RVA provides a measuring device and numerous analysis methods to observe retinal microcirculation offering a wide range of possible applications [65].

This device may be useful in the assessment of the effect of vasoactive substances on the large retinal vessels. RVA, however, may be insensitive to changes in the peripheral vascular tone or changes in blood flow due to altered blood rheology.

2.5.2. Canon Laser Blood Flowmetry

The Canon laser Doppler blood flowmetry (CLDBF) combines a retinal vessels diameter assessment system with the principle of retinal blood speed measurement by the means of laser Doppler Velocimetry [67].

The CLDBF is the only blood flow device currently available that is capable of calculating volumetric blood flow to the retina.

This device uses a modified fundus camera equipped with 2 lasers, the first measuring blood velocity and the second simultaneously measuring vessels diameter while tracking its location [68, 69].

The main limitation of this technique is the fact that there is not single relation between the maximum velocity (measured by CLDBF) and the average velocity (used to calculate flow).

In a laminar flow system, the average velocity is half of the maximum velocity, whereas, in a turbulent flow system, the average velocity is equal to the maximum velocity. The CLDBF system uses something in between these 2 values [29].

2.6. Laser Speckle Phenomenon

In this technique the scattered laser light from the surface of the cortex produces a speckle pattern, which is imaged onto a camera. By analyzing the spatial statistics of the speckle pattern, one determines the speckle contrast, which can be related to a measure of blood flow [70, 71].

Laser speckle imaging (LSI) is an optical technique that can be used to measure local dynamic properties in scattering media both at high temporal and spatial resolution. The underlying principle of LSI is equivalent to the one exploited in LDF. A moving object inside the tissue, such as an erythrocyte, leads to a Doppler shift of the frequency of scattered light, which is directly proportional to the velocity. Rather than analyzing Doppler frequency shifts LSI monitors temporal fluctuations of the scattered light in order to map dynamics.

In LSI a digital camera records the surface intensity pattern of light reflected from a scattering medium. In the absence of movement (or for very short exposure time) there is no detectable fluctuation and the typical granular interference pattern, called speckle, has the same properties in the entire field of view.

There are two basic ways of observing LSI. The first is to image the illuminated area. Whether this is done by the eye or by a camera, a granular speckle pattern will be seen on the surface of the object. This type is known as “image speckle”. The second way is to shine a narrow laser beam at the object and look at the scattered light falling on a screen some distance away. This type of speckle is called “far-filled speckle” [11].

The main disadvantage of this technique is the fact that this device measures blood flow velocities only, since not information of vessels diameters are available.

2.7. Blue Field Entoptic Technique

This technique is based on the flow of leukocytes to assess retinal blood flow [72].

The blue field entoptic phenomenon or Scheerer's phenomenon is the appearance of tiny bright dots moving quickly along squiggly lines in the visual field, especially when looking into blue light (such as the sky) [73]. This is a normal effect that can be perceived by almost everybody. The dots are due to the white blood cells that move in the capillaries in front of the retina of the eye, near the macula [74].

The cellular origin of the entoptically produced bright particles (which often show a dark tail) is controversial. Vierodt first suggested that the particle phenomenon was produced by leukocytes [75] and this was supported by Bauermann who observed in leukemics that variations in the number of particles which passed repeatedly through one of the paths paralleled variations in the peripheral white blood cell count [76].

The entoptic phenomenon is optimally perceived in the deep blue light spectrum at 430 nm, perhaps because hemoglobin has an absorption peak at this wavelength, which may produce relative dark adaptation of the photoreceptors lying beneath capillaries filled with red blood cells.

By comparing and adjusting the number and the mean velocity of the particles in the observed simulated particle field with their own perception an estimated of perimacular white blood cell flux can be obtained.

However, this method is subjective in nature and the quality of the data depends on the patient's full cooperation. In addition, there are large variations between patients and only data from capillaries around the fovea are provided.

Furthermore, it is not clear whether leukocyte flux is proportional to retinal blood flow under all clinical conditions [77].

2.8. Color Doppler Optical Coherence Tomography

Color Doppler Optical coherence tomography (CDOCT) is a non-invasive technique that can be coupled with optical coherence tomography (OCT) to measure the velocity of blood flow within biological tissues.

The technique is based on optical Doppler tomography, which combines Doppler velocimetry with optical coherence tomography to measure blood flow velocity at discrete spatial locations in turbid biological tissue [78, 79].

The flow velocity can be determined by measurement of the Doppler shift of the interference fringe frequency with a short-time Fourier transform or a Hilbert transform [80].

This device offers some additional advantages. Using a broad-band light source in the interferometer enables depth localization of retinal flow with unprecedented axial resolution. In addition to decreasing the spatial resolution to approximately 10 to 20 μm, low-coherence interferometry improves the rejection of light outside the focal volume, resulting in a higher signal-tonoise ratio than confocal detection alone [78].

However, CDOCT has been used only for imaging of large vessels near the optic nerve head. Improvement of both the spatial and velocity resolutions is required for imaging retinal microvasculature, which is composed of smaller-diameter vessels with slower-flow velocities. The velocity resolution depends on the amount of time spent in detecting the Doppler shifts at a given location in the tissue. Therefore, to improve velocity resolution for detecting smaller blood flow velocities, the CDOCT image acquisition time has to be increased, which precludes imaging in a moving sample such as the human retina [78].

2.9. Retinal Oximetry

Although retinal oximetry is not a method for measuring ocular blood flow, the measurements of retinal tissue oxygenation would reveal some aspects of the impact of ischemia on retinal ganglion cell health and function.

Studies of oxygenation of the optic nerve have mainly been studied with invasive techniques in laboratory animals.

Nevertheless, a non-invasive device to measure retinal oxygen levels is needed for the clinical study of oxygen levels in humans. The oxygen saturation of a solution of hemoglobin can be measured by differential spectrometry using two or more wavelengths. Spectro photometric measurements of hemoglobin oxygen saturation in human retinal blood vessels was initiated by Hickam et al [81] in the 1960s but has still not been mastered as a reliable and useful clinical or research tool.

During the past years, there have been developed non-invasive automatic retinal oximeters, which probably will allow studies of human retinal and optic nerve disease in research and clinical settings [85].

Retinal oximetry is composed of a fundus camera coupled with a beam splitter to a digital camera. The beam splitter separates the original image into four optical channels. In each channel, there is a different narrow band-pass filter, through which only light of specific wavelengths can pass. The center wavelengths of the filters are 542, 558, 586, and 605 nm and the half-bandwidth is 5 nm, except for the 542-nm filter, which has a 9-nm half-bandwidth.

With a specialized computer program, optical density can be calculated for every vessel at each of the four wavelengths. Optical density is a measure of the blood's light absorbance and it can be shown that the ratio of optical density at certain wavelengths (OD ratio, ODR) has an inverse and approximately linear relationship to hemoglobin oxygenation [82, 84]. Thus, in theory, hemoglobin oxygenation can be calculated using brightness inside and outside vessels at two wavelengths of light.

The advantages of the new retinal oximeters are that the measurement area is large, and little expertise is needed to acquire a pseudocolor fundus image of retinal vessel oxygenation [85].

The greatest limitation of this technique is that it has not been validated in animal model with a sufficient extent to consider it clinically accurate [29].

In addition, with the current devices, measurement of hemoglobin restricts the analysis to the vessels.

3. The Role of Ocular Blood Flow in Glaucoma

The apparent ability of many eyes to withstand raised pressures without developing glaucomatous damage has caused much speculation on the protective role of the ocular blood supply, particularly to the optic nerve head.

However, assessing the findings of OBF studies in glaucoma is difficult for the following reasons: The studies use different techniques and consequently measuring different aspects of ocular circulation [86]. In addition, the published studies include different types of glaucoma [i.e. normal-tension glaucoma (NTG) vs. high tension glaucoma (HTG)]; glaucoma patients at different stages (i.e. early vs. late glaucoma).

Nevertheless, different studies using different types of instruments point in the same general direction, indicating that on average, blood flow is decreased in some glaucoma patients, especially in primary open-angle glaucoma patients and in patients who progressed despite normalized intraocular pressure [11, 87].

The fact that ocular blood low disturbances can be observed not only in the ocular and retrobulbar vessels, but also in the naildfold capillaries [88], indicates that the reduction in blood flow may be not only secondary either due to IOP increase or due to the glaucomatous optic neuropathy.

Table 3. Summary of the findings of ocular blood flow studies and the method used

Method	Vascular bed	Findings in Glaucoma Patients
Doppler Ultrasound	Retrobulbar vessels	Reduced blood flow velocity Increased resistivity Index
Langham`s pneumotonometer	Choroid	Reduced pulsatile ocular blood flow
Laser Interferometry	Choroid, optic disc	Reduced fundus pulsation amplitude
Laser Doppler flowmetry	Choroid, optic disc	Decreased blood flow in optic disc and choroid
Laser Doppler velocimetry	Retina	Reduced blood velocities
Confocal scanning laser Doppler flowmetry	Optic disc, retina	Reduced blood flow in optic disc and retina
Fluorescein angiography	Retina	Reduced blood flow velocity
Indocyanine green	Choroid	Reduced blood flow velocity (especially in normal-tension glaucoma)
Retinal vessels diameter analyzer	Retina	Narrow arteries and dilated veins
Canon laser Doppler blood flowmetry	Retina	Lack of autorregulation and reduced blood flow and velocities
Laser speckle phenomenon	Retina, optic disc	Lack of autorregulation
Blue field entoptic technique	Foveal retina	Lack of autorregulation
Color Doppler optical coherence tomography	Retina	Lack of autorregulation
Retinal oximetry	Retina	Decreased oxygen saturation (related with the glaucomatous damage)
Nailfold capillary microscopy	Nailfold capillaries	Reduced blood flow velocity
Corneal temperature	Integrative measure of ocular blood flow with overwhelming influence of the choroid	Correlation with retrobulbar blood flow (There is not direct comparisons between glaucoma patients and normal subjects)
Peripheral laser Doppler flowmetry	Peripheral vessels precapillaries, capillaries and shunt-vessels of the skin	Decreased blood flow velocity

Blood flow decreases with increasing damage, but the reduction occurs in both early and late stages of glaucoma [89, 90].

In summary, we have evidence that ocular blood flow is altered independently from IOP or level of damage in patients with progressive glaucoma, which could represent a primary risk factor for disease progression [12-15, 87].

In the following section, some of the studies will be summarized according to the objectives and the assessment methods used (table 3).

3.1. Color Doppler Ultrasound

Several studies have compared the vascular parameters in POAG [11, 91-97]; ocular hypertension [94, 98]; angle-closure glaucoma (ACG) [99, 100]; pseudoexfoliative glaucoma (PXG) [101-107]; and NTG [108-116].

They have found, on average, reduced blood flow velocities and increased resistivity indices in the retrobulbar vessels of glaucoma patients [91-116].

Within individuals, retrobulbar blood flow velocities reductions are greater in the eye with more advance damage [90, 96, 117].

Open-angle glaucoma seems to be associated with a decreased mean flow velocity and an increased mean resistivity index in the retrobulbar vessels. Reduced EDV and increased RI in the OA, reduced maximum and minimum velocities in the central retinal vein (CRV), and reduced PSV and EDV in the CRA and SPCA have been observed in eyes with POAG when compared with normal control eyes [90-98, 110, 116].

Few studies investigated the ocular circulatory changes in angle-closure glaucoma patients [99, 100, 118]. Hou et al [118] reported that eyes during acute attack of primary ACG had significant decrease in PSV in the ophthalmic artery compared with the age-matched normal subjects, whereas eyes in the preclinical stage showed no significant changes.

Cheng et al [100] suggested that as in POAG, the retrobulbar circulation was disturbed in the chronic angle-closure glaucoma. Event with well-controlled IOP, retrobulbar hemodynamics were altered significantly more in chronic angle-closure glaucoma eyes with worse visual field than in those with better visual field.

In addition, significant correlation was found between the severity of glaucomatous visual field defects and the degree of impairment of retrobulbar hemodynamics.

A significant decreased for PSV and EDV and an increase for RI at the OA, SPCA, and CRA in exfoliation syndrome have been reported by previous studies [101-103, 107].

Conversely, our study showed that patients with pseudoexfoliation syndrome, compared with age-matched healthy subjects, had similar peak systolic, end-diastolic and resistivity indices in all the arteries studied [106].

With regards to the comparison between pseudoexfoliative and primary open-angle glaucoma, literature data are still controversial. While Yüksel et al [101] and Detorakis et al [103] found that some retrobulbar hemodynamic parameters were more altered in PXG patients, Martínez & Sánchez [104] reported that color Doppler alterations were more pronounced in POAG than in PXG patients.

A decrease in retrobulbar blood flow has been reported in cases of NTG [108-116, 118]. Harris et al [108] showed that patients with NTG exhibited a low EDV and a high RI in the ophthalmic artery compared with controls.

Kondo et al [112] investigated the retrobulbar hemodynamics by means of color Doppler imaging in NTG patients with asymmetric visual field loss and asymmetric ocular perfusion pressure. The results of this study suggested that there are significant differences in blood velocities and in the RI in the retrobulbar vessels between the eyes with higher ocular perfusion pressure and a better mean deviation, and those with higher ocular perfusion pressure and a worse mean deviation.

Furthermore, Rankin et al [119] found that in both POAG and NTG there is a significant decrease in the mean blood velocity and increase in the mean RI at the level of the CRA and SPCA.

The influence of ocular blood flow disturbances on the progression of the glaucomatous damage has only been recognized more recently [12-15] (table 4).

Table 4. Summary Analysis of Retrobulbar Blood Flow Velocity Studies and Visual Field Progression

Study	Subjects	Time of follow-up	Doppler parameter	Visual field results
Galassi et al [12]	44 POAG	7-years	RI OA≥ 0.78	18/44 patients progressed RI OA≥ 0.78 (14/18 progressed) RI OA< 0.78 (4/18 progressed)
Satilmis et al [13]	20 POAG	4.3 years	Reduced EDV CRA	Multiple r= 0.63 (p=0.0037)
Martínez & Sánchez [14]	51 POAG	3 years	RI OA > 0.72 RI SPCA > 0.65	23/49 patients progressed RI OA > 0.72 & RI SPCA > 0.65 (21/23 progressed) RI OA ≤ 0.72 & RI SPCA ≤ 0.65 (2/23 progressed)
Zeitz et al [15]	114 OAG	1 year	Reduced PSV CRA Reduced PSV SPCA Reduced EDV SPCA	12/114 patients progressed

Abbreviations: POAG= primary open-angle glaucoma; OAG= open-angle glaucoma; OA= ophthalmic artery; SPCA= short-posterior ciliary artery; CRA= central retinal artery; PSV= peak systolic velocity; EDV= end-diastolic velocity; RI= resistivity index.

Galassi and co-workers [12] evaluated the effect of retrobulbar blood flow circulation on the progression of visual field damage in POAG patients. This study included 44 patients with POAG over a period of 7 years. The results of this study suggested that patients with low diastolic velocities and high resistivity indices in the ophthalmic artery had more progressive visual field.

Satilmis and collaborators [13] in a retrospective, observational and case series study evaluate the correlation between progression rate of glaucomatous damage and retrobulbar blood flow. Based on the results of this study, independent of the extend of damage or IOP the visual field deterioration significantly correlates with retrobulbar hemodynamic variables (figure 4).

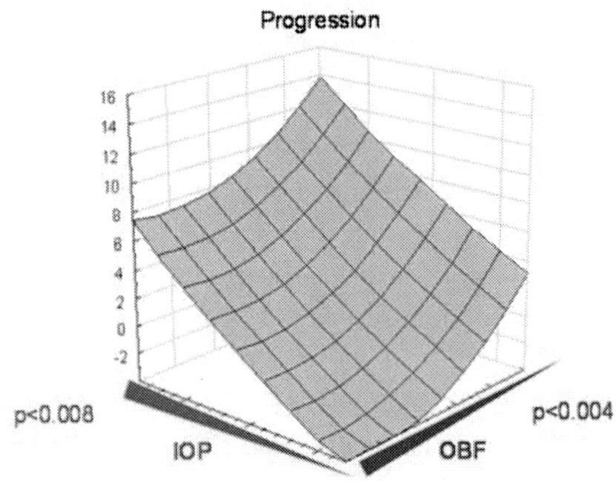

Figure 4. Rate of glaucoma progression correlates with retrobulbar hemodynamic parameters and intraocular pressure. The higher the intraocular pressure, the higher chance of progression. Likewise, the lower the ocular blood flow, the higher the chance of progression. IOP= Intraocular pressure; OBF= Ocular blood flow.

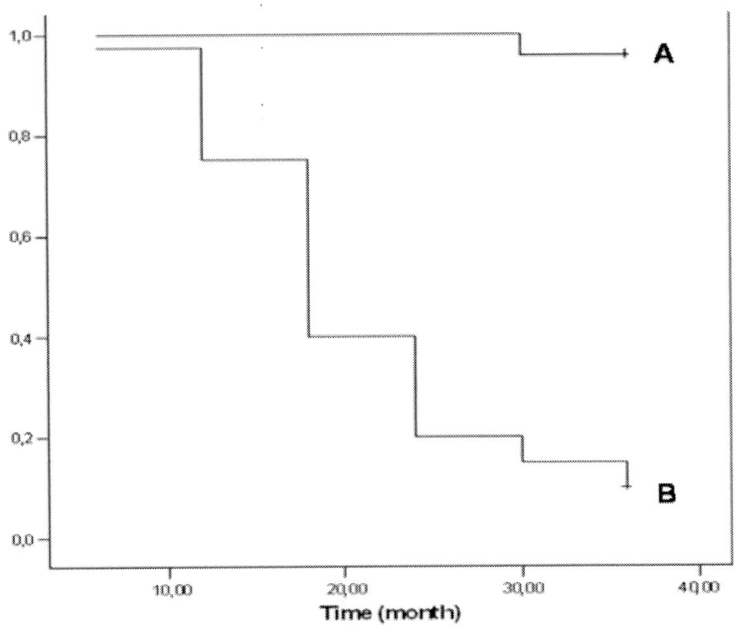

Figure 5. Progression-free survival curve according to the resistivity index (RI) of the ophthalmic artery and short-posterior ciliary arteries. Cut-off values: 1. RI= 0.72 for the ophthalmic artery; 2. RI= 0.65 for the short-posterior ciliary arteries; A= RI below cut-off value in both arteries, rate of progression 4.2%; B= RI above cut-off value in both arteries, rate of progression 90%; Data from Martínez & Sánchez [14].

In addition, Martínez & Sánchez [14], in a prospective cohort study, assessed the value of color Doppler imaging of the ophthalmic artery and short posterior ciliary arteries in prognosis of disease progression in patients with primary open-angle glaucoma. The results of this study suggested that poor blood flow in the retrobulbar vessels is closely link to deterioration in the visual field in patients with POAG and high IOP (figure 5).

3.2. Pulsatile Ocular Blood Flow

Results from pulsatile ocular blood flow analyses in POAG [11, 28, 120-132] patients, pseudoexfoliative glaucoma patients [133], and NTG patients [133-136] show reduced POBF.

Furthermore, although the reductions were more pronounced in patients with visual field loss, they were seen before visual field defects were observed [136].

As regards POAG patients, Kerr et al [126], in a prospective observational study, compared POBF between untreated ocular hypertensive and POAG patients. The results of this study found that POAG and ocular hypertensive patients with an IOP above 25 mm Hg had a significantly lower POBF and pulse volume that ocular hypertensive patients with and IOP below 25 mm Hg. Nevertheless, there were no significant differences between POAG patients and ocular hypertensive patients with an IOP greater than 25 mm Hg.

Similar results were found by Fuchsjäger-Mayrl and co-workers [127] who reported that there was no significant difference in ocular blood flow parameters between patients with POAG and those with OHT.

James & Smith [134] measured the POBF in 22 patients with bilateral NTG and 29 age-matched healthy subjects. The results of this study showed that there was an overall reduction in ocular pulse amplitude, pulse volume, and POBF in subjects with NTG in comparison with a normal volunteer control group.

Aydin et al [125], in a prospective cross sectional study, evaluated POBF analysis in normal subjects and glaucoma patients; and correlated POBF measurements with functional (as determined by visual field [VF]) and structural (as determined by optical coherence tomography). In contrast with previous studies [136, 137], no correlations were found between POBF parameters and either IOP, visual file global indices, or mean retinal nerve fiber layer thickness, with the exception of a significant correlation between POBF and IOP in the glaucoma patients group. The authors concluded that the wide range of normal values and the low discriminating power of POBF between normal and glaucomatous eyes limit the clinical use of the device for glaucoma patients [125].

The laser interferometry [30, 31] was used by Hommer et al [132] for comparing the ocular rigidity. They included in a prospective cross sectional study 70 POAG patients and 70 age matched healthy subjects and assessed the ocular pulse amplitude and POBF with pneumotonometry. The fundus pulsation amplitude was measured by using laser interferometry. Based on tonometric measurements of pulse amplitude and laser interferometric measurements of fundus pulsation amplitude this study indicated that patients with glaucoma have increased ocular structural stiffness [132].

3.3. Laser Doppler Techniques

3.3.1. Laser Doppler Flowmetry

Laser Doppler flowmetry detected circulatory abnormalities consistent with known patterns of glaucomatous loss [138,139].

In subjects with glaucoma, blood flow was significantly lower in the inferotemporal and superotemporal regions of the neuroretinal rim, which are the areas of preferential optic disk damage in glaucoma. Measurements in the nasal rim, which is generally spared from moderate glaucoma damage, did not exhibit any significant alteration in blood flow [140].

As mentioned earlier, because of large inter-patient variations, this method is more suitable for intra-individual comparisons.

Within the clinical applications of LDF, Boehm and collaborators [43] found a decreased blood flow of the temporal neuroretinal rim compared with nasal blood flow in normal healthy subjects, suggesting a potential vulnerability of the temporal neuroretinal rim to ischemic insult.

Zink et al [141] performed a preliminary assessment of the relation between optic nerve circulatory parameters and glaucomatous visual field progression.

This study included 29 eyes of 23 patients with open angle glaucoma (OAG) that had typical glaucomatous nerve fiber bundle visual field defects and increased cup to disc ratios. Laser Doppler flowmetry (Oculix) was used to measure relative optic nerve blood volume velocity and flow in the superior temporal and inferior temporal neuroretinal rim of the optic nerve. In this study patients with lower inferior temporal neuroretinal rim volume tended to have more marked visual field progression. The results of this study suggested that circulatory parameters, assessed by LDF, may have potential for identifying glaucoma patients at risk for future glaucomatous visual field progression [141].

3.3.2. Laser Doppler Velocimetry

Earlier studies by Hamard et al [142, 143] using laser Doppler velocimetry detected decreased velocity of blood in the optic nerve in subjects with glaucoma.

This reduction seems to be associated with rheological alterations [143].

Hamard et al [143] measured the optic disc blood flow velocity in healthy patients, those with primary open angle glaucoma and patients with normal pressure glaucoma. In this study the velocity of the red blood cells (RBCs) in the capillaries of the optic nerve head (ONH) has been measured with a laser Doppler velocimetry, and blood viscosity has been evaluated notably by determining the aggregability of the RBCs with an erythroaggregameter.

The results of this study in POAG patients and normal pressure glaucoma patients showed that their optic nerve blood flow velocity was reduced and that the aggregability of the RBCs was increased [143].

3.3.3. Confocal Scanning Laser Doppler Flowmetry

As it was previously mentioned, the confocal scanning laser Doppler flowmetry or Heidelberg Retinal Flowmeter (HRF) technique combines the principles of laser Doppler flowmetry with confocal scanning laser tomography [48, 49].

A number of studies using HRF have shown that OBF in the optic nerve head and retina of glaucoma patients are reduced [127, 136, 144-152].

Chung et al [153] found reduced blood flow in the peripapillary retina of NTG patients as compared with age-matched healthy subjects.

In another study, Hafez and collaborators [148] found significantly lower blood flow in the neuroretinal rim of the optic nerve head of POAG patients as compared with ocular hypertensive patients and normal subjects. However, No significant differences in ONH blood flow were found between ocular hypertensives and normal volunteers. Furthermore, neuroretinal rim blood flow was significantly inversely correlated to increased C/D ratio. Ocular hypertensives with larger C/D ratios demonstrated significantly lower rim blood flow compared with those with smaller C/D ratios, suggesting that rim perfusion might be reduced in high-risk ocular hypertensives before the manifestation of visual field defects [148].

Similar results were found in a study published by Logan et al [154]. This study aimed to assess retinal blood flow characteristics in subjects with normal tension glaucoma, POAG, and a group of controls using the HRF. This study found no significant differences between POAG and NTG patients. In addition, the glaucoma subjects with normal rim segments had statistically significant lower velocity, flow, and volume measurements than the controls for each location sampled suggesting that differences in the retinal haemodynamics may be able to be detected at an earlier stage than morphological damage [154].

A limited number of papers have evaluated the HRF in pseudoexfoliative glaucoma patients or patients with pseudoexfoliation syndrome [149, 155].

Harju et al [155] compared the optic nerve head and peripapillary retinal blood flow, by using HRF, between the two eyes of patients with unilateral PXG or ocular hypertension with exfoliation syndrome and their fellow normal eyes. This study did not find significant differences in the peripapillary retina between study and control eyes. However, the blood flow of the optic nerve head lamina and rim decreased with increasing glaucomatous damage in the PXG patients. According to the results of this study, advanced glaucomatous damage was associated with reduced flow both in the lamina cribrosa and the rim area but not in the peripapillary retina [155].

In addition there are indications that the reduction precedes the damage in pseudoexfoliative patients [149]. Ocakoglu et al [149] found decreased microvascular perfusion parameters in eyes with clinically detected pseudoexfoliation syndrome without glaucoma [149]. An interesting finding of this paper was the reduced blood flow measurements of fellow eyes with no clinically detected pseudoexfoliation syndrome compared to the age-matched healthy subjects, which may support the idea that pseudoexfoliation syndrome has asymmetric representation with bilateral involvement [149].

The blood flow reductions have been related to larger cup-to-disc ratios [148] and are spatially associated with structural damage to the optic nerve head [154] and to visual field [151].

Sato and co-workers [151] determined the relationship between the blood flow parameters of the optic disc rim and the glaucomatous visual field changes. In an observational cross sectional study the blood flow in the neuroretinal rim within the optic disc was determined with the HRF in 54 eyes of 54 patients with NTG. The results of this study suggested that the blood flow in the neuroretinal rim was found to correspond to the regional visual field defect in eyes with NTG [151].

However, these findings have not been uniform, with some studies showing no reduction [156, 157].

Hollo et al [157] compared the peripapillary blood flow, by means of a HRF, in 40 glaucoma patients and 34 healthy subjects. This study found that the blood flow was significantly reduced in myopia both in controls ($p < 0.05$) and in glaucoma patients ($p < 0.001$). However, there was no difference between both controls and glaucoma patients. The results of this study suggested that capillary perfusion adjacent to the temporal edge of the disc is significantly reduced in myopia but not in glaucoma.

3.4. Angiography

Reduced blood flow in the retina, choroid, and optic nerve head have been observed using angiography in glaucoma patients [158-172].

Different studies assessed the differences between retinal and choroidal hemodynamics in POAG and NTG patients [160, 161, 166].

Whereas retinal circulation is delayed in patients with POAG, choroidal circulation is especially slower in patients with NTG. The choroidal and retinal vascular systems behave differently in primary open-angle and normal-pressure glaucoma, which may be important in the management of glaucoma.

It also has been suggested that areas corresponding to more severe visual field damage have prolonged arteriovenous passage time compared with areas of less damage [162, 173].

In the optic nerve head three types of defects have been described: Local filling defects, slow fillings, and increased leakage [11].

Fluorescein filling defects of the optic nerve head are areas of hypoperfusion, and they have been described in glaucomatous optic neuropathy since the 1970s [174-182]. Absolute filling defects are persistent hypofluorescent areas, and they seem to correspond to capillary dropout in the surface nerve fiber layer of the optic disc [174, 175, 179, 181, 182]. In contrast, relative defects are areas of delayed fluorescence, and they show a slower filling pattern with fluorescein [174, 175, 179]. The filling defects are interpreted as areas of hypovascularity, as they are reproducible, with no consistent correlation with IOP and systemic blood pressure [174, 175, 183].

The number, extent, and topography of fluorescein filling defects correspond to visual field loss, nerve fiber layer defects, and cupping in glaucoma [176, 179, 182, 184, 185].

Absolute fluorescein filling defects of the optic nerve head are statistically significantly larger and are seen more often in patients with POAG and NTG compared with controls [169, 174, 175, 179, 180, 182, 185].

clinical studies [174, 175, 182] dealing with fluorescein angiographic filling defects of the optic nerve head stated that the filling defects, at least in some cases, precede morphologic damage, and vertical studies [182, 185, 186] revealed a strong interrelationship to functional defects.

The few longitudinal follow-up studies available concluded that filling defects emphasized progressive optic nerve damage [159], and new field defects were related to new filling defects in glaucomatous optic neuropathy [172, 187].

Filling defects and delayed filling have also been observed around the optic nerve head, especially when using indocyanine green angiography [165, 182, 185].

3.5. Retinal Vessels Diameter Analyzers

Several studies using different types of instruments point in the same general direction indicating that glaucoma patients have on average relatively narrow arteries and dilated veins [188-190].

Using manual measurements of the vessel diameter from projected images of the retina, Jonas and collaborators [188] demonstrated significantly smaller peripapillary retinal vessel diameters in eyes with OAG than in age-matched normal subjects. Also, Rader et al [189] found general narrowing of retinal artery calibers in 53% (n= 57 patients) of eyes with moderate glaucomatous optic neuropathy and in 71% (n= 56 patients) of eyes with severe glaucomatous optic nerve damage, compared with only 15% (n= 39 subjects) in age-matched healthy subjects. However, these previous studies [188, 189] were limited by use of subjective methods in measuring retinal vessel diameter.

Conflicting results were published about the relationship between OAG and retinal vessels diameter [191, 192].

Mitchell et al [191], in a population-based cross-sectional study, using a reliable computer-assisted method to quantify retinal vessels diameter, eyes with open OAG had significantly narrower adjusted mean retinal arteriolar diameters in a zone outside the immediate peripapillary zone. These eyes were also at least 2 times more likely to have generalized arteriolar narrowing than eyes without glaucoma. In addition, the association was generally similar for high- and low – tension glaucoma. In other words, this study provided data to support an association between narrowing retinal vessel caliber and the presence of glaucomatous optic neuropathy that is independent of blood pressure and other glaucoma risk factors [191].

Conversely, Ikram et al [192], in a population-based, cohort study on chronic diseases in the elderly (part of the Rotterdam Study [193, 194]) found that both retinal arteriolar and venular diameters at baseline were not related to an increased risk of OAG. According with the results of this study, the retinal vessel diameters did not predict incident optic disc changes.

In another paper published by Vlachokosta et al [195] the relation between glaucoma and the variation of vessel diameter by means of advanced image processing algorithms was investigated.

Preliminary results from patients with and without glaucomatous symptoms suggest that glaucoma induces variations of the diameter of retinal vessels [195].

In a retrospective observational case series study Hall et al [196] evaluated the asymmetry of peripapillary retinal vessel caliber between inferior and superior hemispheres in eyes with visual field defects predominantly in one hemifield. The results of this study suggested that the average ratio of the superior temporal artery diameter to inferotemporal artery diameter was significantly greater in the eyes with predominantly superior visual field defects as compared with those with inferior defects. This indicates that the arteriole corresponding to the hemifield with the greater visual field defect was narrower than the arteriole in the other hemifield.

In conclusion, in eyes with POAG, this study reported a strong association between decreased peripapillary arteriole diameter and visual field defects in the corresponding hemifield [196].

3.5.1. Canon Laser Blood Flowmetry

The Canon laser blood flowmetry has been used to assess retinal blood flow rate changes, in response to changes in ocular perfusion pressure resulting from postural changes in OAG patients and compared with those obtained in healthy control subjects [197].

The main finding of this study is that although the control-healthy subjects and glaucoma patients had similar mean arterial pressure, ocular perfusion pressure, and retinal blood flow at baseline, the glaucoma patients, unlike the controls, showed a broad range of retinal hemodynamic responses while reclining compared with sitting [197].

In summary, this study described that lack of autorregulation in a group of OAG patients.

Furthermore, the CLDBF was used to evaluate the relationship between retinal circulatory abnormalities and retinal nerve fiber layer (RNFL) thinning in early-stage open-angle glaucoma [198].

On average, there were significant reductions in retinal blood speed and flow in OAG patients compared to controls. It was odd that there were significant inverse correlations between retinal blood flow and average RNFL thickness and RNFL thickness in the inferior quadrant within the glaucoma group. In other words, the highest retinal blood flow rates were observed in patients with the thinnest RNFL. This finding is consistent with the previous results reported by Feke and associates [199] who found an inverse correlation between optic nerve head capillary blood speed and RNFL thickness at the disc margin in untreated ocular hypertension patients. On the other hand, Plange and associates [97] found a significant positive correlation between central retinal artery blood speed and neuroretinal rim area and volume in patients with more advanced glaucomatous optic neuropathy than in the Berisha et al study [152].

3.6. Laser Speckle Phenomenon

Results available from the literature to date have concentrated mainly on the validation of the technique and study treatment effects [11, 199].

The laser speckle phenomenon has been used to assess the diurnal variations in microcirculation of the ocular fundus in NTG patients and compared with those of normal control eyes [200]. In addition, the correlation between progression of visual field impairment and diurnal variations in ocular circulation was also studied [200].

Diurnal variations of square blur rate (SBR), an index of microcirculation acquired by the laser speckle method, were measured.

It was documented a significant decrease in SBR at night, as compared with the morning value, in the optic nerve head of NTG patients, although no significant diurnal variations were found in SBR either in the choroid-retina or in normal control eyes. In summary, it seems that these findings suggest that diurnal variations in the microcirculation of the optic nerve head may play a role in the progression of NTG [200].

In addition, a different relationship between optic nerve head blood flow velocity and visual field loss in patients with POAG and NTG has been proposed [201].

While there was a significant correlation between a decrease in optic nerve head blood flow velocity, as measured by laser speckle flowgraphy and visual field loss in the normal-tension glaucoma group in the POAG group, such correlation was not found [201].

3.7. Blue Field Entoptic Technique

The blue-field entoptic phenomenon represents a possibility to study leukocyte dynamics in vivo, because only red blood cells and not white blood cells (WBCs) absorb short-wavelength light. When a subject looks into blue light, bright corpuscles are perceived as flying around his or her fovea. Hence, the passage of WBCs within the perimacular retinal capillaries is perceived as a flying corpuscle. A system that allows for the quantification of the blue-field entoptic phenomenon has been realized [72]. There is evidence indicating that perifoveal leukocyte velocity is dependent on mean arterial pressure in healthy subjects, whereas retinal leukocyte density shows only little blood pressure dependence [202].

In glaucoma patients the response to IOP increase is different compared with controls [203].

In addition, significant positive correlations were seen between asymmetry of visual function and asymmetry of retinal leukocyte velocity in the patients with glaucoma. The eye with the higher velocity of retinal leukocyte flow tended to have better visual function as measured by Humphrey mean deviation [204, 205].

However, this technique assesses leukocyte movement, and it is not entirely clear whether results can be directly applied to volumetric blood flow in the retina. There is some evidence that leukocytes move slower in retinal capillaries than erythrocytes [206].

In addition, it is widely accepted that leukocyte velocity can be adequately assessed with the blue-field technique, but it is unclear whether the number of leukocytes as perceived in the blue light is an adequate measure of vascular volume [202].

3.8. Color Doppler Optical Coherence Tomography

A real-time spectral domain Doppler optical coherence tomography has been used to investigate the autoregulatory mechanism of human retinal perfusion [207].

3.9. Retinal Oximetry

Measurement of oxygen saturation in retinal vessels might provide important diagnostic information concerning causative factors other than IOP.

Data obtained with this method suggested that retinal circulation has similar characteristics to brain circulation [208-210].

It seems that oxygen saturation in retinal arterioles of glaucoma patients decreased significantly with increasing glaucomatous damage determined by the rim area. In contrast, no significant correlation was found when glaucomatous damage was quantified according to visual field defect [208].

The decreased in arteriolar oxygen saturation seems to be especially pronounced in NTG patients. However, these changes were not seen in POAG patients [208].

4. Blood Pressure, Ocular Perfusion Pressure, and Glaucoma

The blood flow in the blood vessels can be calculated using the following formula:

Flow= Perfusion Pressure/Resistance to flow (1)

Perfusion pressure is defined as the difference between the arterial and the venous pressure. In the eye, venous pressure is equal or slightly higher than IOP. From this equation, it is evident that the blood flow depends upon:

1. The mean blood pressure
2. The intraocular pressure
3. The vascular resistance in the blood vessels
4. The efficacy of autorregulation

To maintain the blood pressure there must be some contractile tone in most of all the resistance arterioles. In many tissues, flow in the small capillary regions is controlled no only by the resistance arterioles feeding the region, but also by the precapillary sphincters, which are rings of vascular smooth muscle at the point where capillaries branch from the arterioles.

As previously mentioned, tissue perfusion (flow, or Q) from any artery tom its corresponding vein is proportional to the perfusion pressure and inversely proportional to the local vascular resistance of vessels connecting them.

This resistance is made up of arterial resistance distal to the artery under consideration, resistance in the precapillary sphincter (if it exists in this tissue), and resistance in the capillaries leading to the vein.

The principal determinant of the resistance to blood flow through a vessels segment is its caliper. According to the Poiseuille`s law (which applies when the blood flow is relatively steady and laminar, as in vessels larger than arterioles), the flow (Q) is directly proportional to the perfusion pressure ($P_a - P_v$) and to the fourth power of the radius (r) and its inversely proportional to the length (l) of the vessel and to the viscosity of the fluid (h).

$$\mathbf{Q = \pi r^4 (P_a - P_v)/ 8hl} \quad (2)$$

when equations 1 and 2 are combined, it seems clear that the principal determinant of the resistance to blood flow through a vessels is its radius, because the blood viscosity and the length of the segment under consideration can be considered as constant factors.

$$(P_a - P_v)/ R = \pi r^4 (P_a - P_v)/ 8hl$$

$$R= 8hl/\pi r^4$$

Thus a 10% or 25% reduction in the radius of a vessel accounts for, respectively, almost 35% and 70% increase in the resistance in this vessel, demonstrating the powerful influence of the vessel caliper on resistance to blood flow.

Another subject which plays a very important role in the pathogenesis of the glaucomatous damage is the pattern of blood supply to the optic nerve head.

There is universal impression that the pattern of blood supply to the optic nerve head in all eyes is almost identical and that all ischemic lesions are explainable on a standard vascular pattern. It has been demonstrated that there is a marked inter-individual variation in the blood supply of the optic nerve head.

The predominant variability is observed in the arterial supply. The posterior ciliary arteries vary in number, distribution, and caliber. These arteries may be distributed only medially and laterally, or a third superior grouping may be present.

What is a watershed zone? When an organ is supply by an end-arterial system, the border between areas of distribution of any two end-arteries is called a watershed zone (figure 6).

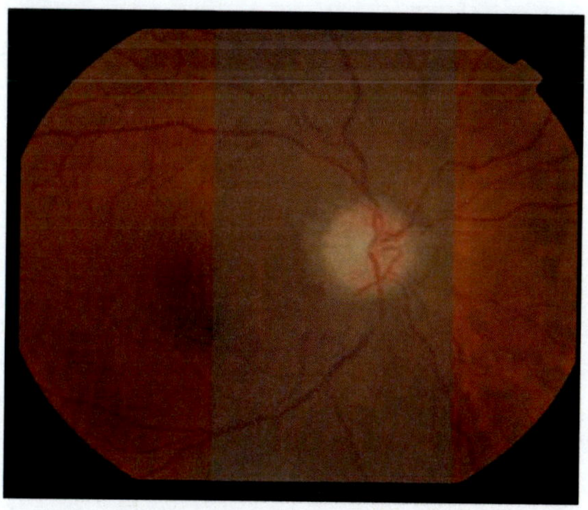

Figure 6. The grey band represents a watershed zone. A watershed zone may be situated anywhere between the fovea and the nasal peripapillary choroid. It may temporal to the disc, or pass through the temporal part of the disc, or the entire disc may lie in the watershed zone, or the watershed zone may pass through the nasal part of the disc or it may be lying nasal to the disc. Data obtained from Hayreh SS [324-326].

The number of posterior ciliary arteries varies between one and five, with most eyes having two or three. The grouping of these vessels into lateral and medial groups could play a role in clinical presentations subsequent to ischemic insults.

The distribution of the posterior ciliary arteries may explain the altitudinal visual filed defects observed following anterior ischemic optic neuropathy, the nasal visual field loss seen in glaucoma, and the arcuate filed loss observed in acute optic nerve infarction (figure 7).

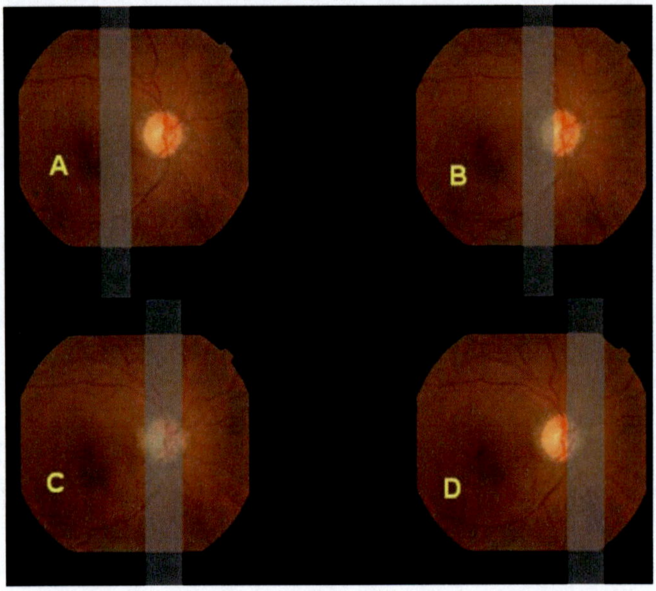

Figure 7. Diagram of some different watershed zones localizations (grey band) between the lateral and medial short-posterior ciliary arteries. A. Temporal to peripapillary choroids; B. Passing through the temporal peripapillary choroid (60% of glaucoma patients have watershed zones located in this region); C. The entire disc lies in the watershed zone (16% of glaucoma patients have watershed zones located in this region); D. The watershed zone passes through the nasal part of the disc (10% of glaucoma patients have watershed zones located in this region); Data obtained from Hayreh SS [324-326].

4.1. Blood Pressure and Intraocular Pressure

Hypertension is a well-recognized risk factor for elevated IOP, and there are consistent cross-sectional associations between systolic blood pressure (SBP) and IOP [211-216] although fewer studies show a similar relationship for diastolic pressure [214, 217, 218]. Both elevated systolic and diastolic blood pressure were positively associated with longitudinal IOP in-creases in the Barbados Eye Study [219], consistent with findings from other cohort studies [220, 221]. These postulates do not, however, satisfactorily explain differences in the associations between systolic and diastolic blood pressure (DBP) with IOP.

In addition, the 4- and 9- year follow-up data from the Barbados Incidence Study of Eye Diseases I and II [219, 222], which examined the surviving cohort of the Barbados Eye Study [212], demonstrated a trend of an increase in IOP with increasing SBP.

Moreover, several studies have consistently demonstrated a positive correlation between SBP and IOP in populations that included glaucoma patients [215, 223- 226]. The Beaver

Dam Study [225] found that there was a mean (Standard deviation) increase of 0.07 (3.14) mm Hg in IOP over the 5 year interval for those whose SBP was within 10 mm Hg of their baseline blood pressure compared to an increase of 0.44 (3.07) mm Hg for those whose SBP increased by 10 mm Hg and a decrease of 0.59 (3.28) mm Hg in IOP for those whose SBP decreased by 10 mm Hg or more.

The positive correlation between SBP and IOP observed in both healthy subjects and OAG patients also seems to be present across all races. The Egna-Neumarkt Study [224], the Rotterdam Study [215], and the Beaver Dam Study [218, 225] were each conducted on populations of predominantly European descent. However, the Barbados Eye Study [212, 219, 222], which had participants of predominantly African ancestry, the Baltimore Eye Survey, in which almost one half of the study population were of African genealogy, and the Tanjong Pagar Study [227], which was conducted on an entirely Asian population, all also suggest a strong correlation between SBP and IOP.

Curiosity, a positive relationship between DBP and IOP was not as evident in normal subjects as was the relationship between SBP and IOP. BISED II [222] suggested a marginally significant association between DBP and IOP. Conversely, in the Nomura et al study [220] and in the Baltimore Longitudinal Study of Aging (BLSA) [221] demonstrated no apparent correlation between DBP and IOP.

Analogous to SBP, DBP is significantly correlated with IOP in OAG patients. The Beaver Dam Study [225] found that there was a mean (Standard deviation) increase of 0.06 (3.06) mm Hg in IOP over the 5 year interval for those whose SBP was within 10 mm Hg of their baseline blood pressure compared to an increase of 0.85 (3.44) mm Hg for those whose SBP increased by 10 mm Hg and a decrease of 0.79 (3.28) mm Hg in IOP for those whose SBP decreased by 10 mm Hg or more.

The pathophysiologic basis for the relationship between blood pressure (BP) and IOP is currently unknown. Increased systemic BP leading to increased production of aqueous humor, by means of elevated ciliary artery pressure, has been postulated as a mechanism linking BP to high IOP [211, 214]. Others have proposed roles for increased sympathetic tone and serum corticosteroids [228]. These postulates do not, however, satisfactorily explain differences in the associations between systolic and diastolic BP with IOP.

4.2. Blood Pressure and Glaucoma

Although controversial, systemic hypertension or high blood pressure (HBP) has been regarded as a possible risk factor for the development and progression of open-angle glaucoma.

Associations between HBP [223, 224, 229] or low perfusion pressure [223, 224] and OAG were found, whereas other studies found a relation with the ratio between blood pressure and IOP [217] or no relation [230-232].

Although there is a positive correlation between BP and IOP, the correlation between BP increase and development of glaucoma is weak. The odds ratio (OR) for developing OAG with each 10 mm Hg increase in SBP ranges from 1.08 to 1.12 [233]. The corresponding OR for the development of OAG with each 10 mm Hg increase in DBP is even weaker, and ranges from 1.00 to 1.09 [233].

Nevertheless, the results from the Baltimore Eye Survey [223] and those from the Rotterdam Eye Study [215] suggested that there is a threshold effect of SBP on glaucoma prevalence. The Baltimore Eye Survey [223] found that the risk of open-angle glaucoma was higher in participants with SBP ≥ 130 mm Hg, compared with those who had lower SBP. Similarly, the prevalence of open-angle glaucoma increased significantly with higher quartiles of SBP, compared with lower quartiles, in the Rotterdam Eye Study [215].

However, the small correlation between higher SBP and increasing OAG prevalence evident in cross-sectional studies is not supported by the results from the longitudinal population-based cohort studies.

Results from the BISED II study [234] indicate that evaluations of SBP, DBP, pulse pressure, and arterial pressure consistently indicated a trend toward negative relationships with OAG risk. The relative risks (RR) per mmHg were all decreased for these four variables (0.89–0.92 per 10 mmHg higher). When data were grouped as high, medium, and low, the lowest categories of SBP and DBP had RR>1, in the direction of an increased risk; results were not as uniform when SBP and DBP were categorized by quartiles, perhaps indicating a minor role of BP, by itself, on open-angle glaucoma risk. A similar pattern was found for arterial pressure and for pulse pressure, which has been found to be an independent cardiovascular risk factor [235].

Recently, the Early Manifest Glaucoma trial has reported lower SBP at baseline as a predictor for glaucomatous damage progression, particularly in patients with baseline IOP < 21 mm Hg [7].

Low blood pressure is a known risk factor in the development and progression of the glaucomatous optic neuropathy [236-239]. A number of studies indicate that in POAG, and especially in NTG, the progression of glaucomatous damage seems to be related to systemic hypotension [224, 237, 240-248]. These studies mainly focused on the relation between low blood pressure and NTG, other groups however have demonstrated that this relationship is not restricted to NTG. Graham and coworkers showed in a case-control setting with a total of 84 patients that blood pressure parameters of NTG and HTG patients did not differ significantly, but that all nocturnal blood pressure parameters were lower in patients with progressive field defects compared with patients whose pressure parameters were stable [249].

Patients have been divided into “dippers” or “nondippers” based on the criteria that both the mean systolic and diastolic day blood pressures fall by more than 10% at night [250]. About two thirds of the normal population is thereby classified as dippers, with the blood pressure fall characterized as a normal physiologic, diurnal event. However, if the nocturnal dip is exaggerated, perfusion pressure in some vascular beds may be compromised.

Large nocturnal dips have been implicated in nocturnal myocardial infarction,

[251] in particular of the subendocardial type (non Q-wave), which is perfusion related rather than thrombotic [252].

The relation between nocturnal BP dip and the progression of the visual damage in POAG and NTG patients was examined in a prospective long-term study in a prospective long-term study [253].

Patients were classified based on the percentage of nocturnal BP dip as "Non-dipper" (dip of < 10%), "dipper" (physiologic dip of 10-20%), and "extreme dipper" (dip of > 20%). Interestingly, there was a tendency for the visual field defect to progress not only in the extreme dipper group, but also in the non-dipper group.

To summarize, some evidence suggests that especially nocturnal drops in blood pressure may play a role in the pathogenesis of glaucoma, possibly by reducing the optic nerve head blood flow below a crucial level.

However, not all patients with low blood pressure develop glaucoma, thus suggest an underlying vascular dysregulation, and no merely low nocturnal BP, as a contributory factor for glaucomatous damage.

4.3. Ocular Perfusion Pressure and Glaucoma

Blood flow in any tissue is generated by the perfusion pressure that is defined as the difference between mean arterial blood pressure (MAP) and venous pressure. In the resting position, MAP is calculated as [254, 255]:

MAP = DBP + 1/3 (SBP-DBP)

The difference between the systolic (SBP) and diastolic (DBP) blood pressures is the pulse pressure [251]. As previously mentioned, in the eye, the venous pressure should be marginally higher than the IOP, to allow for adequate blood circulation. Therefore, for the calculation of the mean ocular perfusion pressure (MOPP), IOP is substituted for venous pressure [256-258] so that the MOPP in the eye is equal to the difference between the MAP and IOP [259-261].

MOPP = 2/3 MAP-IOP

The prevalence of glaucoma was significantly associated with the ocular perfusion pressure (OPP). In the Baltimore Eye Survey, lower perfusion pressure was strongly associated with a higher prevalence of glaucoma [223].

The prevalence of glaucoma remained constant at diastolic perfusion pressure (DPP) above 50 mm Hg but increased substantially with a decrease in DPP to below 50 mm Hg, such that an age-and sex- adjusted OR for open-angle glaucoma was more than 6 times higher in subjects with DPP < 30 Hg [223].

Likewise, the prevalence of glaucoma decreases progressively with increased diastolic perfusion pressure, whereas no correlation is detectable with either systolic or mean perfusion pressure in the Egna-Neumarkt Study [224].

Similar results were shown by the Rotterdam Eye study [215, 226] and the Barbados Eye Study [237, 246].

In the Rotterdam Eye Study those with a low diastolic perfusion pressure (<50 mm Hg) had a significantly lower risk of normal-tension glaucoma, whereas the OR for POAG was

4.68 compared with participants with a diastolic perfusion pressure higher than 65 mmHg [215, 226].

Leske et al reported that open-angle glaucoma incidence was highest with low OPP. Persons with lower systolic OPP (SOPP), i.e., lower than the first quartile (<101.3 mm Hg), had a significant, more than 2.5 times increased RR of developing open-angle glaucoma (RR, 2.6). Persons with moderately low SOPP (101.3-114.4 mm Hg) also tended to have an increased RR (RR, 1.5), whereas persons with moderately high SPP (114.4-129.8mmHg) had similar a RR (RR, 0.9) as those with higher SPP. A similar pattern was found for diastolic OPP (DOPP), where lower DPP (<55 mm Hg) more than tripled the RR of OAG (RR, 3.2) [237].

The disparity among different studies in the cut-off values of DOPP below which it is significantly associate whit open-angle glaucoma may be attributed to different population characteristics, the discrepant definitions of glaucoma, and the small number of participants in some studies. Nevertheless, it is ostensible from these cross-sectional studies that there is an increased risk for open-angle glaucoma with low DOPP.

However, this fact does not appear to be present across all races. The Beijing Eye Study [262], a population-based study conducted on an entirely Asian population, failed to confirm the fact that ocular perfusion pressure is significantly associated with the prevalence of open-angle glaucoma. It also holds true if the whole glaucoma group was differentiated into a normal-pressure glaucoma group and a high-pressure glaucoma group.

In summary, in contrast to earlier population-based studies on western societies, the prevalence of OAG (also when differentiated into normal-pressure and high-pressure glaucomas) was not associated with the ocular perfusion pressure [262].

The perfusion pressure changes during the day, but the tissue blood flow should remain stable, to maintain metabolic activity [254, 255, 263, 264]. Diurnal variation of IOP has been well documented [265-270], and it has been demonstrated that the range of IOP fluctuation is larger than normal in persons with untreated glaucoma [6, 267, 269, 271, 272]. Diurnal variation of SBP has also been well studied [238, 274-276]. However, there are few studies regarding diurnal variation in MOPP [270, 277] and its role as a risk factor for the diagnosis of POAG.

Sehi et al [278] investigated diurnal change and pattern of variation in IOP and systolic and diastolic blood pressures in a group with untreated POAG and compared it with an age-matched, normal group.

This study found that the mean MOPP was significantly lower in patients with POAG than in normal subjects throughout the day, and the absolute diurnal change was greater in the POAG group. The minimum MOPP in the POAG group was recorded at 7 AM and it was significantly lower than normal subjects at this time. In addition, the pattern of diurnal variation in MOPP relative to the 7 AM level was significantly different between patients with POAG and normal subjects. Specifically, the MOPP was elevated at 2 PM and at the end of the day (from 8 PM) in the POAG group, but in the normal group there was only a slight increase. In summary, there was a significant diurnal change in MOPP in both groups, and the pattern of diurnal variation was different between groups.

Similarly, Choi and collaborators [279] reported, in a cohort of 113 Asian normal-tension glaucoma patients, that circadian MOPP fluctuation was the most consistent clinical risk factor in determining glaucoma severity in patients with NTG.

4.4. Hypertension Treatment and Primary Open-Angle Glaucoma

Because hypertension generally is treated with antihypertensive medication, often it is difficult to distinguish whether an increased risk of OAG results from hypertension or from its treatment.

The Rotterdam Eye Study indicated an association between use of systemic beta-blockers and lower IOP, with a protective effect on OAG [222]. Conversely, a recent published paper (a subset of 3842 participants of the Rotterdam Study) suggested that the use of calcium channel antagonist had almost a 2-fold increase in risk of developing open-angle glaucoma [280].

This finding is in agreement with an earlier large-scale case-control study by Langman et al [281], who found a significant risk increase of open-angle glaucoma in users of calcium channel antagonists. While the likelihood of glaucoma being diagnosed was significantly reduced in current users of oral B-blocking agents, odds ratios were significantly raised in current takers of ACE inhibitors, and calcium channel antagonists, and remaining raised in ever users.

However, these results seem to contradict several studies that advocate the use of calcium channel antagonists in normal-tension glaucoma patients [219].

The bases of this recommendation are the results of several human and animal studies that have shown blockade of membrane-bound calcium channels to induce ocular vascular dilatation and to improve optic nerve perfusion [282-284]. There are some reports showing visual field improvements of normal-tension OAG patients after using calcium channel antagonists [285, 286].

Differences between these studies and the Müskens et al study [280] may be the result of patient selection in the aforementioned studies, which could mean that there may be a small, selective group of normal-tension glaucoma patients who may benefit from calcium channel antagonists. However in the present study, no significant interaction between IOP and calcium channel antagonist use was found. Because results of earlier reports are by no means conclusive, and the present results suggest that calcium channel antagonists may have a harmful effect on development of open-angle glaucoma, the treatment of open-angle glaucoma patients with calcium channel antagonists should be handled with caution and in fact may be contraindicated.

Moreover, a positive association between low DOPP and POAG was detected only in subjects with antihypertensive treatment in the Rotterdam Eye Study [226]. The association between low diastolic perfusion pressure and POAG in this study was present only in participants receiving treatment for systemic hypertension, probably because the perfusion in the eye will be more hampered in case of an elevated IOP.

5. Regulation of Ocular Blood Flow

In peripheral tissues, contractile tone of vascular wall (and hence vessel diameter and resistance to blood flow) is under the influence of both local and systemic mechanisms.

Autoregulation is a term we hear applied to the physiologic phenomenon in which the resistance changes dynamically to keep flow at whatever constant level is required by the local metabolic activity despite changes in perfusion pressure, e.g., when arterial pressure changes or when venous pressure is affected by IOP [287-290].

Local regulation or autoregulation is known to have at least three components separated according to the stimulus for flow adjustment: stretch dependent (myogenic), shear dependent, and metabolic dependent [290-292].

Vasoactive substances released in response to stretch of the vascular smooth muscle and sheer stress at the endothelial surface have been identified as mediators of "myogenic" mechanisms behind this regulation, but accumulation or depletion of adenosine, oxygen, carbon dioxide, and other vasoactive substances contribute a "metabolic" component to the local control mechanism. It is important to recognize that not only nutritional flow, but also capillary intraluminal hydrostatic pressure must be controlled in order to avoid either tissue dehydration or edema [287, 290, 293]. This balance of needs may require balanced control of tone (resistance) in the veins, the capillary walls, and the precapillary sphincters, in addition to the arterioles and arteries.

The retina and optic nerve share the feature of exhibiting autoregulation of blood flow with the rest of the central nervous system [287, 288, 290, 293, 294]. In addition, the retina and optic nerve seem to have a constant blood flow despite external challenges (such as IOP or changes in blood pressure), and the flow changes according to metabolic demand [295].

The retinal vessels behave similarly to brain vessels with the exception that they do not have any autonomic innervation [296]. The size of the retinal vessels is regulated by endothelial cells and by the neural retinal tissue providing adaptation to retinal activity. Dissimilarity, choroidal vessels are regulated by a dense autonomic innervation [297, 298].

The circulation in the optic nerve head is somewhat similar to the circulation in the retina with some anatomical and physiological particularities: while the arterial supply is provided through the ciliary circulation, the venous drainage occurs through the retinal veins [299].

The size of the vessels in the optic nerve head, and to some extend also, the vessels around the optic nerve head, are highly influenced by circulating hormones diffusing from the fenestrated choriocapillaries into the optic nerve head and its surroundings [300].

Considering this very extended and sophisticated regulation, it is not surprising that under certain conditions this regulation may be disturbed. To describe this situation Flammer in 1994 introduced the term "Vascular Dysregulation" [301].

6. Vascular Dysregulation

As mentioned early, blood flow through an organ is regulated by perfusion pressure and local resistance to flow. Local resistance in turn is controlled by the radius of the local vessels. Thus, the regulation serves the purpose of ensuring an adequate supply of oxygen and nutrients reaching the tissues, as well as volume regulation and temperature.

Dysregulation is defined as a regulation of circulation that is not properly adapted to the local needs.

There are a number of pathological conditions that interfere locally with vessel size regulation and there are also however, conditions in which dysregulation occur more globally, involving many different organs simultaneously or sequentially.

Flammer et al differentiated between a primary vascular dysregulation (PVD) and a secondary vascular dysregulation (SVD) [302].

Whereas PVD is an inborn predisposition to respond differently to various stimuli, a SVD is a local or systemic dysregulation as a consequence of an underlying disease. A systemic vascular dysregulation can be secondary, as for example, in multiple sclerosis [302, 303] or rheumatoid arthritis [304], lead to a market increase of circulating endothelin.

Primary vascular dysregulation however occurs in otherwise healthy subjects particularly, but not only, in young slim females. Patients with PVD have a compromised autoregulation [305] of ocular perfusion, explaining their increase risk of glaucoma principally normal-tension glaucoma [306].

6.1. Primary Vascular Dysregulation

As mentioned above, PVD is characterized by an inborn tendency to respond differently to a variety of stimuli, such as cold temperatures or emotional or mechanical stress. The symptoms might be already presents in childhood but manifest clearly during puberty and improve as subjects get older, in particular during menopause, but can re-exacerbate when women with PVD receive hormonal-replacement therapy [307].

According to different authors [292, 299, 301, 302] PVD occurs more frequently in women, young adults, slim-built individuals, type A personalities, in academics than in blue collar workers, is associated with a history of cold hands (but not necessarily Raynaud's phenomenon), and in Asian than in Caucasians.

The leading symptom of PVD is cold extremities. Subjects with PVD often state that they suffer from cold hands but, when measured, their feet cold as well [302].

Additionally, they feeling of thirst is reduced [308], and although they normally drink enough this is not because they are thirsty but, rather, because they know that they have to drink.

They also have a prolonged sleep onset time. This is due to the fact that there is a connection between foot temperature and sleep onset time [309]. As these individuals have colder feet, they require longer time to warm them up.

People with PVD syndrome also have altered drug sensitivity and therefore often prefer complementary medicine [292]. This is at least partially due to an altered gene expression of the ABC transport (ATP-binding cassette) proteins [310].

When treating these patients with systemic drugs such as beta-blockers or calcium channel blockers, a much lower dose can achieve a full pharmacological effect while minimizing side effects. However, for other class of drugs, such as painkillers, they need the same or even higher doses to get sufficient effects [292].

It should be noted that although PVD does not cause any significant disability in most cases. They do, however, have a higher chance for certain diseases. This includes the risk of anterior ischemic optic neuropathy [311], vein occlusions [312], central serous chorioretinopathy [313], Susac syndrome [314], and glaucoma [292].

6.2. Secondary Vascular Dysregulation

Secondary vascular dysregulation syndrome occurs concomitantly with other diseases, usually autoimmune disorders (such as rheumatoid arthritis, temporal arteritis, and multiple sclerosis) but also other diseases such as some infection diseases, brain hemorrhages, and tumors (table 5).

Table 5. Diseases that lead to local or systemic Vascular Dysregulation

Autoimmune Diseases	Multiple sclerosis Giant cell arteritis Lupus erythematosus Antiphospholipid syndrome Rheumatoid arthritis Pre-eclampsia
Infectious diseases	Some bacterial infections (i.e. bacterial meningitis) Some viral diseases (i.e. viral liver cirrhosis) AIDS
Other possible causes	Cerebral hemorrhage Head injury Anorexia nervosa Mitochondriopathies Some tumors (i.e. prostate cancer) Ulcerative colitis and Crohns disease
Drugs (in patients having a predisposition)	Adrenaline Alpha II Interferon Sumatriptane

Adapted from Grieshaber et al [292].

It is not necessarily clear in each of these conditions what mechanisms lead to vasospasm, but it is apparent that in most instances there is an increase in the concentration of endothelin-1 (ET-1) [315].

ET-1 constricts vessels not only directly but also indirectly by increasing sensitivity to other vasoconstrictive hormones such as norepinephrine and angiotensin-II. An increase in circulating dramatically reduces blood flow in the eye and in the kidney, whereas brain circulation is less affected, unless the blood barrier is disturbed [292].

The fact that SVD is due to changes of vasoactive substances in the circulating blood, and the fact that these circulating molecules have a major impact on OBF, especially in the choroid and in the optic nerve head, is the reason why SVD is relevant to ophthalmologists.

6.3. Diagnosis of Vascular Dysregulation

In terms of diagnostic testing there are currently no readily available tests that can help with the diagnosis of vascular dysregulation. In the clinical setting, the diagnosis of vascular dysregulation relies mainly on the patient history.

Direct contact of the patient's hands (i.e. shaking hands) often yields a sufficient clue for the clinician, in particular if the patient is not aware of having PVD [292].

Using specialized test performed in some laboratories or clinics, it is possible to identify unclear cases.

Nail-fold capillary microscopy, laser Doppler flowmetry, or even measurement of plasma ET-1 are helpful to confirm the diagnosis in patients with suspect of vascular dysregulation syndrome.

All these test, however, are not routinely available, and their role in diagnosing vascular dysregulation, if any, should be established.

6.4. Vascular Dysregulation and Glaucoma

The question of whether OBF alterations is a secondary effect, caused either by increased IOP or the presence of glaucomatous optic neuropathy or whether changes in OBF are an independent primary factor remains.

There is increasing evidence that ocular blood flow changes are involved in both the pathogenesis of glaucoma [9-11] and in progression of glaucomatous damage [12-15].

For instance, blood flow velocity is, on average slower in the retina, in the choroids, and in the optic nerve head in patients with glaucoma, particularly in normal-tension glaucoma patients or in patient that progress despite normalized intraocular pressure. In addition, blood flow is also reduced in retrobulbar vessels and in peripheral capillaries [292].

In addition blood flow is reduced if reduction in perfusion pressure exceeds the capacity of autoregulation. Consequently, if autoregulation is disturbed already a mild reduction of OPP reduces OBF.

Interestingly, however, there is a component of OBF reduction that is independent of the damage and often precedes the damage [117], and independent of IOP (it is even more pronounced in normal-tension than in high-tension glaucoma [110], and that is not confined to the eye (it can be observed in the nailfold capillaries) [88].

Additionally, different independent studies demonstrated that OBF alterations allows a prediction of future progression of damage [12-15] and is therefore of major clinical relevance.

Since the firsts published studies suggesting an association between vasospasm and glaucoma [88, 319, 320], 2 population-based studies have reported on the prevalence of glaucoma with different results: 1 showed an increased prevalence of migraine among glaucoma patients [321], while the other showed no significant association between the 2 diseases [322].

In an elegant study, Schulzer and collaborators [323] identified 2 distinct populations of glaucoma patients; 1 with signs of vasospasm in the peripheral circulation and the other with disturbed coagulation and biochemical measurements, suggestive of ischemic vascular disease.

Interestingly, in this study the authors found a correlation between the amount of visual field loss (summarized by the mean deviation index of visual field) and the highest recorded IOP only in the vasospastic group, suggesting that this group has a pressure-sensitive disease and, therefore, would more likely benefit from IOP reduction.

Despite considerable evidence that vascular dysregulation is associated with at least some types of glaucoma, it is not clear how this association occurs and what the relevance is of vasospasm in individuals with glaucoma.

We are therefore faced with the seemingly contradictory situation that, whereas in glaucoma blood flow is reduced and this reduction has a relatively strong predictive power, the OBF reduction (as shown in experimental studies and in other clinical conditions), although leading to some atrophy, does not lead to glaucomatous damage.

The OBF alterations can lead to periods of relative ischemia, resulting in what is known as reperfusion in jury, which occurs when normal blood flow is re-established and causes local inflammation an oxidative damage. It has been hypothesized that, in glaucoma, periods of relative ischemia lead to repetitive episodes of reperfusion injury that can contribute to the development or worsening of the disease [299] (figure 8).

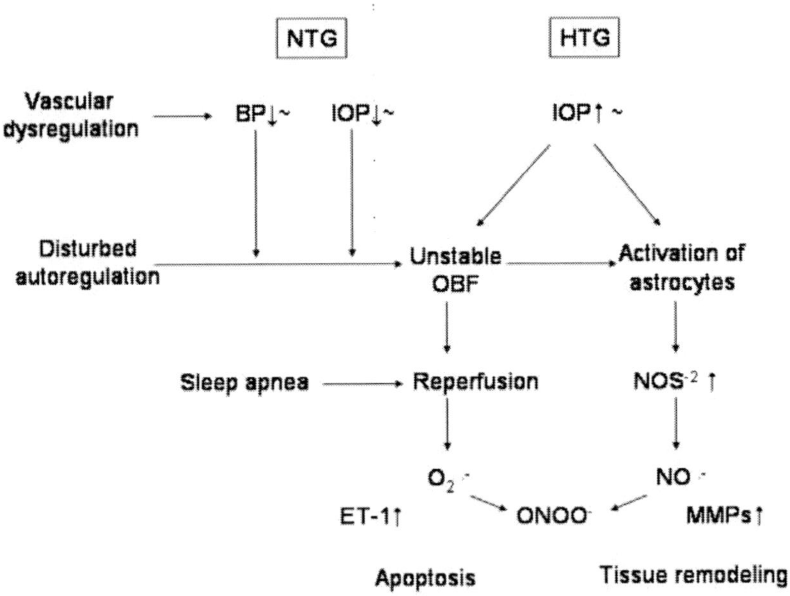

Figure 8. Simplified pathogenic concept of glaucomatous optic neuropathy. Unstable ocular perfusion leads to a reperfusion damage in the retinal ganglion cell axons. In parallel the glial cells are activated leading to an altered micro-environment. Abreviations: NTG= normal-tension glaucoma; HTG= high-tension glaucoma; BP= blood pressure; IOP= intraocular pressure; OBF= ocular blood flow; ET-1= endothelin-1, MMP= metalloproteinases. Adapted from Flammer & Mozzafarieh [309].

Reperfusion injury refers to damage to tissues caused when blood supply returns to the tissue after a period of ischemia. The absence of oxygen and nutrients from tissue creates a condition in which the restoration of circulation results in inflammation and oxidative damage rather than restoration of normal function. The restored blood flow re-introducing oxygen thereby damages proteins, lipids, and the plasma membrane.

The major source of the oxidative stress in reperfusion, therefore, stems from the mitochondria, which are much crowed in the optic nerve head due to the high energy consumption in these nerve fiber lacking myelin sheaths [316].

The assumption of reperfusion injury being involved in the pathogenesis also explains why sleep apnea [317], or reversible shock-like states, can lead to glaucomatous optic neuropathy [318].

In conclusion, the instability of OBF leads to a mild but repeated, reperfusion injury increasing the oxidative stress, especially in the optic nerve head.

7. Conclusions

The development of new instruments now allows for the study of some aspects of ocular hemodynamics under physiological and pathological conditions. However, only a few of these technologies are currently used in routine clinical care and none of these techniques can be regarded as gold standard for the measurement of ocular blood flow.

Many different studies, using different type of instruments point in the same general direction indicating that on average ocular blood flow is decreased in some glaucoma patients, particularly in normal-tension glaucoma patients and in patients that progress despite normalized intraocular pressure.

Further more the decrease in blood flow, although related to the extend of damage, can precede the glaucomatous damage and is not confined to the eye alone. This would indicate that at least one component of the blood flow reduction in glaucoma is of primary nature.

We have evidence suggesting a strong positive association between systolic blood pressure and IOP, and a weaker association between diastolic blood pressure and IOP.

However, the association between the incidence of open-angle glaucoma and systemic hypertension is an inverse one, with hypotension increasing the risk of open-angle glaucoma.

In addition, the prevalence of open-angle glaucoma increases with decreasing ocular perfusion pressure, possibly because of reduction in the ocular blood flow. However, the exact cause of this is not known yet.

There is ample evidence of the involvement of general vascular dysregulation in the pathogenesis of glaucomatous optic neuropathy. Dysregulation is defined as a regulation of circulation that is not properly adapted to the local needs.

The vascular dysregulation, also termed vasospastic syndrome, can be subdivided as primary or secondary. Although primary and secondary vascular dysregulation have many symptoms in common, their influence on eye circulation is distinctively different.

PVD is characterized by an inborn tendency to respond differently to a variety of stimuli, such as cold temperatures or emotional or mechanical stress, whereas the SVD occurs concomitantly with other diseases, usually autoimmune disorders but also other diseases such as some infection diseases, brain hemorrhages, and tumors.

Additionally, it has been suggested that, in glaucoma, periods of relative ischemia lead to repetitive episodes of reperfusion injury that can contribute to the development or worsening of the disease.

The relevance of these findings for the treatment of glaucoma is critically dependent on whether an increase of the ocular blood flow will contribute to retinal ganglion cell survival in glaucoma.

In conclusion, the understanding of the role of ocular blood flow disturbances in the pathogenesis of glaucoma has improved greatly. There is overwhelming evidence that ocular blood flow is altered independently from IOP or level of damage in patients with progressive glaucoma, which could represent a primary risk factor for disease progression.

In looking forward, we need long-term prospective multicenter studies to evaluate the impact of ocular blood flow in glaucoma and the benefit of improving ocular blood flow.

References

[1] European Glaucoma Society. Terminology and Guidelines for Glaucoma. 3 rd ed. Savona, Italy: Dogma; 2008: 95-97.

[2] Kass MA, Kolker AE, Becker B. Prognostic factors in glaucomatous visual field loss. *Arch. Ophthalmol.* 1976; 94: 1274-1276.

[3] Gordon MO, Beiser JA, Brandt JD, et al. The Ocular Hypertension Treatment Study: baseline factors that predict the onset of primary open-angle glaucoma. *Arch. Ophthalmol.* 2002; 120: 714-720.

[4] Kass MA, Heuer DK, Higginbotham EJ et al. The Ocular Hypertension Treatment Study: a randomized trail determines that topical ocular hypotensive medication delays or prevents the onset of primary open-angle glaucoma. *Arch. Ophthalmol.* 2002; 120:701-713.

[5] AGIS investigators: The Advance Glaucoma Intervention Study (AGIS) 7. The relationship between control of intraocular pressure and visual field deterioration. *Am. J. Ophthalmol.* 2000; 130: 429-440.

[6] Heijl A, Leske MC, Bengtsson B et al. Reduction of intraocular pressure and glaucoma progression: results from the Early Manifest Glaucoma Trial. *Arch. Ophthalmol.* 2002; 120: 1268-1279.

[7] Leske MC, Heijl A, Hyman L et al. Predictors of long-term progression in the Early Manifest Glaucoma Trial. *Ophthalmology.* 2007; 114: 1965-1972.

[8] Collaborative Normal-Tension Glaucoma Study Group. Comparison of glaucomatous progression between untreated patients with normal-tension glaucoma and patients with therapeutically reduced intraocular pressures. *Am. J. Ophthalmol.* 1998; 126: 487-497.

[9] Carter CJ., Brooks DE., Doyle DL., Drance SM. Investigation into a vascular aetiology for low tension glaucoma. *Ophthalmology.* 1990; 97:49-55.

[10] Hayreh SS Progress in the understanding of the vascular aetiology of glaucoma. *Curr. Opin. Ophthalmol.* 1994; 5:26-35.

[11] Flammer J., Orgül S., Costa VP., et al The impact of ocular blood flow in glaucoma. *Prog. Retin. Eye Res.* 2002; 21: 359-393.

[12] Galassi F, Sodi A, Ucci F, et al Ocular hemodynamics and glaucoma prognosis: a color Doppler imaging study. *Arch. Ophthalmol.* 2003; 121: 1711-5.

[13] Satilmis M, Orgül S, Doubler B, Flammer J Rate of progression of glaucoma correlates with retrobulbar circulation and intraocular pressure. *Am. J. Ophthalmol.* 2003; 135: 664-9.

[14] Martinez A, Sanchez M (2005). Predictive Value of Color Doppler Imaging in a Prospective Study of Visual Field Progression in Primary Open-Angle Glaucoma. *Acta Ophthalmol. Scand.* 83: 716-723.

[15] Zeitz O., Galambos P., Weirmann A., et al. Glaucoma progression is associated with decreased blood flow velocities in the short posterior ciliary artery. *Br. J. Ophthalmol.* 2006; 90: 1245-1248.

[16] Flammer J, Orgül S, Costa VP et al. The impact of ocular blood flow in glaucoma. *Prog. Retin Eye Res.* 2002; 21: 359-393.

[17] Lieb WE, Cohen SM, Merton DA et al. Color Doppler Imaging of the eye and orbit. Technique and normal vascular anatomy. *Arch. Ophthalmol.* 1991; 109: 527-531.

[18] Joseph F. Polak, Joseph P. Polak. Peripheral Vascular Sonography: A Practical Guide 1st ed. Lippincott Williams & Wilkins, 2004 pages 23-25.

[19] Schmetterer L, Garhofer G. How can blood flow be measured? *Surv. Ophthalmol.* 2007; 52 Sppl: S134-S138.

[20] Evans DH, Barrie WW, Asher MJ, Bentley S, Bell PR. The relation ship between ultrasonic pulsatility index and proximal arterial stenosis in a canine model. *Circ. Res.* 1980; 46: 470-475.

[21] Pourcelot L. Applications clinique de l`examen Doppler transcutané. *INSRM.* 34; 1974: 213-240.

[22] Polska E, Kircher K, Ehrlich P et al. RI in central retinal artery as assessed by CDI does not correspond to retinal vascular resistance. *Am. J. Phisiol. Heart Cir. Physiol.* 2001; 280: H1442-7.

[23] Williamson TH, Harris A, Martin BJ. Reproducibility of color Doppler imaging assessment of blood flow velocity in orbital vessels. *J. Glaucoma.* 1995; 4: 281-286.

[24] Kaiser HJ, Schoetzau A, Flammer J. The frequency distribution of blood flow velocities in the extraocular vessels. *Graefes Arch. Clin. Exp. Ophthalmol.* 1996; 234: 537-541.

[25] Quaranta L, Harris A, Donato F et al. Color Doppler imaging of ophthalmic artery blood flow velocity: a study of repeatability and agreement. *Ophthalmology.* 1997; 104: 653-658.

[26] Langham ME. Farrel RA, O'Brien V, Silver DM, Schilder P. Blood flow in the human eye. *Acta Ophthalmol.* 1989; 191: 9-13.

[27] Langham ME. Ocular blood flow and vision in normal healthy and glaucomatous eyes. *Surv. Ophthalmol.* 1994; 38(Suppl): S161-S168.

[28] Silver DM, Farrel RA, Langham ME et al. Estimation of pulsatile ocular blood flow from intraocular pressure. *Acta Ophthalmol.* 1989; 191: 25-9.

[29] Harris A, Kagemann L, Ehrlich R, Rospigliosi C, Moore D, Siesky B. Measuring and interpreting ocular blood flow and metabolism in glaucoma. *Can. J. Ophthalmol.* 2008; 43: 328-36.

[30] Schmetterer L, Lexer F, Unfried C et al. Topical measurements of fundus pulsations. *Opt. Eng.* 1995; 34: 711-16.

[31] Schmetterer L, Woltz M, Salomon A et al. Effect of isoproterenol, phenylefrine, and sodium nitroprusside on fundus pulsation in healthy volunteers. *Br. J. Ophthalmol.* 1996; 80: 217-23.

[32] Schmetterer L, Dallinger S, Findl O, Eichler HG, Woltz M. A comparison between laser interferometric measurement of fundus pulsation and pneumotonometric measurement of pulsatile ocular blood flow. Baseline considerations. *Eye*. 2000; 14: 39-52.

[33] Riva C, Ross B, Benedek GB. Laser Doppler measurements of blood flow in capillary tubes and retinal arteries. *Invest. Ophthalmol.* 1972; 11: 936-944.

[34] Riva CE, Grunwald JE, Sinclair SH. Laser Doppler measurement of relative blood velocity in the human optic nerve head. *Invest. Ophthalmol. Vis. Sci.* 1982; 22: 241-48.

[35] Bonner R, Nossal R. Principles of laser-Doppler flowmetry, in Shepard AÖ, PA (ed.): Developments in cardiovascular medicine: Laser Doppler Blood Flowmetry. Boston, MA Kluwer Academic Publisher, 1990, pp. 17-65.

[36] Riva CE, Harino S, Petrig BL, Shonat RD. Laser Doppler flowmetry in the optic nerve. *Exp. Eye Res.* 1992; 55: 499-506.

[37] Riva CE, Granstoun SD, Grunwald JE, Petrig BL. Choroidal blood flow in the foveal region of the human ocular fundus. *Invest. Ophthalmol. Vis. Sci.* 1994; 35: 4273-81.

[38] Osusky R, Schoetzau A, Flammer J. Variations in the blood flow of the human optic nerve head. *Eur. J. Ophthalmol.* 1997; 7: 364-369.

[39] Koelle JS, Riva CE, Petrig BL, Cranstoun SD. Depth of tissue sampling in the optic nerve head using laser Doppler flowmetry. *Las. Med. Sci.* 1993; 8: 49-54.

[40] Straubhaar M, Orgül S, Gugleta K, Schoutzau A, Erb C, Flammer J. Choroidal laser Doppler flowmetry in healthy subjects. *Arch. Ophthalmol*. 2000; 118: 211-215.

[41] Polska E, Polak K, Luksch A et al. Twelve hours reproducibility of choroidal blood flow parameters in healthy subjects. *Br. J. Ophthalmol.* 2004; 88: 533-537.

[42] Gugleta K, Orgül S, Flammer I, Ghergel D, Flammer J. Reliability of confocal choroidal laser Doppler flowmetry. *Invest. Ophthalmol. Vis. Sci.* 2002; 34:3609-3613.

[43] Boehm AC, Pillunat LE, Koeller U et al. Regional distribution of optic nerve head blood flow. *Graefes Arch. Clin. Exp. Ophthalmol*. 1999; 237: 484-8.

[44] Petrig BL, Riva CE, Hayreh SS. Laser Doppler flowmetry and optic nerve head blood flow. *Am. J. Ophthalmology.* 1999; 127:413-425.

[45] Riva CE, Feke GT, Eberli B, Benary V. Bidirectional LDV system for absolute measurements of blood speed in retinal vessels. *Appl. Opt.* 1979; 18: 2301-6.

[46] Mendel MJ, Toi VV, Riva CE, Petrig BL. Eye-tracking laser Doppler velocimeter stabilized in two dimensions: principle, design, and construction. *J. Opt. Soc. Am. A.* 1993; 10: 1663-1669.

[47] Riva CE, Grunwald JE, Sinclair SH et al. Blood velocity and volumetric flow rate in human retinal vessels. *Invest. Ophthalmol. Vis. Sci.* 1985; 26: 1124-32.

[48] Michelson G, Schmauss B, Langhans MJ, Harazny J, Groh MJ. Principle, validity, and reliability of scanning laser Doppler flowmetry. *J. Glaucoma*. 1996; 5: 99-105.

[49] Chauhan BC, Smith FM. Confocal scanning laser Doppler flowmetry: experiments in a model flow system. *J. Glaucoma.* 1997; 6: 237-245.

[50] Hollo G, Greve EL, van den Berg TJ, Vargha P. Evaluation of the peripapillary circulation in healthy an glaucoma eyes with scanning laser Doppler flowmetry. *Int. Ophthalmol.* 1996; 20: 71-77.

[51] Kagemann L, Harris A, Chung HS, Evans D, Buck S, Martin B. Heidelberg retinal flowmetry: factors affecting blood flow measurement. *Br. J. Ophthalmol.* 1998; 82: 131-6.

[52] Michelson G, Welzenbach J, Pal I, Harazny J. Automatic full field analysis of perfusion images gained by scanning laser Doppler flowmetry. *Br. J. Ophthalmol.* 1998; 82: 1294-1300.

[53] Hosking SL, Embleton S, Kagemann L, Chabra A, Jonescu-Cuypoers C, Harris A. Detector sensitivity influences blood flow sampling in scanning laser Doppler flowmetry. *Graefes Arch. Clin. Exp. Ophthalmol.* 2001; 239: 407-410.

[54] Strenn K, Menapace R, Rainer G et al. Reproducibility and sensitivity of scanning laser Doppler flowmetry during graded changes in PO2. *Br. J. Ophthalmol.* 1997; 81: 360-364.

[55] Wolf S, Jung F, Kiesewetter H et al. Video fluorescein angiography: method and clinical application. *Graefes Arch. Clin. Exp. Ophthalmol.* 1989; 227: 145-51.

[56] 56. Prünte C, Niessel P. Quantification of choroidal blood flow parameters using indocyanine green video-fluorescence angiography and statistical picture analysis. *Graefes Arch. Clin. Exp. Ophthalmol.* 1988; 226: 55-58.

[57] Arend O, Harris A, Martin BJ, Remky A. Scanning laser ophthalmoscopy-based evaluation of epipapillary velocities: method and physiologic variability. *Surv. Ophthalmol.* 44 (Suppl 1): S3-S9.

[58] Preussner PR, Richard G, Darrelmann O et al. Quantitative measurements of retinal blood flow in humans beings by application of digital image-processing methods to television fluorescein angiograms. *Graefes Arch. Clin. Exp. Ophthalmol.* 1983; 221: 110-112.

[59] Tanaka T, Muraoka K, Shimizu K. Fluorescein fundus angiography with scanning laser ophthalmoscope. Visibility of leukocytes and platelets in perifoveal capillaries. *Ophthalmology.* 1991; 98: 1824-29.

[60] Wolf S, Arend O, Toonen H et al. Retinal capillary blood flow measurements with a scanning laser ophthalmoscope. Preliminary results. *Ophthalmology.* 1991; 98:996-1000.

[61] Webb RH, Hughes GW, Pomerantzeff O. Flying spot T.V. ophthalmoscope. *Applied Optics.* 1980; 19: 1991-1997.

[62] Wolf S, Remky A, Elsner AE, Arend O, Reim M. Indocyanine green video-angiography in patients with age-related maculopathy-related retinal pigment detachments. *Ger. J. Ophthalmol.* 1994; 3: 224-227.

[63] Arend O, Remky A, Elsner AE, Wolf S, Reim M. Indocyanine green angiography in traumatic choroidal rupture: clinicoangiography case report. *Ger. J. Ophthalmol.* 1995; 4: 257-63.

[64] Wolf S, Arend O, Reim M. Measurement of retinal hemodynamics with scanning laser ophthalmoscopy: reference values and variation. *Surv. Ophthalmol.* 1994; 38 (Suppl): S95-S100.

[65] Seifert U, Vilser W. Retinal Vessel Analyzer (RVA) - *Design and Function Biomed. Tech.* 2002; 47 (Suppl.1): 678-681.

[66] Polak K., Dorner G., Kiss B. et al. Evaluation of the Zeiss retinal vessel analyzer. *Br. J. Ophthalmol.* 2000; 84: 1285-1290.

[67] Feke GT, Goger DG, Tagawa H et al. Laser Doppler technique for absolute measurement of blood speed in retinal vessels. *IEEE Trans. Biomed. Eng.* 1987; 34: 673-80.

[68] Yoshida A, Feke GT, Mori et al. Reproducibility and clinical application of a newly developed stabilized retinal laser Doppler instrument. *Am. J. Ophthalmol.* 2003; 135: 356-61.

[69] Feke GT. Laser Doppler instrumentation for the measurement of retinal blood flow: Theory and practice. *Bull. Soc. Belge.* 2006: 171-184.

[70] Tamaki Y, Araie M, Kawamoto E, Eguchi S, Fujii H. Noncontact, two-dimensional measurement of retinal microcirculation using laser speckle phenomenon. *Invest. Ophthalmol. Vis. Sci.* 1994; 3825-3834.

[71] Tamaki Y, Araie M, Kawamoto E, Eguchi S, Fujii H. Noncontact, two-dimensional measurement of tissue circulation in choroid and optic nerve head using laser speckle phenomenon. *Exp. Eye Res.* 1995; 60: 373-383.

[72] Riva CE, Petrig B. Blue field entoptic phenomenon and blood velocities in the retinal capillaries. *J. Opt. Soc. Am.* 1980; 70: 1234-1238.

[73] Scheerer R., "Die entoptische Sichtbarkeit der Blutbewegungen im Auge und ihre klinische Bedeutung." *Klinisches Monatsblatt Augenheilkunde.* 1924;73:67-107.

[74] Sinclair SH, Azar-Cananagh M, Soper KA, Tuma RF, Mayroviz HN. Investigation of the source of the blue field entoptic phenomenon. *Invest. Ophthalmol. Vis. Sci.* April 1989; 30(4):668-673.

[75] Vierodt K: Grundries der Physiologic Frankfurt, *Meideinger,* 1860, p. 234.

[76] Bauermann VM: Uberdas Phanomen derentoptish sichtbaren Blutbewegrung. *Klin. Monatsbl. Augenheilkd.* 1980; 137:621.

[77] Fuchsjäger-Mayrl G, Malec M, Polska E et al. Effects of granulocyte colony stimulating factor on retinal leukocyte and erythrocyte flux in the human retina. *Invest. Ophthalmol.Vis. Sci.* 2002; 43: 2720-29.

[78] Yazdanfar S, Rollins AM, Izatt JA. In vivo imaging of human retinal flow dynamics by color Doppler optical coherence tomography. *Arch. Ophthalmol.* 2003; 121: 145-51.

[79] Yazdanfar S, Rollins AM, Izatt JA. Imaging and velocimetry of the human retinal circulation with color Doppler optical coherence tomography. *Optics Letters.* 2000; 25: 1448-50.

[80] Meng J, Ding Z. Optical Doppler tomography with short-time Fourier transform and Hilbert transform. *Proc. SPIE,* Vol. 6826, 682602 (2007); DOI:10.1117/12.757243.

[81] Hickam JB, Frayser R, Ross JC. A study of retinal venous blood oxygen saturation in human subjects by photographic means. *Circulation.* 1963;27:375–385.

[82] Beach JM, Schwenzer KJ, Srinivas S, Kim D, Tiedeman JS. Oximetry of retinal vessels by dual-wavelength imaging: calibration and influence of pigmentation. *J. Appl. Physiol.* 1999; 86:748–758.

[83] Delori FC. Noninvasive techniques for oximetry of blood in retinal vessels. *Appl. Opt.* 1988;27:1113–1125.

[84] Harris A, Dinn RB, Kagemann L, Rechtman E. A review of methods for human retinal oximetry. *Ophthalmic Surg. Lasers Imaging.* 2003; 34:152–164.

[85] Hardarson S H, Harris A, Karlsson RA et al. Automatic retinal oximetry. *Invest. Ophthalmol. Vis. Sci.* 2006; 47: 5011–5016.

[86] Carter CJ, Brooks DE, Doyle DL, Drance SM. Investigations into a vascular etiology for low-tension glaucoma. *Ophthalmology.* 1990; 97: 49-55.

[87] Martinez A, Sanchez M. Ocular blood flow and glaucoma. *Br. J. Ophthalmol.* 2008 Sep; 92(9):1301.

[88] Gasser P, Flammer J. Blood-cell velocity in the nailfold capillaries of patients with normal tension and high tension glaucoma. *Am. J. Ophthalmol.* 1991; 111: 585-588.

[89] Michelson G, Langhans MJ, Harazny J, Dichtl A. Visual field defect and perfusion of the juxtapapillary retina and the neuroretinal rim area in primary open-angle glaucoma. *Graefes Arc. Clin. Exp. Ophthalmol.* 236: 80-85.

[90] Martinez A, Gonzalez F, Capeans C, Perez R, Sanchez-Salorio M. Dorzolamide effect on ocular blood flow. *Invest. Ophthalmol. Vis. Sci.* 40: 1270-75.

[91] Galassi F, Nuzzaci G, Sodi A, Casi P, Vielmo A. Color Doppler imaging in evaluation of optic nerve blood supply in normal and glaucomatous subjects. *Int. Ophthalmol.* 1992; 16: 273-276.

[92] Trible JR, Costa PV, Sergott RC et al. The influence of primary open-angle glaucoma upon the retrobulbar circulation: baseline, postoperative and reproducibility analysis. *Trans. Am. Soc.* 1994; 245-265.

[93] Birinci H, Danaci M, Oge I, Erkan ND. Ocular blood flow in healthy and primary open-angle glaucomatous eyes. *Ophthalmologica.* 2002; 216(6):434-7.

[94] Akarsu C, Bilgili MY. Color Doppler imaging in ocular hypertension and open-angle glaucoma. *Graefes Arch. Clin. Exp. Ophthalmol.* 2004; 242(2):125-9.

[95] Grieshaber MC, Flammer J. Blood flow in glaucoma. *Curr. Opin. Ophthalmol.* 2005; 16(2):79-83.

[96] Plange N, Kaup M, Arend O, Remky A. Asymmetric visual field loss and retrobulbar haemodynamics in primary open-angle glaucoma. *Graefes Arch. Clin. Exp. Ophthalmol.* 2006; 244(8):978-83.

[97] Plange N, Kaup M, Weber A, Arend KO, Remky A. Retrobulbar haemodynamics and morphometric optic disc analysis in primary open-angle glaucoma. *Br. J. Ophthalmol.* 2006; 90(12):1501-4.

[98] Nicolela MT, Wolman BE, Buckley AR, Drance SM. Ocular hypertension and primary open-angle glaucoma: a comparative study of their retrobulbar blood flow velocity. *J. Glaucoma.* 1996; 5(5):308-10.

[99] Nong T, Ninghua F. Color Doppler imaging in the study of retrobulbar hemodynamic changes of primary angle-closure glaucoma. *Yan Ke Xue Bao.* 1997; 13(3):113-5.

[100] Cheng CY, Liu CJ, Chiou HJ, Chou JC, Hsu WM, Liu JH. Color Doppler imaging study of retrobulbar hemodynamics in chronic angle-closure glaucoma. *Ophthalmology.* 2001; 108(8):1445-51.

[101] Yüksel N, Karabaş VL, Arslan A, Demirci A, Cağlar Y. Ocular hemodynamics in pseudoexfoliation syndrome and pseudoexfoliation glaucoma. *Ophthalmology.* 2001; 108(6):1043-9.

[102] Yüksel N, Karabaş VL, Demirci A, Arslan A, Altintaş O, Cağlar Y. Comparison of blood flow velocities of the extraocular vessels in patients with pseudoexfoliation or primary open-angle glaucoma. *Ophthalmologica.* 2001; 215(6):424-9.

[103] Detorakis ET, Achtaropoulos AK, Drakonaki EE, Kozobolis VP. Hemodynamic evaluation of the posterior ciliary circulation in exfoliation syndrome and exfoliation glaucoma. *Graefes Arch. Clin. Exp. Ophthalmol.* 2007; 245(4):516-21.

[104] Martinez A, Sanchez M. Ocular haemodynamics in pseudoexfoliative and primary open-angle glaucoma. *Eye.* 2008; 22(4):515-20.

[105] Dayanir V, Topaloğlu A, Ozsunar Y, Keceli M, Okyay P, Harris A. Orbital blood flow parameters in unilateral pseudoexfoliation syndrome. *Int. Ophthalmol.* 2008 23. [Epub ahead of print]

[106] Martinez A, Sanchez M. Retrobulbar hemodynamic parameters in pseudoexfoliation syndrome and pseudoexfoliative glaucoma. *Graefes Arch. Clin. Exp. Ophthalmol.* 2008 Sep; 246(9):1341-9.

[107] Galassi F, Giambene B, Menchini U. Ocular perfusion pressure and retrobulbar haemodynamics in pseudoexfoliative glaucoma. *Graefes Arch. Clin. Exp. Ophthalmol.* 2008; 246(3):411-6.

[108] Harris A, Sergott RC, Spaeth GL, Katz JL, Shoemaker JA, Martin BJ. Color Doppler analysis of ocular vessel blood velocity in normal-tension glaucoma. *Am. J. Ophthalmol.* 1994 15; 118(5):642-9.

[109] Yamazaki Y, Hayamizu F. Comparison of flow velocity of ophthalmic artery between primary open angle glaucoma and normal tension glaucoma. *Br. J. Ophthalmol.* 1995; 79(8):732-4.

[110] Kaiser HJ, Schoetzau A, Stümpfig D, Flammer J. Blood-flow velocities of the extraocular vessels in patients with high-tension and normal-tension primary open-angle glaucoma. *Am. J. Ophthalmol.* 1997 Mar; 123(3):320-7.

[111] Rankin SJ. Color Doppler imaging of the retrobulbar circulation in glaucoma. *Surv. Ophthalmol.* 1999 Jun; 43 Suppl 1:S176-82.

[112] Kondo Y, Niwa Y, Yamamoto T, Sawada A, Harris A, Kitazawa Y. Retrobulbar hemodynamics in normal-tension glaucoma with asymmetric visual field change and asymmetric ocular perfusion pressure. *Am. J. Ophthalmol.* 2000; 130(4):454-60.

[113] Plange N, Remky A, Arend O. Colour Doppler imaging and fluorescein filling defects of the optic disc in normal tension glaucoma. *Br. J. Ophthalmol.* 2003; 87(6):731-6.

[114] Emre M, Orgül S, Gugleta K, Flammer J. Ocular blood flow alteration in glaucoma is related to systemic vascular dysregulation. *Br. J. Ophthalmol.* 2004; 88(5):662-6.

[115] Plange N, Kaup M, Weber A, Harris A, Arend KO, Remky A. Performance of colour Doppler imaging discriminating normal tension glaucoma from healthy eyes. *Eye.* 2007 10. [Epub ahead of print].

[116] Katamay R, Grieshaber MC, Weich C, Flammer J, Orgül S. Central corneal thickness and retrobulbar blood flow in glaucoma patients. *Klin. Monatsbl. Augenheilkd.* 2008; 225(5):346-8.

[117] Nicolela MT, Drance SM, Rankin SJ, Buckley AR. Walman BE. Color Doppler imaging in patients with asymmetric glaucoma and unilateral visual field loss. *Am. J. Ophthalmol.* 1996; 121: 502-510.

[118] Hou Q, Li X, Zhang X. Measurement of velocity of ophthalmic arterial blood flow in normal persons with color Doppler sonography. *Chung Hua Yen Ko Tsa Chich.* 1995; 31: 288-290.

[119] Rankin SJA, Walman BE, Buckley AR, Drance SM. Color Doppler imaging and spectral analysis of the optic nerve vasculature in glaucoma. *Am. J. Ophthalmol.* 1995; 119: 685-693.

[120] Langham ME. Ocular blood flow and vision in healthy and glaucomatous eyes. *Surv. Ophthalmol.* 1994; 38 Suppl:S161-8.

[121] Schmidt KG, von Rückmann A, Mittag TW. Ocular pulse amplitude in ocular hypertension and open-angle glaucoma. *Ophthalmologica.* 1998; 212(1):5-10.

[122] James CB. Pulsatile ocular blood flow. *Br. J. Ophthalmol.* 1998; 82(7):720-1.

[123] Kuba GB, Austermann P, Kroll P. Ocular blood flow in patients with asymmetric glaucoma. *Ophthalmologe.* 2002; 99(11):835-8.

[124] Agarwal HC, Gupta V, Sihota R, Singh K. Pulsatile ocular blood flow among normal subjects and patients with high tension glaucoma. *Indian J. Ophthalmol.* 2003; 51(2):133-8.

[125] Aydin A, Wollstein G, Price LL, Schumann JS. Evaluating pulsatile ocular blood flow analysis in normal and treated glaucomatous eyes. *Am. J. Ophthalmol.* 2003; 136(3):448-53.

[126] Kerr J, Nelson P, O'Brien C. Pulsatile ocular blood flow in primary open-angle glaucoma and ocular hypertension. *Am. J. Ophthalmol.* 2003; 136(6):1106-13.

[127] Fuchsjäger-Mayrl G, Wally B, Georgopoulos M, et al. Ocular blood flow and systemic blood pressure in patients with primary open-angle glaucoma and ocular hypertension. *Invest. Ophthalmol. Vis. Sci.* 2004; 45(3):834-9.

[128] Zhang MZ, Fu ZF, Liu XR, Zheng C. A comparison study of pulsatile ocular blood flow in normal eyes and primary open angle glaucoma. *Zhonghua Yan Ke Za Zhi.* 2004; 40(4):250-3.

[129] Mrugacz M, Sredzińska-Kita D, Bakunowicz-Lazarczyk A, Pawłowski P. Pulsatile ocular blood flow in patients with juvenile glaucoma. *Klin. Oczna.* 2004; 106(1-2 Suppl):209-10.

[130] Weigert G, Findl O, Luksch A, Rainer G, Kiss B, Vass C, Schmetterer L. Effects of moderate changes in intraocular pressure on ocular hemodynamics in patients with primary open-angle glaucoma and healthy controls. *Ophthalmology.* 2005; 112(8):1337-42.

[131] Kim SK, Cho BJ, Hong S, Kang SY, Kim JS, Kim CY, Seong GJ. Pulsatile ocular blood flow in healthy Koreans. *Korean J. Ophthalmol.* 2008; 22(1):6-9.

[132] Hommer A, Fuchsjäger-Mayrl G, Resch H, Vass C, Garhofer G, Schmetterer L. Estimation of ocular rigidity based on measurement of pulse amplitude using

pneumotonometry and fundus pulse using laser interferometry in glaucoma. *Invest. Ophthalmol. Vis. Sci.* 2008; 49(9):4046-50.

[133] Mistlberger A, Gruchmann M, Hitzl W, Grabner G. Pulsatile ocular blood flow in patients with pseudoexfoliation. *Int. Ophthalmol.* 2001; 23(4-6):337-42.

[134] James CB, Smith SE. Pulsatile ocular blood flow in patients with low tension glaucoma. *Br. J. Ophthalmol.* 1991; 75(8):466-70.

[135] Quaranta L, Manni G, Donato F, Bucci MG. The effect of increased intraocular pressure on pulsatile ocular blood flow in low tension glaucoma. *Surv. Ophthalmol.* 1994; 38 Suppl:S177-81

[136] Fontana L, Poinoosawmy D, Bunce CV, O'Brien C, Hitchings RA. Pulsatile ocular blood flow investigation in asymmetric normal tension glaucoma and normal subjects. *Br. J. Ophthalmol.* 1998; 82(7):731-6.

[137] Kerr J, Nelson P, O'Brien CA. A comparison of ocular blood flow in untreated primary open-angle glaucoma and ocular hypertension. *Am. J. Ophthalmol.* 1998; 126: 42-51.

[138] Trew DR, Smith SE. Postural studies in pulsatile ocular blood flow: II. Chronic open-angle glaucoma. *Br. J. Ophthalmol.* 1991; 75: 71-75.

[139] Grunwald JE, Piltz JE, Hariprasad SM, DuPont J: Optic nerve and choroidal circulation in glaucoma. *Invest. Ophthalmol. Vis. Sci.* 1998; 39:2329–2336.

[140] Grunwald JE, Piltz JR, Hariprasad SM, et al: Optic nerve blood flow in glaucoma: Effect of systemic hypertension. *Am. J. Ophthalmol.* 1999; 127:516–522.

[141] Piltz-Seymour JR. Laser Doppler flowmetry of the optic nerve head in glaucoma. *Surv. Ophthalmol.* 1999; 43 Suppl 1:S191-8.

[142] Zink JM, Grunwald JE, Piltz-Seymour J, Staii A, Dupont J. Association between lower optic nerve laser Doppler blood volume measurements and glaucomatous visual field progression. *Br. J. Ophthalmol.* 2003; 87(12):1487-91.

[143] Hamard P, Hamard H, Dufaux J: Blood flow rate in the microvasculature of the optic nerve head in primary open angle glaucoma: A new approach. *Surv. Ophthalmol.* 1994; 38:S87– S94.

[144] Hamard P, Hamard H, Dufaux J, Quesnot S: Optic nerve head blood flow using a laser Doppler velocimeter and haemorheology in primary open-angle glaucoma and normal pressure glaucoma. *Br. J. Ophthalmol.* 1994; 78:449–453.

[145] Findl O, Rainer G, Dallinger S et al. Assessment of optic disk blood flow in patients with open-angle glaucoma. *Am. J. Ophthalmol.* 2000; 130(5):589-96.

[146] Ciancaglini M, Carpineto P, Costagliola C, Matropasqua L. Perfusion of the optic nerve head and visual field damage in glaucomatous patients. *Graefes Arch. Clin. Exp. Ophthalmol.* 2001; 239(8):549-55.

[147] 146. Ben Simon GJ, Moroz I, Goldenfeld M, Melamed S. Scanning laser Doppler flowmetry of non perfused regions of the optic nerve head in patients with glaucoma. *Ophthalmic. Surg. Lasers Imaging.* 2003; 34(3):245-50.

[148] Yaoeda K, Shirakashi M, Fukushima A, Funaki S, Funaki H, Abe H, Tanabe N. Relationship between optic nerve head microcirculation and visual field loss in glaucoma. *Acta Ophthalmol. Scand.* 2003; 81(3):253-9.

[149] Hafez AS, Bizzarro RL, Lesk MR. Evaluation of optic nerve head and peripapillary retinal blood flow in glaucoma patients, ocular hypertensives, and normal subjects. *Am. J. Ophthalmol.* 2003; 136(6):1022-31.

[150] Ocakoglu O, Koyluoglu N, Kayiran A, Tamcelik N, Ozkan S. Microvascular blood flow of the optic nerve head and peripapillary retina in unilateral exfoliation syndrome. *Acta Ophthalmol. Scand.* 2004; 82(1):49-53.

[151] Lam A, Piltz-Seymour J, Dupont J, Grunwald J. Laser Doppler flowmetry in asymmetric glaucoma. *Curr. Eye Res.* 2005; 30(3):221-7.

[152] Sato EA, Ohtake Y, Shinoda K, Mashima Y, Kimura I. Decreased blood flow at neuroretinal rim of optic nerve head corresponds with visual field deficit in eyes with normal tension glaucoma. *Graefes Arch. Clin. Exp. Ophthalmol.* 2006; 244(7):795-801.

[153] Berisha F, Feke GT, Hirose T, McMeel JW, Pasquale LR. Retinal blood flow and nerve fiber layer measurements in early-stage open-angle glaucoma. *Am. J. Ophthalmol.* 2008; 146(3):466-472.

[154] Chung HS, Harris A, Kagemann L, Martin B. Peripapillary retinal blood flow in normal tension glaucoma. *Br. J. Ophthalmol.* 1999; 83:466–469.

[155] Logan JF, Rankin SJ, Jackson AJ. Retinal blood flow measurements and neuroretinal rim damage in glaucoma. *Br. J. Ophthalmol.* 2004; 88(8):1049-54.

[156] Harju M, Vesti E. Blood flow of the optic nerve head and peripapillary retina in exfoliation syndrome with unilateral glaucoma or ocular hypertension. *Graefe`s Arch. Clin. Exp. Ophthalmol.* 2001; 271-277.

[157] Holló G, van den Berg TJ, Greve EL. Scanning laser Doppler flowmetry in glaucoma. *Int. Ophthalmol.* 1996-1997; 20(1-3):63-70.

[158] Holló G, Greve EL, van den Berg TJ, Vargha P. Evaluation of the peripapillary circulation in healthy and glaucoma eyes with scanning laser Doppler flowmetry. *Int. Ophthalmol.* 1996-1997; 20(1-3):71-7.

[159] Hitchings RA, Spaeth GL. Fluorescein angiography in chronic simple and low-tension glaucoma. *Br. J. Ophthalmol.* 1977; 61: 126-132.

[160] Talusan ED, Schwartz B, Wilcox LM Jr. Fluorescein angiography of the optic disc. A longitudinal follow-up study. *Arch. Ophthalmol.* 1980; 98(9):1579-87

[161] 160. Huang LN, Zhou WB. Comparison of optic disc damages and fluorescein filling defect of the disc between low tension and primary open angle glaucoma. *Zhonghua Yan Ke Za Zhi.* 1992; 28(4):209-13.

[162] Tanaka Y. Color-fluorescein relationship in glaucomatous optic nerve damage. *Jpn. J. Ophthalmol.* 1995; 39(2):180-6.

[163] Yamazaki S, Inoue Y, Yoshikawa K. Peripapillary fluorescein angiographic findings in primary open angle glaucoma. *Br. J. Ophthalmol.* 1996; 80(9):812-7.

[164] Ulrich A, Ulrich C, Barth T, Ulrich WD. Detection of disturbed autoregulation of the peripapillary choroid in primary open angle glaucoma. *Ophthalmic. Surg. Lasers.* 1996; 27(9):746-57.

[165] Duijm HF, van den Berg TJ, Greve EL. Choroidal haemodynamics in glaucoma. *Br. J. Ophthalmol.* 1997; 81:735–742.

[166] O'Brart DP, de Souza Lima M, Bartsch DU, Freeman W, Weinreb RN. Indocyanine green angiography of the peripapillary region in glaucomatous eyes by confocal scanning laser ophthalmoscopy. *Am. J. Ophthalmol.* 1997; 123(5):657-66.

[167] Duijm HF, van den Berg TJ, Greve EL. A comparison of retinal and choroidal hemodynamics in patients with primary open-angle glaucoma and normal-pressure glaucoma. *Am. J. Ophthalmol.* 1997; 123(5):644-56.

[168] Yin ZQ, Vaegan, Millar TJ, Beaumont P, Sarks S. Widespread choroidal insufficiency in primary open-angle glaucoma. *J. Glaucoma.* 1997; 6(1):23-32.

[169] Hitchings RA. Intraocular pressure and circulation at the disc in glaucoma. *Acta Ophthalmol. Scand. Suppl.* 1997; 220:15-20.

[170] Plange N, Kaup M, Weber A, Remky A, Arend O. Fluorescein filling defects and quantitative morphologic analysis of the optic nerve head in glaucoma. *Arch. Ophthalmol.* 2004; 122(2):195-201.

[171] Arend O, Remky A, Plange N, Kaup M, Schwartz B. Fluorescein leakage of the optic disc in glaucomatous optic neuropathy. *Graefes Arch. Clin. Exp. Ophthalmol.* 2005; 243:659-64.

[172] Wu LL, Chen W, Chen ZQ, Yin JF, Zhou H, Liu J, Su ZA. Indocyanine green and fluorescein angiography study of glaucomatous peripapillary atrophy. *Zhonghua Yan Ke Za Zhi.* 2006; 42(11):967-71.

[173] Plange N, Kaup M, Remky A, Arend KO. Prolonged retinal arteriovenous passage time is correlated to ocular perfusion pressure in normal tension glaucoma. *Graefes Arch. Clin. Exp. Ophthalmol.* 2008 Aug; 246(8):1147-52.

[174] Shulte K, Wolf S, Arend O, Harris A, Henle C, Reim M. Retinal hemodynamics during increased intraocular pressure. *Ger. J. Ophthalmol.* 1996; 5:1-5.

[175] Spaeth GL. Fluorescein angiography: its contributions towards understanding the mechanisms of visual field loss in glaucoma. *Trans. Am. Ophthalmol. Soc.* 1975; 73:491-553.

[176] Schwartz B. Circulatory defects of the optic disc and retina in ocular hypertension and high pressure open-angle glaucoma. *Surv. Ophthalmol.* 1994; 38(suppl): S23-S34.

[177] Francois J, De Laey JJ. Fluorescein angiography of the glaucomatous disc. *Ophthalmologica.* 1974; 168:288-298.

[178] Raitta C, Sarmela T. Fluorescein angiography of the optic disc and the peripapillary area in chronic glaucoma. *Acta Ophthalmol.* (Copenh). 1970; 48:303-308.

[179] Oosterhuis JA, Gortzak-Moorstein N. Fluorescein angiography of the optic disc in glaucoma. *Ophthalmologica.* 1970; 160:331-353.

[180] Schwartz B, Rieser JC, Fishbein SL. Fluorescein angiographic defects of the optic disc in glaucoma. *Arch. Ophthalmol.* 1977; 95:1961-1974.

[181] Loebl M, Schwartz B. Fluorescein angiographic defects of the optic disc in ocular hypertension. *Arch. Ophthalmol.* 1977; 95:1980-1984.

[182] Hayreh SS, Walker WM. Fluorescent fundus photography in glaucoma. *Am. J. Ophthalmol.* 1967; 63:982-989.

[183] Plange N, Remky A, Arend O. Papilla¨re fu¨ llungsdefekte in fluoreszeinangiographien bei glaukom: eine retrospektive klinische studie. *Klin. Monatsbl. Augenheilkd.* 2001; 218:214-221.

[184] Arnold AC. Fluorescein angiographic characteristics of the optic disc in ischemic and glaucomatous optic neuropathy. *Curr. Opin. Ophthalmol.* 1995; 6:30-35.

[185] Fishbein SL, Schwartz B. Optic disc in glaucoma: topography and extent of fluorescein filling defects. *Arch. Ophthalmol.* 1977; 95:1975-1979.

[186] Nanba K, Schwartz B. Nerve fiber layer and optic disc fluorescein defects in glaucoma and ocular hypertension. *Ophthalmology.* 1988; 95:1227-1233.

[187] Tsukahara S, Nagataki S, Sugaya M, Yoshida S, Komuro Y. Visual field defects, cup-disc-ratio and fluorescein angiography in glaucomatous optic atrophy. *Adv. Ophthalmol.* 1978; 35:73-93.

[188] Tuulonen A, Nagin P, Schwartz B, Wu D. Increase of pallor and fluoresceinfilling defects of the optic disc in the follow-up of ocular hypertensives measured by computerized image analysis. *Ophthalmology.* 1987; 94:558-563.

[189] Jonas JB, Nguyen XN, Naumann GO. Peripapillary retinal vessels diameter in normaland glaucoma eyes. I. Morphometric data. *Invest. Ophthalmol. Vis. Sci.* 1989; 30:1599-1603.

[190] Rader J, Feuer WJ, Anderson DR. Peripapillary vasoconstriction in the glaucomas and the anterior ischemic optic neuropathies. *Am. J. Ophthalmol.* 1994; 117: 72-80.

[191] Sugiyama T, Schwartz B, Takamoto T, Azuma I. Evaluation in the circulation in the retina, peripapillary choroid and optic disk in normal-tension glaucoma. *Ophthalmic Res.* 2000; 32: 79-86.

[192] Mitchell P, Leung H, Wang JJ et al. Retinal vessel diameter and open-angle glaucoma: the Blue Mountains Eye Study. *Ophthalmology.* 2005; 112(2):245-50.

[193] Ikram MK, de Voogd S, Wolfs RC et al. Retinal vessel diameters and incident open-angle glaucoma and optic disc changes: the Rotterdam study. *Invest. Ophthalmol. Vis. Sci.* 2005; 46(4):1182-7.

[194] Hofman A, Grobbee DE, de Jong PT, van den Ouweland FA. Determinants of disease and disability in the elderly. The Rotterdam Elderly Study. *Eur. J. Epidemiol.* 1991; 7:403–422.

[195] Wolfs RC, Borger PH, Ramrattan RS, et al. Changing views on open-angle glaucoma: definitions and prevalences. The Rotterdam Study. *Invest. Ophthalmol. Vis. Sci.* 2000; 41:3309–3321.

[196] Vlachokosta AA, Asvestas PA, Matsopoulos GK, Uzunoglu N, Zeyen TG. Preliminary study on the association of vessel diameter variation and glaucoma. *Conf. Proc. IEEE Eng. Med. Biol. Soc.* 2007; 2007:888-91.

[197] Hall JK, Andrews AP, Walker R, Piltz-Seymour JR. Association of retinal vessel caliber and visual field defects in glaucoma. *Am. J. Ophthalmol.* 2001; 132(6):855-9.

[198] Feke GT, Pasquale LR. Retinal blood flow response to postural change in glaucoma patients compared with healthy subjects. *Ophthalmology.* 2008; 11%: 246-252.

[199] Feke GT, Schwartz B, Takamoto T, et al. Optic nerve head circulation in untreated ocular hypertension. *Br. J. Ophthalmol.* 1995; 79:1088 –1092.

[200] Tamaki Y, Araie M, Hasegawa T, Nagahara M. Optic nerve head circulation alter intraocular pressure reduction achieved by trabeculectomy. *Ophthalmology.* 2001; 108: 627-632.

[201] Okuno T, Sugiyama T, Kojima S, Nakajima M, Ikeda T. Diurnal variation in microcirculation of ocular fundus and visual field change in normal-tension glaucoma. *Eye*. 2004; 18(7):697-702.

[202] Yaoeda K, Shirakashi M, Fukushima A et al. Relationship between optic nerve head microcirculation and visual field loss in glaucoma. *Acta Ophthalmol. Scand.* 2003; 81(3):253-9.

[203] Fuchsjäger-Mayrl G, Polak K, Luksch A et al. Retinal blood flow and systemic blood pressure in healthy young subjects. *Graefe's Arch. Clin. Exp. Ophthalmol.* 2001; 239:673–677.

[204] Grunwald J, Riva CE, Stone RA, Keates EU, Petrig BL. Retinal autorregulation in open-angle glaucoma. *Ophthalmology.* 1984; 91: 1690-1694.

[205] Sponsel WE, DePaul KL, Kaufman PL. Correlation of visual function and retinal leukocyte velocity in glaucoma. *Am. J. Ophthalmol.* 1990 15; 109(1):49-54.

[206] Sponsel WE, Kaufman PL, Blum FG Jr. Association of retinal capillary perfusion with visual status during chronic glaucoma therapy. *Ophthalmology.* 1997; 104(6):1026-32.

[207] Ben-Nun J (1996) Comparative flow velocity of erythrocytes and leukocytes in feline retinal capillaries. *Invest. Ophthalmol. Vis. Sci.* 37:1854–1859.

[208] Bower BA, Zhao M, Zawadzki RJ, Izatt JA. Real-time spectral domain Doppler optical coherence tomography and investigation of human retinal vessel autoregulation. *J. Biomed. Opt.* 2007; 12(4):041214.

[209] Michelson G, Scibor M. Intravascular oxygen saturation in retinal vessels in normal subjects and open-angle glaucoma subjects. *Acta Ophthalmol. Scand.* 2006: 84: 289–295.

[210] Kim MB, Ward DS, Cartwright CR, Kolano J, Chlebowski S, Henson LC. Estimation of jugular venous O2 saturation from cerebral oximetry or arterial O2 saturation during isocapnic hypoxia. *J. Clin. Monit. Comput.* 2000; 16: 191–199.

[211] Torella F, Haynes SL, McCollum CN. Cerebral and peripheral oxygen saturation during red cell transfusion. *J. Surg. Res.* 2003; 110: 217–221.

[212] Shiose Y, Kawase Y. A new approach to stratified normal intraocular pressure in a general population. *Am. J. Ophthalmol.* 1986; 101:714–21.

[213] Wu SY, Leske MC. Associations with intraocular pressure in the Barbados Eye Study. The Barbados Eye Study Group. *Arch. Ophthalmol.* 1997;115:1572-6.

[214] Bengtsson B. Some factors affecting the distribution of intraocular pressures in a population. *Acta Ophthalmol.* (Copenh) 1972;50:33–46.

[215] Bulpitt CJ, Hodes C, Everitt MG. Intraocular pressure and systemic blood pressure in the elderly. *Br. J. Ophthalmol.* 1975; 59:717–20.

[216] Dielemans I, Vingerling JR, Algra D, Hofman A, Grobbee DE, de Jong PT. Primary open-angle glaucoma, intraocular pressure, and systemic blood pressure in the general elderly population. *Ophthalmology.* 1995;102:54–60.

[217] Carel RS, Korczyn AD, Rock M, Goya I. Association between ocular pressure and certain health parameters. *Ophthalmology.* 1984;91:311–4.

[218] Leske MC, Pogdor MJ. Intraocular pressure, cardiovascular risk variables, and visual field defects. *Am. J. Epidemiol.* 1983; 118: 280-287.

[219] Klein BEK, Klein R, Linton KLP. Intraocular pressure in an American community: the Beaver Dam Eye Study. *Invest. Ophthalmol. Vis. Sci.* 1992;33:2224–8.
[220] Hennis A, Wu SY, Nemesure B, Leske MC for the Barbados Eye Study Groups. Hypertension, diabetes, and longitudinal changes in intraocular pressure. *Ophthalmology.* 2003;110:908–914.
[221] Nomura H, Shimokata H, Ando F, et al. Age-related changes in intraocular pressure in a large Japanese population. A cross-sectional and longitudinal study. *Ophthalmology.* 1999; 106:2016–22.
[222] McLeod SD, West SK, Quigley HA, Fozard JL. A longitudinal study of the relationship between intraocular and blood pressures. *Invest. Ophthalmol. Vis. Sci.* 1990;31:2361–6.
[223] Wu SY, Nemesure B, Hennis A, Leske MC for the Barbados Eye Study Groups. Nine-year changes in intraocular pressure: The Barbados eye Studies. *Arch. Ophthalmol.* 2006; 124: 1631-36.
[224] Tielsh JM, Katz J, Sommer A, Quigley HA, Javitt JC. Hypertension, perfusion pressure, and primary open-angle glaucoma: a population-based assessment. *Arch. Ophthalmol.* 1995; 113: 216-221.
[225] Bonomi L, Marchini G, Marrafa M et al. Vascular risk factors for primary open-angle glaucoma: The Egna-Neumarkt study. *Ophthalmology.* 2000; 107: 1287-1293.
[226] Klein BEK, Klein R, Knudtson MD. Intraocular pressure and systemic blood pressure: Longitudinal perspective: The Beaver Dam Eye Study. *Br. J. Ophthalmol.* 2005; 89: 284-7.
[227] Hulsman CA, Virgerling JR, Hofman A, Witteman JC, de Jong PT. Blood pressure, arterial stiffness and open-angle glaucoma: The Rotterdam Study. *Arch. Ophthalmol.* 2007; 125: 805-12.
[228] Yip JL, Aung T, Wong TY, et al. Socioeconomic Status, systolic blood pressure and intraocular pressure: The Tanjong Pagar Study. *Br. J. Ophthalmol.* 2007; 91: 56-61.
[229] Carel RS, Korczyn AD, Rock M, Goya I. Association between ocular pressure and certain health parameters. *Ophthalmology.* 1984;91:311–4.
[230] Wilson MR, Hertzmark E, Walker AM, Childs-Shaw K, Epstein DL. A case-control study of risk factors in open-angle glaucoma. *Arch. Ophthalmol.* 1987; 105: 1066-1071.
[231] Quigley HA, Enger C, Katz J et al. Risk factors for the development of glaucomatous visual field loss in ocular hypertension. *Arch. Ophthalmol.* 1994; 112: 644-649.
[232] Jonas JB, Grundler AE. Prevalence of diabetes mellitus and arterial hypertension in primary and secondary open-angle glaucomas. *Graefes Arch. Clin. Exp. Ophthalmol.* 1998; 236: 202-206.
[233] Kurita N, Tomidokoro A, Mayama C, Aihara M, Araie M. No apparent association between ocular perfusion pressure and visual field damage in normal tension glaucoma patients. *Jpn. J. Ophthalmol.* 2006; 50: 547-549.
[234] Deokule S, Weinreb RN. Relationships among systemic blood pressure, intraocular pressure, and open-angle glaucoma. *Can. J. Ophthalmol.* 2008; 43: 302-307.
[235] Leske MC, Wu SY, Hennis A, Honkanen R, Nemesure B, for the BESs Study Group. Risk factors for incident open-angle glaucoma: the Barbados Eye Studies. *Ophthalmology.* 2008; 115: 85-93.

[236] Safar ME. Systolic blood pressure, pulse pressure and arterial stiffness as cardiovascular risk factors. *Curr. Opin. Nephrol. Hypertens.* 2001;10:257– 61.
[237] Bonomi L, Babighian S, Bonadimani N et al. Correlation between glaucoma and vascular factors, and circumstances leading to the diagnosis of glaucoma. *Acta Ophthalmol. Scand. Suppl.* 2000; 232: 34-35.
[238] Leske MC, Wu SY, Nemesure B et al. Incident open-angle glaucoma and blood pressure. *Arch. Ophthalmol.* 2002; 120: 954-959.
[239] Hayreh SS, Zimmerman MB, Podhajsky P, Alward WL. Nocturnal arterial hypotension and its role in optic nerve head and ocular ischemic disorders. *Am. J. Ophthalmol.* 1994; 117: 603-624.
[240] Hayreh SS. Role of nocturnal arterial hypotension in the development of ocular manifestations of systemic arterial hypertension. *Curr. Opin. Ophthalmol.* 1999; 10: 474-482.
[241] Drance SM: Some factors in the production of low tension glaucoma. *Br. J. Ophthalmol.* 1972; 56:229-42.
[242] Demailly P, Cambien F, Plouin PF, et al: Do patients with low tension glaucoma have particular cardiovascular characteristics? *Ophthalmologica.* 1984;188: 65-75.
[243] Gramer E, Leydhecker W: Glaukom ohne Hochdruck. Eine klinische Studie. *Klin. Monatsbl. Augenheilkd.* 1985; 186:262-7.
[244] Kaiser HJ, Flammer J: Systemic hypotension: a risk factor for glaucomatous damage? *Ophthalmologica.* 1991; 203:105-8.
[245] Kaiser HJ, Flammer J, Graf T, et al: Systemic blood pressure in glaucoma patients. *Graefes Arch. Clin. Exp. Ophthalmol.* 1993; 231:677-80.
[246] Bechetoille A, Bresson-Dumont H: Diurnal and nocturnal blood pressure drops in patients with focal ischemic glaucoma. *Graefes Arch. Clin. Exp. Ophthalmol.* 1994; 232:675-9.
[247] Leske MC, Connell AM, Wu SY, Hyman LG, Schachat AP. Risk factors for open-angle glaucoma. The Barbados Eye Study. *Arch. Ophthalmol.* 1995; 113:918-24.
[248] Leske MC, Nemesure B, He Q, et al: Patterns of open-angle glaucoma in the Barbados Family Study. *Ophthalmology.* 2001; 108:1015-22.
[249] Pache M, Flammer J. A sick eye in a sick body? Systemic findings in patients with primary open-angle glaucoma. *Surv. Ophthalmol.* 2006; 51:179-212.
[250] Graham SL, Drance SM, Wijsman K, et al: Ambulatory blood pressure monitoring in glaucoma. The nocturnal dip. *Ophthalmology.* 1995; 102:61-69.
[251] Verdecchia P, Schillaci G, Porcellati C: Dippers versus nondippers. *J. Hypertens.* 1991; 9 (Suppl 8):S42–S44.
[252] Floras J: Antihypertensive treatment, myocardial infarction, and nocturnal myocardial ischaemia. *Lancet.* 1998; 2:994–996.
[253] Hosaka O, Kashiwagi F et al. Systemic circulatory parameters. comparison between patients with normal tension glaucoma and normal subjects using ambulatory monitoring. *Jpn. J. Ophthalmol.* 2001; 45(4):388-96.
[254] Tokunaga T, Kashiwagi K, Tsomura T. Association between nocturnal blood pressure reduction and progression of visual field defect in patients with primary open-angle glaucoma or normal-tension glaucoma. *Jpn. J. Ophthalmol.* 2004; 48: 380-385.

[255] Anderson DR. Introductory comments on blood flow autorregulation in the optic nerve head and vascular risk factors in glaucoma. *Surv. Ophthalmol.* 2004;43:S5–S9.

[256] Sherwood L. Human Physiology: from Cells to Systems. 5th ed. Pacific Grove, CA: Brooks Cole; 2004.

[257] Flammer J, Orgül S. Optic nerve blood-flow abnormalities in glaucoma. *Prog. Retin. Eye Res.* 1998;17:267–289.

[258] Anderson DR. Introductory comments on blood flow autorregulation in the optic nerve head and vascular risk factors in glaucoma. *Surv. Ophthalmol.* 2004;43:S5–S9.

[259] Hayreh SS. Blood flow in the optic nerve head and factors that may influence it. *Prog. Retin. Eye Res.* 2001;20:595–624.

[260] Hayreh SS. The blood supply of the optic nerve head and the evaluation of it: myth and reality. *Prog. Retin. Eye Res.* 2001;20: 563–593.

[261] Gherghel D, Orgül S, Gugleta K, Gekkieva M, Flammer J. Relationship between ocular perfusion pressure and retrobulbar blood flow in patients with glaucoma with progressive damage. *Am. J. Ophthalmol.* 2000;130:597–605.

[262] Bisantis C. Ocular blood flow and its autoregulation. In: Bucci MG, ed. Glaucoma: Decision Making in Therapy. Milan: Springer- Verlag, 1996:37–40.

[263] Xu L, Wang YX, Jonas JB. Ocular perfusion pressure and glaucoma: *the Beijing Eye Study.* doi:10.1038/eye.2008.342.

[264] Pillunat LE, Anderson DR, Knighton RW, Joos KM, Feuer WJ. Autoregulation of human optic nerve head circulation in response to increased intraocular pressure. *Exp. Eye Res.* 1997;64:737–744.

[265] Riva CE, Hero M, Titze P, Petrig B. Autoregulation of human optic nerve head blood flow in response to acute changes in ocular perfusion pressure. *Graefes Arch. Clin. Exp. Ophthalmol.* 1997;235: 618–626.

[266] Drance SM. Diurnal variation of intraocular pressure in treated glaucoma. Significance in patients with chronic simple glaucoma. *Arch. Ophthalmol.* 1963;70:302–311.

[267] Drance SM. The value of diurnal tension studies in the early diagnosis and management of treatment in chronic simple glaucoma. *Trans. Can. Ophthalmol. Soc.* 1963;26:210–224.

[268] Asrani S, Zeimer R, Wilensky J, Gieser D, Vitale S, Lindenmuth K. Large diurnal fluctuations in intraocular pressure are an independent risk factor in patients with glaucoma. *J. Glaucoma.* 2000;9: 134–142.

[269] Hughes E, Spry P, Diamond J. 24-hour monitoring of intraocular pressure in glaucoma management: a retrospective review. *J. Glaucoma.* 2003;12:232–236.

[270] Liu JH, Zhang X, Kripke DF, Weinreb RN. Twenty-four-hour intraocular pressure pattern associated with early glaucomatous changes. *Invest. Ophthalmol. Vis. Sci.* 2003;44:1586–1590.

[271] Liu JH, Gokhale PA, Loving RT, Kripke DF, Weinreb RN. Laboratory assessment of diurnal and nocturnal ocular perfusion pressures in humans. *J. Ocul. Pharmacol. Ther.* 2003;19:291–297.

[272] Fontana L, Armas R, Garway-Heath DF, Bunce CV, Poinoosawmy D, Hitchings RA. Clinical factors influencing the visual prognosis of the fellow eyes of normal tension glaucoma patients with unilateral field loss. *Br. J. Ophthalmol.* 1999;83:1002–1005.

[273] Hughes E, Spry P, Diamond J. 24-hour monitoring of intraocular pressure in glaucoma management: a retrospective review. *J. Glaucoma.* 2003;12:232–236.

[274] Sacca SC, Rolando M, Marletta A, Macri A, Cerqueti P, Ciurlo G. Fluctuations of intraocular pressure during the day in open-angle glaucoma, normal-tension glaucoma and normal subjects. *Ophthalmologica.* 1998;212:115–119.

[275] Bresson-Dumont H, Bechetoille A. Role of arterial blood pressure in the development of glaucomatous lesions (in French). *J. Fr. Ophthalmol.* 1996;19:435–442.

[276] Claridge KG, Smith SE. Diurnal variation in pulsatile ocular blood flow in normal and glaucomatous eyes. *Surv. Ophthalmol.* 1994; 38(suppl):S198 –S205.

[277] Hayreh SS, Podhajsky P, Zimmerman MB. Beta-blocker eyedrops and nocturnal arterial hypotension. *Am. J. Ophthalmol.* 1999;128: 301–309.

[278] Liu CJ, Ko YC, Cheng CY, et al. Changes in intraocular pressure and ocular perfusion pressure after latanoprost 0.005% or brimonidine tartrate 0.2% in normal-tension glaucoma patients. *Ophthalmology.* 2002;109:2241–2247.

[279] Sehi M, Flanagan JG. Zeng L, Cook RJ, Trope GE. Relative change in diurnal mean ocular perfusion pressure: A risk factor for the diagnosis of primary open-angle glaucoma. *Invest. Ophthalmol. Vis. Sci.* 2005;46: 561–567.

[280] Choi J, Lim KH, Jeong J, Cho HS, Lee CH, Kook MS. Circadian fluctuations of mean ocular perfusion pressure is a consistent risk factor for normal tension glaucoma. *Invest. Ophthalmol. Vis. Sci.* 2007; 48: 104-111.

[281] Müskens RP, Voogd S, Wolfs RC et al. Systemic antihypertensive medication and incident open-angle glaucoma. *Ophthalmology.* 2007; 114: 2221-6.

[282] Langman MJ, Lancaster RJ, Cheng KK, Stewart PM. Systemic hypertension and glaucoma: mechanisms in common and co-occurrence. *Br. J. Ophthalmol.* 2005; 89:960 –3.

[283] Yu DY, Su EN, Cringle SJ, et al. Systemic and ocular vascular roles of the antiglaucoma agents b-adrenergic antagonists and Ca2+ entry blockers. *Surv. Ophthalmol.* 1999; 43(suppl):s214 –22.

[284] Takayama J, Tomidokoro A, Tamaki Y, Araie M. Time course of changes in optic nerve head circulation after acute reduction in intraocular pressure. *Invest. Ophthalmol. Vis. Sci.* 2005;46: 1409–19.

[285] Orgül S, Gugleta K, Flammer J. Physiology of perfusion as it relates to the optic nerve head. *Surv. Ophthalmol.* 1999;43(suppl):s17–26.

[286] Kitazawa Y, Shirai H, Go FJ. The effect of Ca2(□)-antagonist on visual field in low-tension glaucoma. *Graefes Arch. Clin. Exp. Ophthalmol.* 1989;227:408–12.

[287] Netland PA, Chatuverdi N, Dreyer EB. Calcium channel blockers in the management of low-tension and open-angle glaucoma. *Am. J. Ophthalmol.* 1993;115:608 –13.

[288] Anderson DR: Glaucoma, capillaries and pericytes: 1. Blood flow regulation. *Ophthalmologica.* 1996; 210:257–262.

[289] Anderson DR: Optic nerve blood flow, in Drance SM, Anderson DR (eds): Optic Nerve in Glaucoma. New York, Kugler Publications, 1995, pp 311–331.

[290] Guyton AC: Textbook of Medical Physiology. Philadelphia, W. B. Saunders, 1986, ed 7, pp 230–235.

[291] Haefliger IO, Anderson DR: Blood flow regulation in the optic nerve head, in Ritch R, Shields MB, Krupin T (eds): *The Glaucomas,* Vol. 1. St. Louis, Mosby, 1996, pp 189–197 .

[292] Granger HJ. Local regulation of blood flow by resistance vessels sensitive to shear rate, stretch, and tissue metabolites. In Weinreb RN, Joyner WL, Wheeler LA, ed: *Biology of ocular microcirculation,* Amsterdam, 1992, Elsevier.

[293] Grieshaber MC, Mozaffarieh M, Flammer J. What is the link between vascular dysregulation and glaucoma? *Surv. Ophthalmol.* 2007; 52: S144-S154.

[294] Berne RM, Levy MN: *Physiology.* St. Louis, Mosby Year Book, 1993, ed 3, pp 472, 481–494.

[295] Drance SM, Anderson DR (eds): *Optic Nerve in Glaucoma.* New York, Kugler Publications, 1995, pp 243–330.

[296] Riva CE, Harino S, Shonat RD, Petrig BL: Flicker evoked increase in optic nerve head blood flow in anesthetized cats. *Neurosci. Lett.* 1991; 128:291–296.

[297] Metea MR, Newman EA. Signaling within the neurovascular unit in the retina. *Exp. Physiol.* 2007; 92: 635-640.

[298] Albrecht MC, Kaufman PL, Lutjen-Drecoll E et al. Choroidal innervation and optic neuropathy in macaque monkeys with laser or anterior chamber perfusion-induced short-term elevation of intraocular pressure. *Exp. Eye Res.* 2006; 82: 1060-67.

[299] Lutjen-Drecoll E. Choroidal innervation in primate eyes. *Exp. Eye Res.* 2006; 82: 357-361.

[300] Flammer J, Mozaffarieh M. What is the present pathogenetic concept of glaucomatous optic neuropathy? *Surv. Ophthalmol.* 2007; 52: S162-173.

[301] Sossi N, Anderson DR. Blockage of axonal transport in optic nerve head induced by elevation of intraocular pressure. Effect of arterial hypertension induced by angiotensin I. *Arch. Ophthalmol.* 1983; 101: 94-97.

[302] Flammer J. The vascular concept of glaucoma. *Surv. Ophthalmol.* 1994; 38: S3-S6.

[303] Flammer J, Pache M, Resink T. Vasospasm, its role in the pathogenesis of diseases with particular reference to the eye. *Prog. Retin Eye Res*. 2001; 20: 319-349

[304] Haufschild T, Shaw SG, Kesselring J et al. Increased endothelin-1 plasma levels in patients with multiple sclerosis. *J. Neuroophthalmol.* 2001; 21: 37-38.

[305] Pache M, Schwarz HA, Kaiser HJ et al. Elevated plasma endothelin-1 levels and vascular dysregulation in patients with rheumatoid arthritis. *Med. Sci. Monit.* 2002; 8: CR616-619.

[306] Ghergel D, Orgül S, Dubler B, Lubeck P, Gugleta K, Flammer J. Is vascular regulation in the central retinal artery altered in persons with vasospasm? *Arch. Ophthalmol.* 1999; 117: 1359-62

[307] Flammer J, Haefliger IO, Orgül S et al. Vascular dysregulation: a principal risk factor for glaucomatous damage? *J. Glaucoma.* 1999; 8: 212-19.

[308] Kaiser HJ, Meinberg O. Deterioration or onset of migraine under oestrogen replacement therapy in the menopause. *J. Neurol.* 1993; 240: 195-96.

[309] Teuchner B, Orgul S, Ulmer H, Haufschild T, Flammer J. Reduced thirst in patients with vasospastic syndrome. *Acta Ophthalmol. Scand.* 2004; 82: 738-40.

[310] Flammer J, Mozaffarieh M. Autoregulation, a balancing act between supply and demand. *Can. J. Ophthalmol.* 2008; 43: 317-21.

[311] Wunderlich K, Zimmerman C, Gutmann H, Teuchner B, Flammer J, Drewe J. Vasospastic persons exhibit differential expression of ABC-transport proteins. *Mol. Vis.* 2003; 9: 756-61.

[312] Kaiser HJ, Flammer J, Messerli J et al. Vasospasm- a risk factor for nonarteric anterior ischemic optic neuropathy? *Neuro Ophthalmol.* 1996; 16: 5-10.

[313] Messerli J, Flammer J. Central vein thrombosis in younger patients. *Klim. Monatsbl. Augenheilkd.* 1996; 208: 303-305.

[314] Prünte C, Flammer J. Choroidal capillary and venous congestion in central serous chorioretinopathy. *Am. J. Ophthalmol.* 1996; 121:26-34.

[315] Flammer J, Kaiser H, Haufschild T. Susac syndrome : a vasospastic disorder? *Eur. J. Ophthalmol.* 2001; 11: 175-79.

[316] Nicolela MT. Clinical clues of vascular dysregulation and its association with glaucoma. *Can. J. Ophthalmol.* 2008; 43: 337-41.

[317] Andrews RM, Griffiths PG, Johnson MA et al. Histochemical localization of mitochondrial enzyme activity in human optic nerve and retina. *Br. J. Ophthalmol.* 1999; 83: 231-235.

[318] Mojon DS, HessCW, Goldblum D et al. High prevalence of glaucoma in patients with sleep apnea syndrome. *Ophthalmology.* 1999; 106: 1009-12.

[319] Drance SM. The visual field of low tension glaucoma and shock-induced optic neuropathy. *Arch. Ophthalmol.* 1977; 95: 1359-61.

[320] Phelps CD, Corbett JJ. Migraine and low tension glaucoma. A case-control study. *Invest. Ophthalmol. Vis. Sci.* 1985; 26: 1105-8.

[321] Gaser P, Flammer J, Guthauser U, Mahler F. Do vasospasms provoke ocular diseases? *Angiology.* 1990; 41: 213-20.

[322] Wang JJ, Mitchel P, Smith W. Is there any association between migraine headache and open-angle glaucoma? Findings from the Blue Mountains Eye Study. *Ophthalmology.* 1997; 104: 1714-19.

[323] Klein BE, Klein R, Meuer SM, Goetz LA. Migraine headache and its association with open-angle glaucoma: The Beaver-Dam Eye Study. *Invest. Ophthalmol. Vis. Sci.* 1993; 343024-27.

[324] Schulzer M, Drance SM, Carter CJ, Brooks DE, Douglas GR, Lau W. Biostatistical evidence for two distinct chronic open-angle glaucoma populations. *Br. J. Ophthalmol.* 1990; 74: 196-200.

[325] Hayreh SS. Inter-individual variation in blood supply of the optic nerve head. Its importance in various ischemic disorders of the optic nerve head, and glaucoma, low-tension glaucoma and allied disorders. *Doc. Ophthalmol.* 1985; 59: 217-246.

[326] Hayreh SS. Optic nerve head blood supply in health and disease. In Lambrou GN, Geve EL, eds: Ocular blood flow in glaucoma: means, methods, and measurements, Amsterdam, 1989, Kluger & Ghedini.

[327] Hayreh SS. In vivo choroidal circulation and its watershed zones. *Eye.* 1990; 4: 273-289.

In: Eye Research Developments
Editor: Alan N. Westerhouse

ISBN: 978-1-60741-177-2

Chapter XIV

Ahmed Drainage Implant in the Treatment of Refractory Paediatric Glaucoma

***Mohamed Ali El Afrit**, *Hela Mazlout*,**
Mejda Bouladi and Abdelhafidh Kraiem
Department of Ophthalmology. Habib Thameur University Hospital 1008.
Tunis, Tunisia

Abstract

Purpose: To evaluate the efficacy and safety of the Ahmed glaucoma valve implant in children with refractory glaucoma in the early, intermediate and long term follow up period.

Patients & Methods: A retrospective study included 57 eyes (of 52 patients with refractory paediatric glaucoma, age range at surgery 1 year to 16 years, average 10± 4.7 years) treated with the Ahmed glaucoma valve implant (model S3, FP8 or FP7) between January 1995 and January 2008.We reviewed the final intraocular pressure (IOP), the need for postoperative antiglaucoma medications and the incidence of complications in all patients.

In 54 eyes, it was a secondary intention surgery after failure of one or more glaucoma surgery procedures many. In 3 eyes, it was a first intention.

The success was defined as an average intraocular pressure less than 22 mm Hg for at least 2 follow-ups in eyes with preoperative intraocular pressure greater than 22 mm Hg, without additional glaucoma surgery or a visually devastating complication.

Results: The most common aetiology of refractory glaucoma was primary congenital glaucoma (68.4%) and aphakic glaucoma (17.5 %). After a mean follow-up period of 68.2 months (range, 8 to 156 months), the mean intraocular pressure decreased from 35.66± 6,5 mm Hg before surgery to 14 ± 5,3 mm Hg at the last follow-up visit after surgery. Thus, the procedure was successful with or without medications in 92%, 82%, 73%, 47% and 37.5% of cases after 12,24,36,48 and 68 months respectively. The average number of medications used decreased from 3.1 ± 1.9 to 1.9 ± 1.1.

Complications occurred in 27 eyes (47%). Transient postoperative hypotony (less than 5 mm Hg) occurred in 12 of 52 patients (57 eyes). This was, with transient hyphaema, the most common postoperative complication. The other complications were less common: exposed tube, tenon cyst,

* Email:ali.elafrit@rns.tn

choroidal detachment, tube corneal touch, endophtalmitis, retracted tube or tube migration. Two patients had severe visual loss and an other eye demonstrated tube obstruction.

Conclusion: Refractory paediatric glaucoma requires urgent surgery in the aim to save remaining visual function. The Ahmed glaucoma valve implant is an effective treatment for paediatric refractory glaucoma. However, the success rate decreases with the follow up.

Introduction

Paediatric glaucomas are defined as glaucomas between 0 and 16 years. It's a potentially blinding disease. The first aetiology is congenital/infantile glaucoma, but also Aphakic/Pseudophakic and Juvenile glaucoma[1].

The success rate after traditional surgery like trabeculotomy or trabeculectomy with or without adjunctive antimetabolite therapy, decreases very quickly with the follow up and paediatric glaucoma requires other kind of surgery to save remaining visual acuity.

For refractory glaucoma, we must choose between cycloablative techniques with limited success rate and higher rate of phtysis; and aqueous drainage devices.

In children, the majority of authors prefer this second alternative[2,3].

Glaucoma drainage implants that have been used frequently include the non restrictive implants like Schocket tube shunt, Molteno implant, Baerveldt implant, and the restrictive devices like Ahmed Glaucoma valve implants. The theoretical advantage of Ahmed GDD is to prevent postoperative hypotony.

The aim of this study was to evaluate the surgical outcome of this procedure in patients with paediatric refractory glaucoma in the Department of Ophthalmology at Habib Thameur University Hospital of Tunisia.

Material and Methods

A retrospective analysis of 57 eyes of 52 patients aged between 1 and 16 years, average age 10 ± 4, 7 years with uncontrolled glaucoma by medications and previous surgery undergoing procedure with the Ahmed Glaucoma valve implant (model S3 and FP8: age less than 8 years and model S2 or FP7 age over 8 years), New World Medical, USA at Habib Thameur Hospital Tunisia between January 1995 and January 2008.

All procedures were performed by only one surgeon and in 54 eyes like a secondary procedure after failure of one or several classic surgeries. In 3 eyes, it was a first intention procedure.

For all patients, the following information was noted: age, gender, clinical history, and ocular examination including if possible the best corrected visual acuity, IOP measurement with Goldmann applanation tonometre or Perkins tonometre, a gonioscopy with Possner mirror and wherever possible (in 12 eyes) visual fields using automated perimetry by Octopus 100.

Surgical Procedure

The Ahmed Glaucoma Valve implantation was performed in all cases under general anaesthesia. The first choice of site implantation was superotemporal quadrant (in all 57 eyes).After conjunctiva dissection, the Ahmed valve was inserted 8-10 mm from the limbus and fixed to the sclera by mersilene 6/0 through two holes in the valve. Previously, we must improve and open the valve mechanism by irrigating with saline solution through the tube of the valve. Then a scleral flap is dissected like for a trabeculectomy (because we can't have pericardium or other tissue to cover the tube). A 23 gauge needle was used to enter the anterior chamber at the surgical limbus. The tube was cutted (only 1-2 mm in the anterior chamber). The tube was secured to the sclera with a preplaced 10-0 nylon suture. Then, the flap is sutured with nylon 10-0.Conjunctiva was reapposed with 8-0 vicryl sutures. Subconjunctival injection of gentamycin and dexamethasone were done inferiorly at the end of the procedure.

Postoperatively, the patients received topical antibiotic-steroid drops for 6 to -10 weeks. Each patient was reviewed daily the first week. All eyes were examined at 1 day, 1 week, 1 month, 3 months, 6 months and more periodically depending on the patient IOP and clinical status. Examination with or without sedation was performed to measure IOP and detect some happening complication like major hypotony, choroidal detachment, endophtalmitis…

The use of one or several antiglaucomatous medications was possible to control the IOP.

Absolute success rate was defined as an IOP between 5-21 mm Hg without additional glaucoma surgeries or devastating complications postoperatively .Relative success was defined by adjunction of antiglaucomatous medications.

Table 1. Demographic Data

	Patients Number (%) (n=52)	Eyes Number (%) (n=57)
Mean age in years	10 ± 4, 4	
	2 to 16 years	
Male	32 (61. 5)	
Diagnosis		
Congenital/infantile glaucoma	35 (61.6)	39 (68.4)
Aphakia	9 (17.3)	10 (17.5)
Rieger	1 (1.9)	1 (1.7)
ICE syndrome	2 (3.8)	2 (3.5)
Uveitic glaucoma	2 (3.8)	2 (3.5)
Juvenile glaucoma	3 (5.7)	3 (5.2)
Previous surgery		
Trabeculotomy	7 (13.4)	8 (14)
Trabeculectomy	30 (57.6)	32 (56.1)
Trabeculectomy with Antimetabolites	38 (73)	39 (68. 4)

Some patients underwent more than one surgery.

Results

This retrospective study included 57 eyes of 52 patients who underwent Ahmed Glaucoma Valve Implantation.

Table 1 summarizes the demographic data of our study population. Patients ranged in age from 1to 16 years with a mean age of 10 years.

Male gender predominates in our study population (32 of 52 patients: 61.5 %)

All refractory glaucomatous eyes had undergone at least one previous glaucoma surgery before Ahmed Valve Implantation except in 3 eyes where the Device was performed like first procedure. The previous surgery was usually trabeculectomy without (57. 6%) or with (73%) antimetabolites. There is any case of goniotomy in previous surgery.

Most of these patients had congenital/infantile glaucoma (39 of 57, 68. 4%), aphakic glaucoma(10 of 57,17.5%), Rieger syndrome(1 of 57,1.7%), ICE syndrome (2 of 57, 3.5%), uveitic glaucoma (2 of 57,3.5%), and juvenile glaucoma(3 of 57,5.2%).

The follow up was 68.2 months (range 8 to 156 months). Figure 1 represents the cohort of patients with different follow up periods.

The mean preoperative IOP was 35.66 ± 6, 5 mm Hg with 3.1± 1.9 antiglaucoma medications. The preoperative antiglaucoma medications used usually comprised timolol maleate 0.25%, latanoprost 0.005% and dorzolamide.

The mean post operative IOP at last follow up for all eyes was 14.0 ± 5.3 mmHg with 1.9 ± 1.1 glaucoma medications.

Thus, the procedure was successful with or without medications in 92%, 82%, 73%, 47% and 37.5% of cases after 12,24,36,48 and 68 months respectively (figure 4).

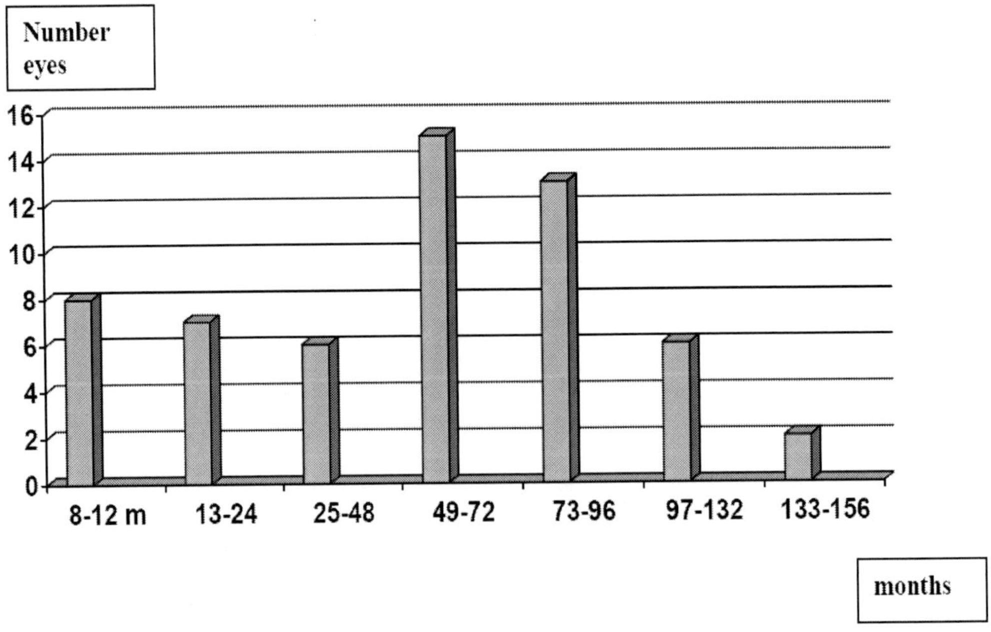

Figure 1. Eyes number according to follow up periods.

Figure 2 presents average number of antiglaucomatous medications used during the follow up period.

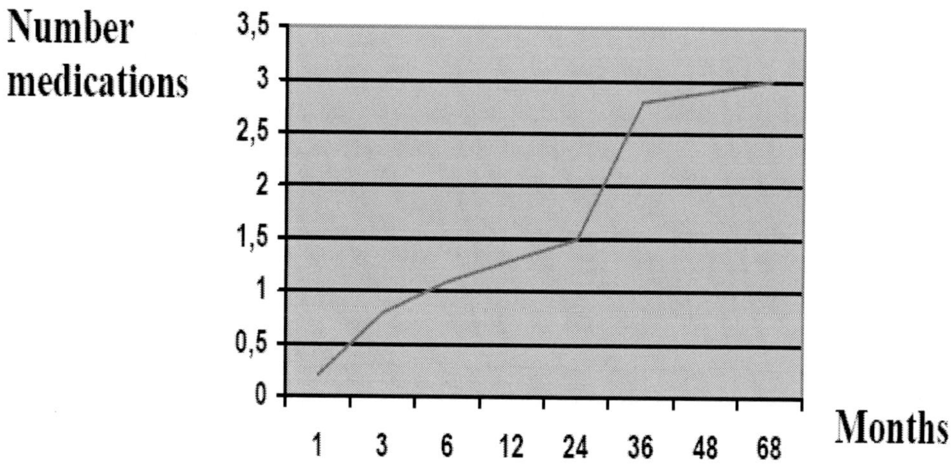

Figure 2. Average number of glaucoma medications during the follow up period.

Figure 3 presents IOP measurements during the entire follow-up period. In early post operative period (2-4 weeks), IOP was relatively low. Between 4 and 8 weeks, there is an increase of IOP and after values reached values of 18 to 22 mm Hg during the follow up.

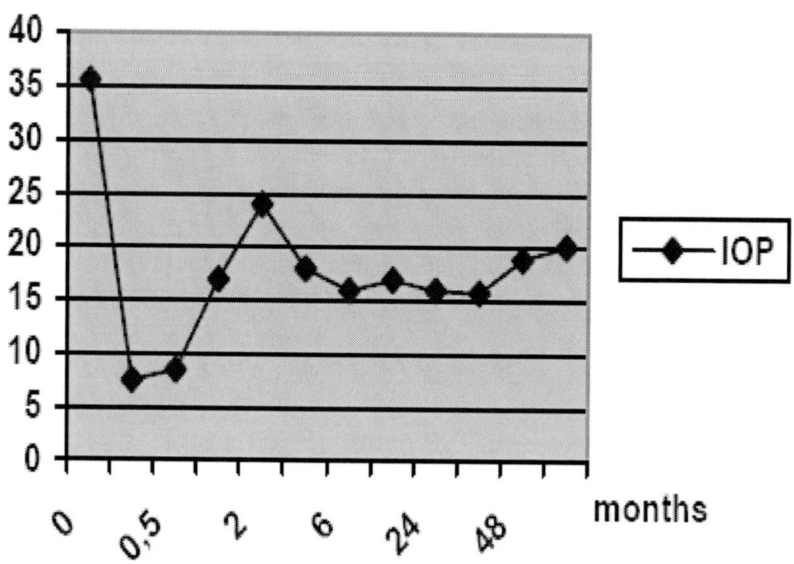

Figure 3. IOP measurements during the follow-up.

Complications occurred in 27 of 57 eyes (47%) and are presented in table 2.

Table 2. Complications after Ahmed valve implantation

Complication	Eyes Number (%) N=57	Average time from surgery (months)	treatment (number of cases)
Hypotony <5 mm Hg	12 (21%)	1.2 ± 0.5	resolute (12)
Hyphaema	9 (15.7%)	0.6 ± 0.4	resolute (9)
Choroidal detachment	1 (1.7%)	0.9	spontaneous resolution
Tube extrusion	2 (3.5%)	6.0 ±1.0	scleral patch (2)
Wound leak	2 (3.5%)	1.75 ±1.5	new surgery (2)
Tube retraction	1 (1.7%)	17.5	tube reinsertion
Tube migration	2 (3.5%)	12.3 ± 2.5	anchoring sutures
Tenon cyst	3 (5.2%)	3.0 ± 1.3	needling
Complication	Eyes Number (%) N=57	Average time from surgery (months)	treatment (number of cases)
Tube obstruction	1 (1.7%)	24	new surgery
Cataract	1 (1.7%)	28	phacoextraction
Failure of membrane	2 (3.5%)	25.5 ± 5.7	removal and new valve
Endophtalmitis	1 (1.7%)	2.7	implantation vitrectomy + antibiotics

Two patients had severe visual loss more than 2 lines of Snellen visual acuity after 32 and 45 months follow up because of agonizing visual field.

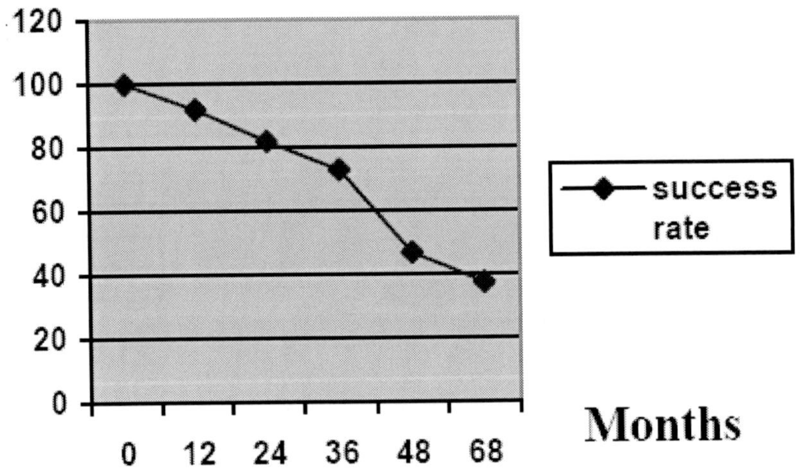

Figure 4. Success rate with the follow-up.

The most common complication was transient hypotony 12 of 57 eyes, 21 %.Usually, it occurred in the first post-operative week and resolved in 2 to 3 weeks. In one patient with uveitic glaucoma, a choroidal detachment occurred. Transient hyphaema occurred in 9 eyes (15.7%) and spontaneously resolved in 3 to 6 days.

Two patients had tube extrusion, which required repositioning and reinforcement with scleral patch. Two cases of wound leak and dehiscence required additional surgery. Tube migration occurred in 3 cases: one case of tube retraction and in 2 cases further into the anterior chamber, reestablishment of anchoring sutures was required. Tenon cyst occurred in three eyes (5.2%) and resolved by needling. Two patients required tube removal and insertion of new Ahmed valve implant.

One patient had a resolutive streptococcus endophtalmitis in eye with corneal graft.

Any case of phtysis, malignant glaucoma and motility disorder was seen.

Discussion

The management of paediatric refractory glaucoma has improved last years with advances in glaucoma drainage devices especially with the Ahmed glaucoma implant. [4] This device is valved propylene which contains an elastomere membrane and the tube that will be inserted in anterior chamber. This type of valve is designed to provide resistance to aqueous flow and prevent excessive drainage and chamber collapse.

The valve is implanted in a single stage procedure.S3 and FP8 models had little surface area (96.00 mm^2) and are used in our group cohort (33 eyes) in patients aged between 10 and 16 years. After, this age we used the FP7 model with 184.00mm^2 areas (24 eyes).

In all eyes, it was a secondary surgery after failure of one or several trabeculectomies with or without antimetabolites, except in three eyes, where the valve was implanted in first intention because of the severity of the disease. When the visual acuity is still good, we prefer Ahmed GDD to cyclodestruction which is reserved with very poor visual acuity.

Most series involving glaucoma drainage implants, like our series, have used IOP ranges of greater than 5 mm Hg and less than 22 mm Hg as their success criteria. The Ahmed valve has been investigated extensively by Coleman and associates and in children they reported an overall success rate of 78% and 61% [2, 5, 6, and 7]. Englert and associates reported an overall success rate of 91% and 58% during the same follow up but the latter group had at least one cycloablation before Ahmed implantation [3]. Djodeyre and all reported a success rate of 70% and 63% at 12 and 24 months [4]. Morad and associates in a retrospective chart review in 60 eyes and 44 patients with paediatric glaucoma reported an overall success rate of 71% and 46% after 36 and 48 months, respectively [8]. These results are very similar to our results (47% at 48 months) .In our study, this success rate decreased at 68 months to 37.5%.These results are similar at Denis's results(30-40% at 48 months) [9].The main potential weakness of Ahmed valve surgery is perhaps long term encapsulation, failure of valve membrane and long term fibrosis [4,10]. Syed, in a case-controlled comparison, reported that the Baerveldt-350 mm implant and the Ahmed valve had similar control and surgical outcomes in patients with refractory glaucoma at 1 year follow-up.[11] Adjunction of mitomycin C not increases the short and intermediate success rates of Ahmed glaucoma valve implantation (Costa, Kook, Susanna...) [12, 13, 14].

We have seen a transient period of IOP elevation in the early postoperative phase (between 4 and 10 weeks).It's the classic "hypertensive phase" which characterizes the bleb encapsulation. [6, 15]

Post operative hypotony was the most common complication but with spontaneously resolution in 21% of surgery. Eisenberg in a vitro study of several glaucoma implant devices (Baerveldt, Optmed, Joseph, and Krupin) reported that only the Ahmed valve device had consistent valve behaviour.[16] None of the devices created enough resistance to explain long term clinical failure of glaucoma drainage device surgery.

Hypotony was reported in 11% to 14% in Coleman series, 23% in Morad's series and 25% in Djodeyre series (21% in our series). [4, 5, 7]

Transient hyphaema was the second common complication but also with spontaneously resolution. We observed only one case of choroidal detachment(1.7%).In Morad's series18% were seen especially in Sturge Weber syndrome. [7,17]

Tube extrusion was seen in 2 eyes (3.5%) of our series, and in 13% in Morad's series. This complication increases the risk of endophtalmitis. The management of tube exposure needs scleral patch or human pericardium. Wound leak dehiscence occurred in 2 cases and required additional surgery. The incidence of wound leaks in glaucoma shunt surgery is reported at an average of 1.5% for all types of implants.

Endophtalmitis is relatively rare (5% Morad's series). [8]

Tube migration has been reported in several series. It was seen into the anterior chamber in 2 cases and one case of retraction in our series and required additional sutures. It is associated with somatic growth of paediatric patients.

Morad and associates reported 7% of tenon cyst, 5.2% in our series treated by needling or excision.

At long term follow up (19.8 at 31.2 months) we have seen two cases of failure of drainage membrane that required a replacement of Ahmed valve implant.

In our series, we didn't see any case of motility disorder, found in 3% in Morad's series and 5% in Coleman's series. Transient diplopia can occur resolving with decreased postoperative periocular swelling. Strabismus had also low incidence in Coleman's series (4%) with Ahmed valve. However, with the Baerveldt implant, with its larger plate size had a high incidence of strabismus (77%). [18, 19,20,21,22]

We think that Ahmed valve implant in refractory paediatric glaucoma is a good alternative with relatively good success rate without touching ciliary's body.

However the success rate decreases with the long term follow-up period.

Nevertheless, it's important, especially in children, to keep useful visual function for psychological developing in early period of life .In spite of the improvement of the valve material, the Ahmed valve implant is a foreign body and the conjunctiva tolerance is required for surgery success. We think that previous surgery is a high failure risk factor for device implantation because of decreasing conjunctiva reserves.

References

[1] Schneider C, Mermoud A. Glaucome. *Les glaucomes développementaux.* 181-194.

[2] Coleman AL,Smyth RJ,Wilson MR,Tam M. Initial clinical experience with the Ahmed Glaucoma Valve Implant in pediatric patients. *Arch. Ophtalmol.* 1997;115:186-191.

[3] Englert JA, Freedman SF, Cox TA. The Ahmed valve in refractory paediatric glaucoma. *Am. J. Ophtalmol.* 1999;127:34-42.

[4] Djodeyre MR, Calvo JP, Gomez JA. Clinical evaluation and risk factors of time to failure of Ahmed glaucoma valve implant in paediatric patients. *Ophtalmology.* 2001; 108:614-620.

[5] Coleman A,Hill R,WilsonNM et al.Initial experience with the Ahmed glaucoma valve implant. *Am. J. Ophtalmol.* 1995; 120:23-31.

[6] JC Das, Z Chaudhuri, P Sharma and S Bhomaj: The Ahmed Glaucoma Valve in Refractory Glaucoma: experiences in Indian eyes. *Eye.* (2005)19,183-190

[7] Topouzis F, Coleman AL, Coplin N, Bethlem MM, Hill R,Yu F et al. Follow-up of the original cohort with the Ahmed Glaucoma Valve implant. *Am. J. Ophtalmol.* 1999;128(2):198-204.

[8] Yair Morad, MD, Craig E.Donaldson, Fraco, Fracs,Yuri M.Kim,MD,Mohamed Abdolell, MSc, and Alex V. Levin. *American Journal of Ophthalmology.* Vol.135, No.6, June 2003, 821-9

[9] Denis P, Rouland JF, Ousmane laoual: La chirurgie du glaucome de l'enfant. 385-397 Chirurgie des glaucomes. *BSOF.* Lamy, Nov 2005.

[10] Huang MC,Netland PA,Coleman AL,Seigner SW,Moster MR, Hill RA.Intermediate-term clinical experience with the Ahmed glaucoma valve implant. *Am. J. Ophtalmol.* 1999;127(1):27-33.

[11] Hasan M Syed BS,Simon K Law,MD,Sok H.Nam,MD,Gang Li PhD,Joseph Caprioli MD and Anne Coleman MD. Barveldt-350 Implant versus Ahmed Valve for Refractory Glaucoma. *J. Glaucoma.* *Volume 13, Number 1, February 2004, 38-45.

[12] Vital P.Costa,Augusto Azuara-Blanco,Peter A.Netland,Mark R.Lesk,Enyr S.Arcieri Efficacy and safety of adjunctive Mitomycin C during Ahmed Glaucoma Valve Implantation. *A prospective Randomzed Clinical Trial. Ophtalmology.* Vol 111, Number 6, June 2004, 1071-1076.

[13] Kook MS,Yoon J,Kim J, Lee MS.Clinical results of Ahmed Glaucoma Valve implantation in Refractory Glaucoma with adjunctive Mitomycin C. *Ophtlmic. Surg. Lasers.* 2000.31(02):100-106.

[14] Susanna R.Latin American Glaucoma Society Investigators.Partial Tenon's capsule resection with adjunctive mitomycin C in Ahmed Glaucoma Valve implant surgery. *Br. J. Ophtalmol.* 2003; 87(8):994-998.

[15] Netland PA ,Watson DS.Glaucoma drainage implants in pediatric patients. *Ophtalmic surg.* 1993 ;24 :723-729.

[16] Eisenberg DL, Koo EY, Hafner G, et al. In vitro flow properties of glaucoma implant devices. *Ophtalmic Surg. Lasers.* 1999.30:662-667.

[17] Hamush NG, Coleman AL, Wilson MR. Ahmed glaucoma valve implants for management of glaucoma in Sturge Weber syndrome. *Am. J. Ophtalmol.* 1999; 128:758-760.

[18] Smith SL,Starita RJ,Fellman RL,Lynn JR.Early clinical experience with the Baerveldt 350 mm glaucoma implant and associated extraocular muscle imbalance. *Ophtalmology*. 1993;109:914-918.

[19] Munoz M,Tomey FK,Traverso C,et al.Clinical experience with the Molteno implant in advanced glaucoma. *J. Paediatric Ophtalmol. Strabismus*. 1991; 28:68-72.

[20] Donahue SP, Keech RV, Munden P, Scott WE. Baerveldt implant surgery in the treatment of advanced childhood glaucoma. *J. AAPOS*. 1997; 1:41-45.

[21] Johnson CC,Dietrich M,Tsai JC.Baerveldt shunt vs.Ahmed shunt for refractory glaucoma:a single surgeon comparison of outcome. *IVOS*. 2001;42:S552.

[22] Ayyala RS,Zurakowski D,Monshizadeh R,Hong CH,Richards D,Layden WEet al.Comparison of double-plate Molteno and Ahmed glaucoma valve in patients with advanced uncontrolled glaucoma. *Ophtalmic Surg. Lasers*. 2002;33(2):94-101.

In: Eye Research Developments
Editor: Alan N. Westerhouse

ISBN: 978-1-60741-177-2

Short Communication A

Bacterial Eye Infections

Michael O'Keefe and Fiona D'Arcy
Children's Univ. Hospital, Dublin, Ireland

Introduction

Infection of the eye and the periocular region account for the vast majority of ophthalmic emergencies. In the primary care setting acute bacterial conjunctivitis is estimated to represent approximately 1% of all consultations[1]. Infections can occur in any structure of the eye or orbit and vary in severity from benign self limiting to causing rapid blindness.

Most infections affect the external eye; infections of the orbit and ocular adnexae most often arise due to spread from surrounding structures, usually from sinuses or infected skin lesions. Intraocular bacterial eye infections are rare and are categorized as exogenous or endogenous.

This chapter reviews ocular and periocular infections; their aetiology, pathogenesis, investigations and treatment.

Skin Infections

Impetigo is a superficial skin infection characterised by erythematous macules which develop into vesicles. These produce a golden crust on rupturing. The most common offending organisms are *Staphylococcus Aureus* and *Streptococcus. Pyogenes*. Treatment is with oral flucloxacillin. This infection is most commonly seen in children aged 2-6 yrs. See figure 1 Below:

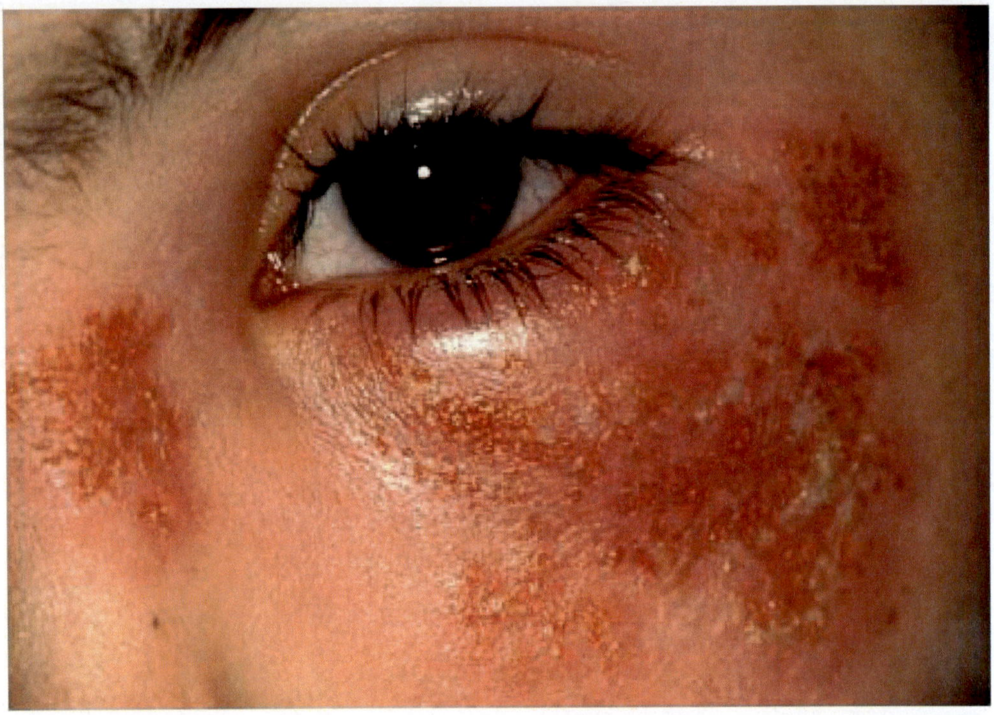

Figure 1. Impetigo.

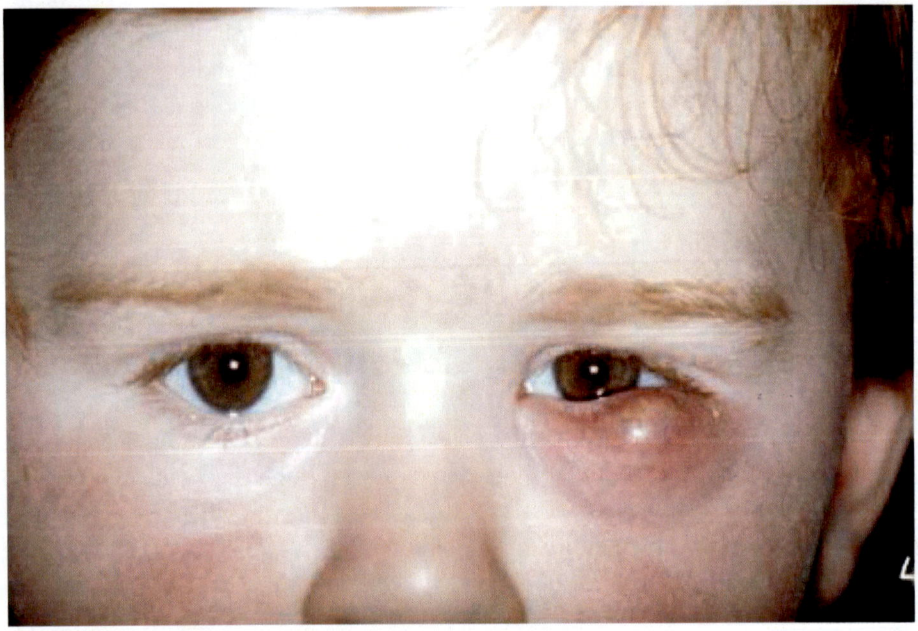

Figure 2. Infected Meibomiam Cyst.

Erysipelas is an acute subcutaneous cellulitis characterised by a red rash with well defined borders. It usually arises from an infection due to minor skin trauma, and has a well defined crusting plaque. *Streptococcus pyogenes* is the usual cause and treatment is with oral penicillin.

Necrotising Fasciitits – This is an extremely rare but potentially devastating infection of the subcutaneous tissue, usually caused by *Staphylococcus Aureus* or *Streptococcus Pyogenes*. It is characterised by rapid progression from periorbital redness and swelling to black skin discolouration. This is secondary to necrosis of skin due to underlying thrombosis. Death may result if not treated aggressively with intravenous (IV) benzylpenicillin and skin debridement.

Internal Hordolem – This is a localised lid inflammation due to an acute Staphylococcal infection of a meibomiam gland. This is also referred to as an infected meibomiam cyst. Presentation is with a localised painful red lid swelling. Treatment is with hot compresses to help discharging of infected contents. If infection is slow to resolve a course of oral antibiotics is necessary. Incision and curetteage is usually required after the acute phase to prevent re-infection. See figure 2:

External Hordoleum - Also known as a 'Stye', this is an acute Staphylococcal infection of a lash follicle. It is located on the lash margin and points anteriorly towards skin surface. Treatment is with hot compresses to encourage discharge of contents and lash epilation.

Blepharitis

Blepharitis describes inflammation of the eyelid margins. This can generally be detected without slit lamp examination as patients have a characteristic red rim around the eyelid margins. It is a chronic condition with relapses and remissions, and it is important to advise patients that while it may not be permanently cured symptomatic relief is possible.

It is divided broadly into anterior (affecting anterior lid margin and eyelashes) and posterior (affecting meibomiam glands) forms.

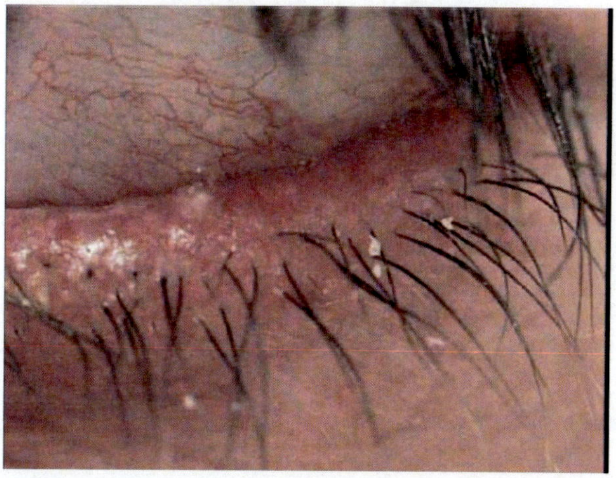

Figure 3. Staphylococcal Blepharitis.

Anterior blepharitis may be caused by seborrhoea or Staphylococcal infection. Staphylococcal blepharitis is characterised by lid margin hyperaemia, telangletasia and crusts at lash bases known as 'collarettes'. Seborrhoeic blepharitis is associated with lid irritation secondary to breakdown of excessive lipids into irritating fatty acids. Crusting of lashes anywhere along its length and lid hyperemia is typical. (figure 3)

Posterior blepharitis describes meibomiam gland dysfunction, and is sometimes referred to as ocular rosacea and is associated with facial rosacea.

Symptoms of blepharitis range from asymptomatic to burning, 'gritty', itchy eyes. Up to 50% of people with blepharitis have an associated dry eye. This is secondary to tear film instability.

The most common organisms isolated from patients with chronic blepharitis include *Staphylococcus epidermidis, Proprionibacterium acnes, Corynebacteria, and Staphylococcus aureus[2]*

Treatment of blepharitis involves a 'lid hygiene' regime, topical and systemic antibiotics, and in certain cases topical anti-inflammatory agents.

Lid hygiene involves applying warm compresses to lids in order to enhance flow of meibomiam gland secretion. Scrubbing of the base of the eyelashes with cotton tips helps to remove encrusted secretions. Application of topical antibiotics, foe example fusidic acid twice daily for 10 days helps in flare ups. In cases not responding to the above measures a course of oral doxycycline 100mg bd for a week, then 100mg od for 3-4 months. The benefit of doxycycline treatment is noted with concurrent remission of facial rosacea, and tetracyclines are known to decrease the production of lipase by *Staphylococcus epidermidis* and *Staphylococcus aureus*. Clarithromycin can be used as an alternative in paediatric blepharitis and in those intolerant to tetracyclines.

Blepharitis is usually a bilateral condition. The appearance of a constant unilateral blepharitis, especially if associated with madarosis (loss of eyelashes) should alert the clinician to the possibility of an infiltrating lid tumor.

Lacrimal System

Acute Dacrocystitis

Infection of the lacrimal sac is usually due to obstruction of the nasolacrimal duct. This is most commonly a Staphylococcal infection[3].

Presentation is with the onset of pain, redness and swelling of the medial canthus, with associated epiphora. The swelling is typically exquisitely tender, and in extreme cases spreads to become a pre-septal cellulitis. The condition can affect any age group. (figure 4)

The infection may extend to outside the sac to form a lacrimal abscess. This is noted by an obvious point to the swelling. This may rupture spontaneously or may be incised to drain pus and alleviate symptoms. The complication of this occurring is the formation of a lacrimal fistula, so that tears drain from the lacrimal sac to the skin surface.

Treatment is admission for intravenous antibiotics – co-amoxiclav, and topical chloromyceitin.

Once infection has resolved a dacrocystorhinostomy (DCR) is usually indicated as re-infection is highly likely.

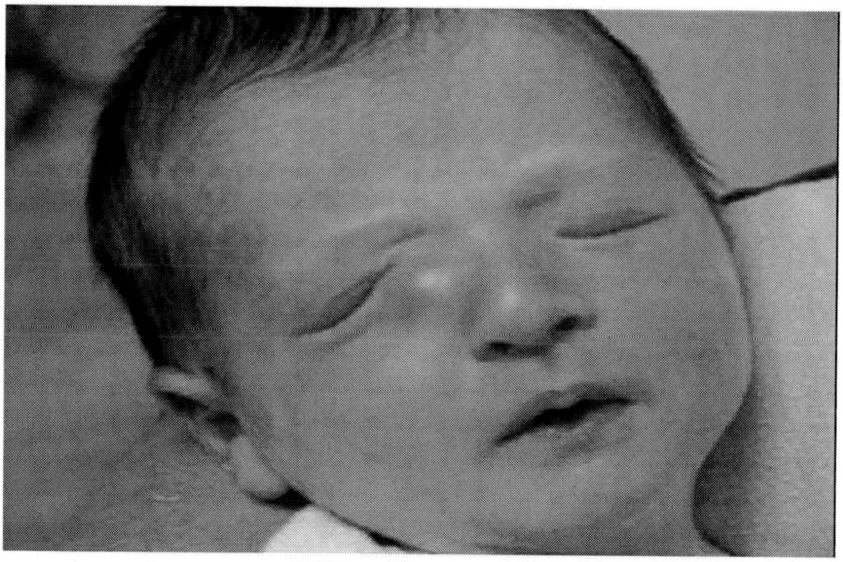

Figure 4. Right Acute Dacrocystitis.

Chronic Dacrocystitis

This presents with epiphoria and may be associated with a recurrent unilateral conjunctivitis. Painless swelling is noted on pressure over the lacrimal sac and very often reflux of mucopurulent material through the canaliculus is noted. (figure 5)

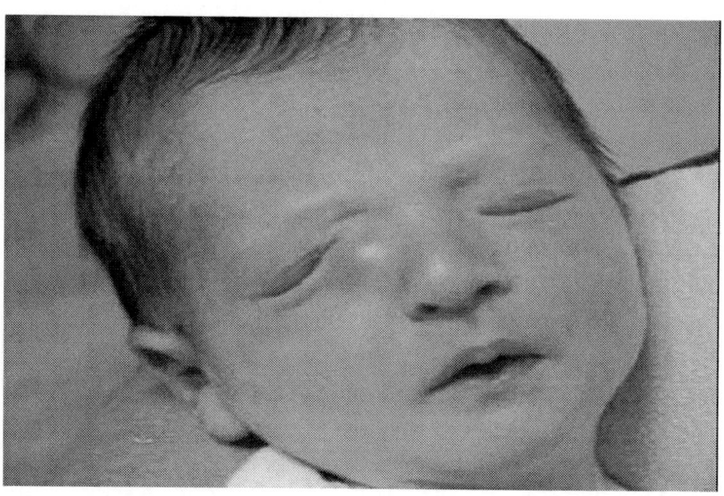

Figure 5. Chronic Left Dacrocystitis – Non tender, non-inflamed swelling over medial canthus.

Chronic Canaliculitis

This is a relatively uncommon chronic condition, frequently caused by *Actinomyces* (anaerobic gram +ve bacteria). Presentation is with epiphora, and a chronic nasal conjunctivitis. Slit lamp examination reveals the characteristic 'pouting' punctum. This is secondary to pericanalicular inflammation. Definitive treatment is opening of the canaliculus and expression of concretions, which consist of sulphur granules.

Conjunctivitis

Simple Bacterial Conjunctivitis

This is a self-limiting condition more often affecting children. It is the most common eye infection seen by general practioners, representing approximately 1% of all consultations in primary care[4].

Symptoms include 'eyes stuck together in the morning', redness, watering and discharge. Infection can spread to the fellow eye and to family members easily, therefore a strict hygiene regime of hand washing and not sharing face cloths apply.

The spread is from direct contact with infected secretions.

The most common offending organisms are *Staphylococcus epidermidis, Staphylococcus aureus, and Streptococcus pneumonia.* Treatment for bacterial conjunctivitis remains controversial. There is a high frequency of spontaneous remission after 10-14 days, whereas treatment with topical antibiotics shortens the course of disease allowing earlier remittance into nursery/school[5]. Topical treatment consists of a broad spectrum antibiotic for example chloramphenicol qid and ointment at night for a week.

It must be remembered that viral conjunctivitis is more common in adults and has a self limiting course. Without slit lamp examination the distinction between viral and bacterial conjunctivitis can be challenging.

Adult Chlamydia Conjunctivitis

Adult Chlamydia conjunctivitis is a sexually transmitted disease, caused by serotypes D-K of *Chlamydia trachomatis,* a gram –ve obligate intracellular bacteria. It is most common in young adults and conjunctivitis occurs in 2% of people infected with Chlamydia.

Presentation is generally with a unilateral red eye, mucopurulent discharge, and an intense follicular reaction. Often the patient has the condition for a few weeks and has not responded to treatment for bacterial conjunctivitis. The cornea may have very fine peripheral infiltrates and subepithelial opacities in later stages of infection.

A tender pre-auricualr lymphadenopathy may be present (this is not exclusive to Chlamydial infections and is present in viral conjunctivitis). There are often no genitor-urinary symptoms.

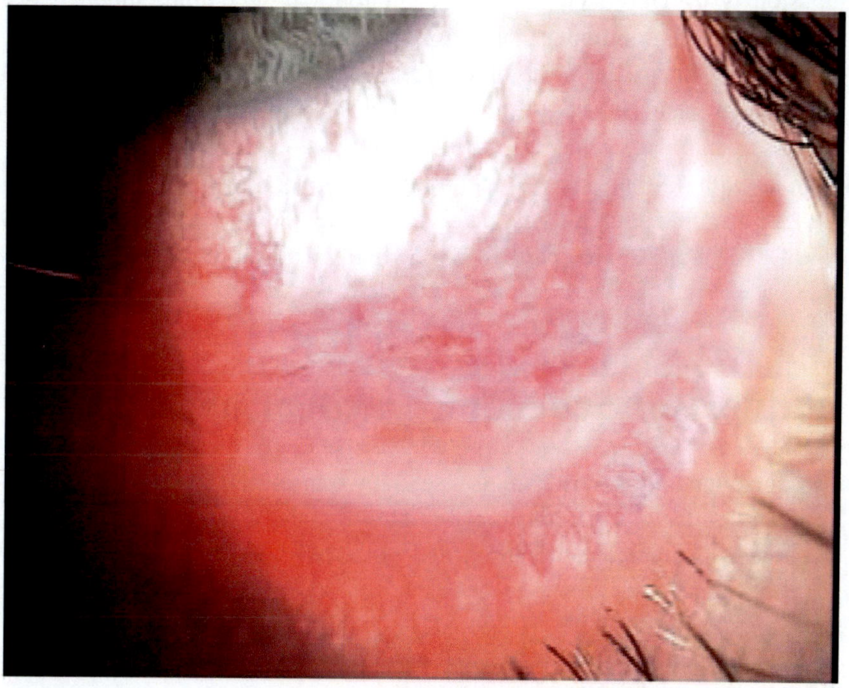

Figure 6. Conjunctival hyperaemia noted in inferior fornix in acute conjunctivitis.

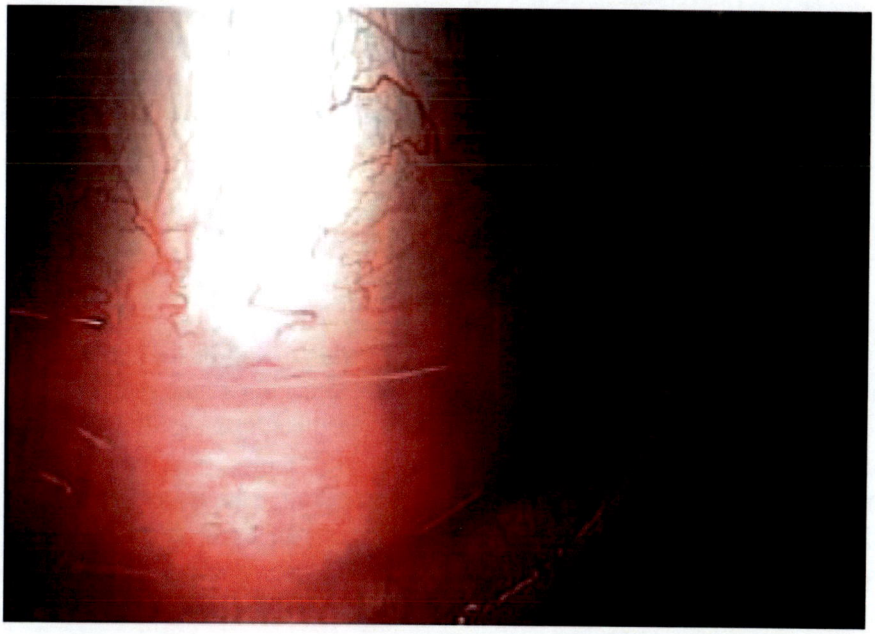

Figure 7. Inferior fornix pseudomembrane (paler area) in severe conjunctivitis.

Transmission is by autoinoculation from genitourinal secretions although eye to eye spread may occur. Inoculation time is approximately one week

Investigation is Chlamydial swabs for immunofluorescent staining. Polymerase Chain Reaction (PCR) may also be used. Smears should be sent for gram staining to look for inclusion bodies.

Treatment is with 1 gram stat of azithromycin and occ tetracycline qid for 6 weeks. Alternatively, for example in pregnancy, po erythromycin 250mg qid is used for 2 weeks.

Referral of patient and sexual partner to a Sexually Transmitted Disease (STD) clinic is essential.

Adult Gonococcal Keratoconjunctivitis

Gonococcal conjunctivitis, now rare, is a sexually transmitted disease caused by the gram negative diplococcus, *Neisseria gonorrhoeae.* This infection, if not treated promptly, can progress to corneal involvement (keratitis) and potentially perforate the cornea from deep involvement.

Transmission is from infected genitourinal secretions and incubation period is 3-5 days.

Presentation is with severe purulent discharge, tender lid oedema and extreme conjunctival injection and chemosis, with occasional conjunctival pseudomembranes. However pseudomemranes can be found in any form of infective conjunctivitis when severe.

Investigation is with gram stain and swabbing for cultures.

Treatment is admission for intensive topical antibiotics, usually ciprofloxacin 2 hourly and frequent saline irrigation of discharge. Systemic antibiotic, usually 1 gram of ceftriaxone stat is administered.

Referral to a sexually transmitted diseases (STD) clinic is essential.

Neonatal Conjunctivitis (Ophthalmia Neonatorum)

This term is used to describe conjunctivitis in the first month of life. It chiefly refers to Gonococcal or Chlamydial infection that follows contamination of the fetus during vaginal delivery, however simple bacterial conjunctivitis may also be the cause. It affects up to 12% of infants in the western world.

The time of onset may indicate the cause. Gonococcal infection typically occurs 2-5 days post delivery whereas Chlamydial infection occurs after a week of life.

Gonococcal conjunctivitis presentation is similar to the adult form with severe mucopurulent discharge, lid oedema and chemosis. Investigation is with gram stain and swabs for culture and sensitivity.

Treatment is with intravenous ceftriaxone and topical bacitracin.

Chlamydia is most common cause of neonatal conjunctivitis. Clinical features are not as acute as Gonococcal conjunctivitis, and a mucopurulent discharge is noted with mild lid odema.The investigations are the same as for adult chladymiae conjunctivitis and treatment is with systemic erythromycin and referral to paediatrician to outrule Chladymiae *pneumonia*. Parents must be referred to a sexually transmitted diseases (STD) clinic.

Table 1 below illustrates the causes and signs of neonatal conjunctivitis

Table 1. Neonatal Conjunctivitis

	Chlamydial	Gonococcal	Simple Bacterial
Presentation (days post partum)	4-28	1-3	4-28
Signs	Mild lid oedema, discharge,	Purulent discharge, severe injection +/- corneal involvement	Mild lid oedema, discharge
Treatment	Oral erythromycin	Intravenous ceftrioxine	Mild-moderate no treatment, if severe broad spectrum topical drops

Pre-Septal Cellulitis

Pre-septal cellulitis is infection of the subcutaneous tissue anterior to the orbital septum. Occasionally this can spread rapidly to cause an orbital cellulitis and should therefore be observed very closely. The cause is usually from spread from a local infection or skin trauma; however it may also arise from haematogenous spread from a systemic infection for example an upper respiratory tract infection. The main causative organisms are Staphylococcus and Streptococcus.

Presentation is with unilateral red swollen lids +/- fever and malaise. A local site of infection may be present. It is differentiated from orbital cellulitis by the absence of proptosis, no pain on eye movement and no deficit in optic nerve function.

In the paediatric setting treatment is admission for intravenous co-amoxiclav. In mild adult forms oral co-amoxiclav and close observation is appropriate.

Bacterial Orbital Cellulitis

This is a serious life threatening condition. The soft tissue behind the orbital septum becomes infected. The most frequent causative organisms are *Streptococcus pyogenes, Haemophilus influenzae and Staphylococcus aureus.*

The most common cause is from direct spread from a sinusitis and very often the symptoms of sinusitis are not obvious. Other causes include spread from a pre-septal cellulitis, spread through the maxillary sinus post dental infection, post traumatic/surgical or haematogenous spread.

Presentation is with a painful tense unilateral lid swelling. This is usually associated with fever and malaise. Proptosis may be present and if so it is more commonly laterally and downwards. There is pain on eye movement and often restriction of eye movements. Optic nerve function must be frequently assessed (Visual acuity, presence of a relative afferent papillary defect – RAPD-, and colour vision) as compression of the optic nerve from inflammation is possible.

Complications include formation of a subperiosteal abscess, usually located along the medial orbital wall – without drainage this may rapidly spread intracranially.

Local complications include optic neuropathy, raised intraocular pressure and central retinal artery occlusion.

Intracranial complications include cavernous sinus thrombosis, brain abscess and meningitis.

Treatment is with urgent admission for intravenous antibiotics, usually benzylpenicillin and metronidazole, CT of orbits, sinuses and brain, and ENT review to outrule sinusitis

In severe cases regular testing (six hourly) of optic nerve function is necessary.

Surgical intervention is necessary when there is a decrease in vision or an orbital or subperiosteal abscess is present.

Table 2 illustrates the main clinical differences in pre-septal and orbital cellulitis.

Table 2.

	Pre Septal Cellulitis	Orbital Cellulitis
Eye Movements	Normal	Painful and/or reduced movement
Proptosis	Absent	Often Present
Optic Nerve Function	Normal	Abnormal if severe

Bacterial Keratitis

Bacterial keratitis describes bacterial infection of the cornea. Whereas viral keratitis can infect a cornea with an intact epithelium, bacterial keratitis generally arises after entry of pathogens through a break in the epithelium.

Due to the risk of deep ulceration and corneal perforation a corneal ulcer is considered an ophthalmic emergency.

Risk factors for the development of bacterial keratitis include contact lens wear, post trauma, post surgical causes, for example a suture abscess after surgery or a post LASIK keratitis. Pre existing corneal disease is another risk factor, for example cases of dry eye or diminished corneal sensation are at increased risk of developing infection. In individuals with poor lid closure, in facial nerve palsies or ectropian, the risk of infection is increased due to corneal exposure.

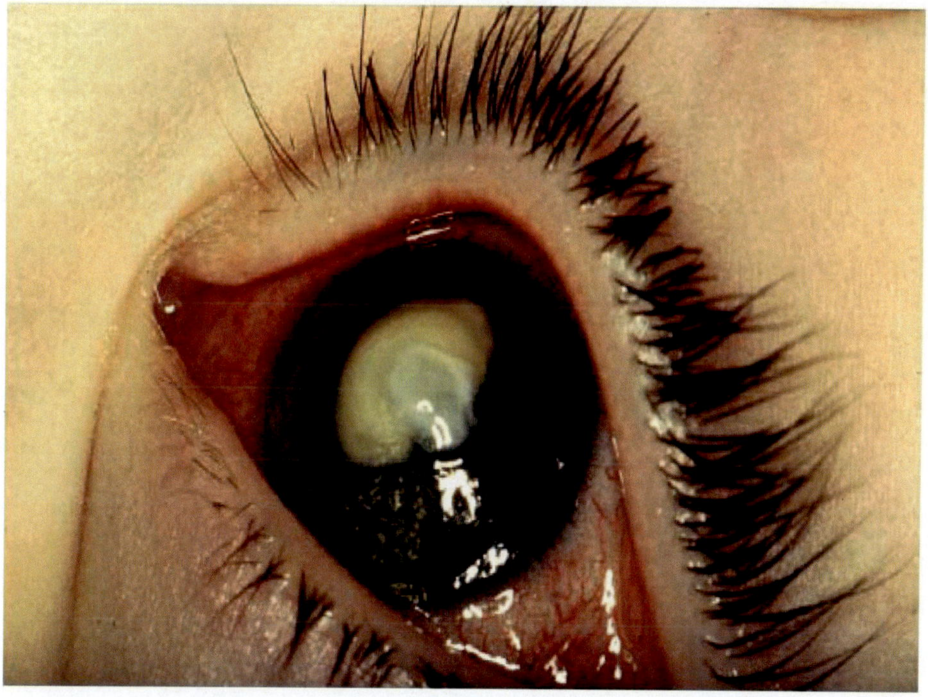

Figure 8. Large Corneal Ulcer Secondary to penetrating eye injury.

Contact Lens Related Keratitis

It is very important to establish if a patient presenting with a corneal ulcer is a contact lens wearer, as most contact lens related infections are due to *Pseudomonas aerigenosa,* which is a highly virulent and potentially rapidly destructive pathogen.

Symptoms include photophobia, foreign body sensation, epiphoria. The main sign is an injected conjunctiva and a visible corneal opacity. An epithelium defect is visible on fluorescein staining and in advanced cases a hypopyon (level of pus in anterior chamber) is evident.

Investigations include culture and gram staining of corneal scrapings, cultures from contact lenses and contact lens cases, and culture from any suture material.

Treatment is admission for hourly broad spectrum topical antibiotics and oral ciprofloxacin. Cycloplegic dilation of the pupil helps with pain from ciliary spasm and prevents the formation of synichae.

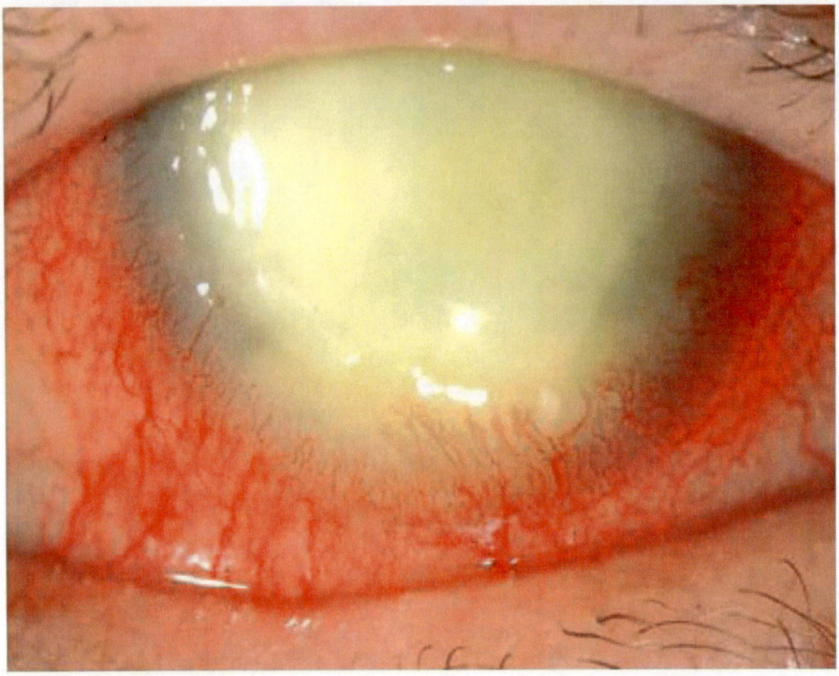

Figure 9a. Devastating Pseudomonas Ulcer in Contact lens wearer, I week history of painful eye.

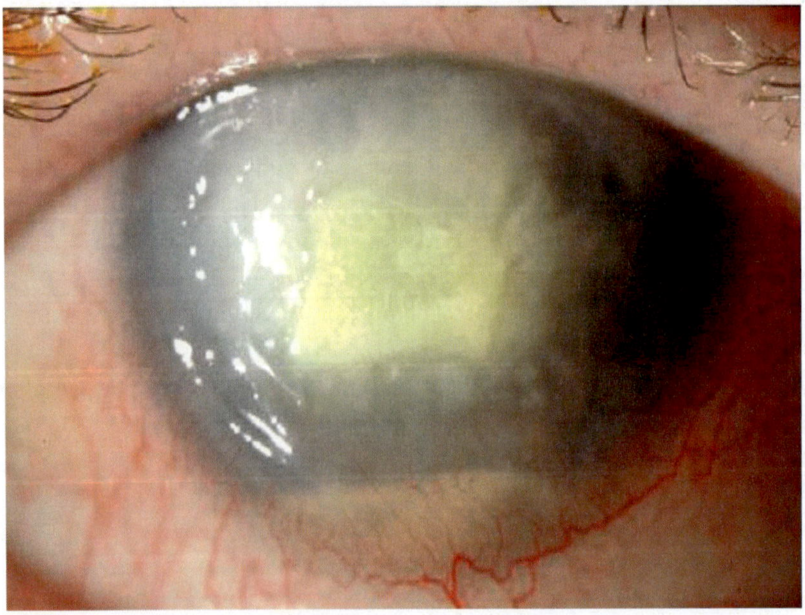

Figure 9b. Same patient two weeks post admission. Note staining of central epithelial defect centrally with fluorescin and hypopyon in anterior chamber.

Acanthomoeba Keratitis

When there has been a lack of response to conventional antibiotic treatment for keratitis, and when repeated sampling reveals no cultures, the diagnosis of acanthomoeba keratitis must be considered.

Acanthomoeba are free living ubiquitous protozoa existing in active or dormant forms. Risks for development of infection include contact lens wear, hot tubs, jacuzzis and swimming pool usage.

Presentation is with an exquisitely painful red eye; typically the pain is disproportionate to clinical signs. A high index of clinical suspicion helps as diagnosis is difficult and often delayed. Initially the infection may mimic a viral keratitis as it presents with a pseudo-dendritic pattern. Later infiltrates form with coalesce to form paracentral 'ring abscesses'. On slitlamp examination of the cornea perineural infiltrates are characteristic. If diagnosis is delayed the infection may progress to leave devastating corneal scarring.

Diagnosis is with specific culture of corneal scrapings and if nothing is isolated a corneal biopsy is performed to look for cysts.

Treatment is with topical anti-amoebic agents, usually polyhexamethylene biguanide (PHMB) or chlorhexidine, propamidine isethionate (Brolene), and cycloplegia. Topical steroids are used cautiously in an attempt to reduce corneal scarring.

Post Lasik Keratitis

Infection post LASIK is a rare potentially sight threatening complication of surgery. A Survey carried out by the American Society of Cataract and Refractive Surgery (ASCRS) Corneal Clinical Committee in 2001 and again in 2004 found the incidence of post LASIK infectious keratitis to be approximately 1:2000[6]. The most common organisms isolated from culture were gram positive bacteria and opportunistic infections, specifically atypical Mycobacteria.

Onset of infection varies from a few days post operatively to several months later. Bacterial infection tends to present earlier whereas atypical organisms such as mycobacteria tend to present later.[7]

Delayed diagnosis of Mycobacterial keratitis can lead to poor clinical outcomes with flap amputation +/- keratoplasty being necessary.

Presentation is with a painful red eye and photophobia with blurred vision, and slit lamp examination reveals white infiltrates in the interface between flap and stromal bed.

If infectious keratitis is suspected the flap needs to be lifted and scrapings taken for culture and sensitivity. The use of acid fast staining techniques and plating on Lowenstein-Jensen culture medium is necessary to detect Mycobacterial infection.

Treatment for suspected bacterial keratitis is with intensive topical fluoroquinlolnes (eg ofloxacin) and fortified vancomycin drops. In the case of suspected Mycobacterial infection topical amikacin and moxifloxacin and oral clarithromycin is the current recommended regime[8]

Interstitial Keratitis

Interstitial keratitis is inflammation of the middle layer of the cornea (stroma). The cause is usually, but not exclusively infectious.

During the acute phase there is bilateral pain with blurring of vision. Clinically there is a whitish haze in the stroma of the cornea which varies in severity and blood vessels are noted to invade the cornea. In the inactive stage a corneal scar of varying severity is left, and ghost vessels are present in stroma.

Diagnosis is by clinical examination and serological testing. The most common cause is congenital Syphilis but other causes include Lyme disease, Epstein Barr virus, and autoimmune causes.

Treatment for active syphilitic interstitial keratitis is with systemic penicillin, topical steroid and cycloplegics.

Bacterial Uveitis

Uveitis is inflammation of the uveal tract. This may affect only the anterior uvea (iritis or iridocyclitis, the posterior uvea (choroiditis +/- vitritis) or there may br a panuveitis where the entire uveal tract is involved in an inflammatory process.

By far the most common cause of uveitis is an autoimmune basis and this may or may not be associated with a systemic autoimmune disease, for example, sarcoidosis.

Infestations with protozoa, for example toxoplasmsis, is another common cause.

Bacterial causes of uveitis are relatively rare, and the offending organism is usually Tuberculosis (TB) or Syphilis. Of note in recent years there has been an upsurge in the number of sexually transmitted diseases, and syphilitic uveitis is becoming more frequently diagnosed. The comeback of tuberculosis and the increasing incidence of HIV infection have lead to a raised awareness of TB as a cause of uveitis and a high degree of clinical suspicion is necessary.

TB causes a chronic granulomatous uveitis. Diagnosis is usually clinical and presumptive, and is considered when there is an intractable uveitis not responding to steroid therapy. Polymerase Chain Reaction (PCR) analysis of intraocular fluid may help in definitive diagnosis. Often there may be no other systemic evidence of TB infection, again making diagnosis challenging.

TB may affect the anterior uveal tract causing a granulomatous anterior uveitis characterised by 'mutton fat' keratitic precipitates (KP's). It may affect the entire uveal tract causing a panuveitis.It may also cause a focal or multifocal choroiditis and rarely a solitary choroidal granuloma which may be mistaken for a choroidal tumor.

Treatment is with anti-tuberculous drugs.

Ocular syphilis must also be considered in intraocular inflammation not responding to steroids. Syphilis is caused by the spirochaete Treponema Pallidum, and is transmitted sexually or transplacentally. Eye involvement usually occurs during secondary or tertiary syphilis. Syphilis is the commonest bacterial intraocular infection in HIV infected patients[9]. Features include iritis, which is inflammation of the anterior uveal tract.

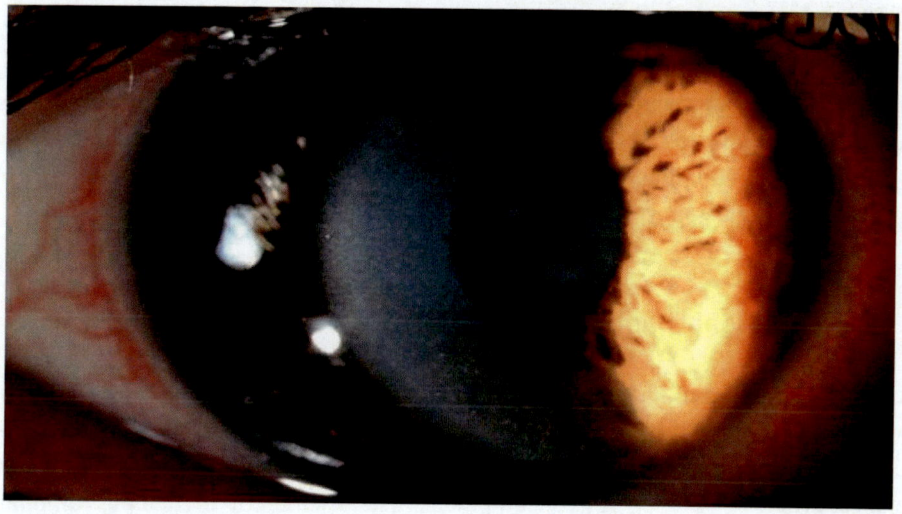

Figure 10. TB Uveitis. Note red injected scleral vessels, Keratitic Precipitates on corneal endothelium and cataract.

Multifical choroiditis is another manifestation where there are multiple foci of inflammation in the choroid. Neuroretinitis can occur whereby there is inflammation involving the retina and optic nerve head, eventually leading to optic atrophy if untreated. Neuro-ophthalmic manifestations include optic neuropathy , oculomotor nerve palsies and visual field defects.

Treatment is the same for neurosyphilis with high dose IV penicillin G.

Lyme Disease

Lyme disease is a systemic disease caused by the spirochete Borrelia burgdorferi. This is similar to the treponeme that causes syphilis. It is usually transmitted from the bite of a tic, these are commonly found in deer in North America or in donkeys and sheep in the west of Ireland.

Early systemic features include malaise, a rash and lymphadenopathy. This is followed by multiple neurological and cardiac complications. Later the disease is associated with a chronic arthritis of large joints.

Ocular manifestations include periorbital oedema, conjunctivitis, scleritis, uveitis, retinal vasculitis and multifocal choroiditis. Neuro-ophthalmological features include optic neuritis, neuroretinitis and ocular motor nerve palsies.

Serologic testing is unpredictable with high rates of false positive and false negative results.

Treatment is with oral doxycycline for 2-4 weeks in early Lyme disease or where there is mild cardiac and neurological manifestations. Intravenous benzylpenecillin or cefotaxime is recommended for late Lyme disease and Lyme arthritis. There may be frequent relapses of the condition and in certain cases long term antibiotic therapy is necessary.

Endophthalmitis

Endophthalmitis is infection of the entire intraocular contents. It progresses rapidly and occasionally even with treatment can result in blindness and loss of eye. It is one of the most feared postoperative complications of cataract surgeons. Broadly, endophthalmitis may be divided into post surgical, post traumatic and endogenous causes.

Post Surgical Endophthalmitis

Acute postoperative endophthalmitis occurs in approximately 1:1000 cases of intraocular surgery. Causative organisms are *Staphylococcus epidermidis, Staphylococcus aureus, Streptococcus and Pseudomonas.* The source of infection is considered to be the patients own flora and occasionally the operative equipment. The routine of meticulous draping and cleaning of the eye and periocular area with povidone-iodine solution ensures minimal contamination. The results of the Endophthalmitis Study Group carried out by the European Society of Cataract and Refractive Surgeons concluded that the use of intracameral cefuroxime at the end of surgery reduced the occurrence of postoperative endophthalmitis. This is now the common practice in most European countries for cataract surgery[10].

Presentation is with severe pain and deteriorating vision. On examination a hypopyon is present with much fibrinous exudate and in advanced cases the red reflex diminishes with a poor view of the posterior chamber. Intraocular pressure is typically low. Treatment is with urgent vitreous sampling, ideally taken from a vitrector and samples sent for gram staining and culture and sensitivity. This is followed by the administration of intravitreal antibiotic injection. Intravitreal ceftazidine and vancomycin is the current treatment. When the vision is less than light perception a full three port vitrectomy is indicated.

Despite aggressive therapy results of acute postoperative endophthalmitis are poor with over 50% of eyes having a final visual acuity of 6/60 or less.

Chronic Postoperative Endophthalmitis

This presents weeks to months post surgery. It is typically associated with cataract surgery and is due to the presence of bacteria on the capsular bag. The most common offending organism is *Propionibacterium acnes.* The patient complains of gradual visual deterioration with floaters. Clinically there is a white plaque on the capsular bag and a low grade anterior uveitis. There is sometimes an associated vitritis causing the symptom of floaters. Topical antibiotics have limited efficacy as the bacteria is sequestered in the capsular bag. Topical steroids help reduce the inflammation but definitive treatment is removal of the intraocular lens and capsular bag. A secondary intraocular lens can be inserted at a later date.

Post-Traumatic Endophthalmitis

Approximately 6-8% of open globe injuries result in endophthalmitis. The most common organisms identified from culture are *Staphylococcus, Streptococcus and Bacillus cerelus.* However the possibility of fungal infection must be considered especially after injury involving soil or other organic material. The risk factors for development of post traumatic endophthalmitis are delayed wound closure, dirty wounds and lens rupture[11]. In the case of an intraocular foreign body delayed removal may be associated with an increased risk of endophthalmitis[12].

Endogenous Endophthalmitis

This results from the haematogenous spread of microorganisms. Endogenous bacterial endophthalmitis accounts for 2-8% of all endophthalmitis and is bilateral in 14-50% of cases[13].Predisposing factors are immunosuppression for example HIV, Leukaemia patients, and intravenous drug abuse. The primary presenting symptom is usually blurred vision. Fungi and bacteria cause endogenous endophthalmitis with the same frequency[14]

Investigation is with sampling of intraocular fluid for culture and sensitivity and Polymerase Chain Reaction (PCR) analysis. Treatment depends on causative organism and is usually with systemic antibiotics or antimycotics, and in some cases vitrectomy with intravitreal injection of antibiotics or antifungals is indicated. Prognosis is variable and usually depends on the pathogen involved.

Methicillin Resistant Staphylococcus Aureus and the Eye

Methicillin-Resistant Staphylococcus Aureus (MRSA) infections of the eye and orbit remain as yet relatively rare. It occurs in approximately 3% of all Staphylococcal infections of the eye.[15] The more common areas affected are the external eye and ocular adnexae. Patients typically have underlying ocular risk factors or are medically debilitated.[16] In a study in San Francisco published in the American Journal of Ophthalmology August 2007, approximately 80% of patients with MRSA eye infections had blepharoconjunctivitis, 14.6% with keratitis, 2.4% had cellulitis and 2.4% had endophthalmitis[17]. The treatment of choice is vancomycin.

Conclusion

The severity of bacterial eye infections varies according to the offending organism. In the case of corneal ulceration, intraocular infection or orbital cellulitis, prompt aggressive treatment is necessary to prevent blindness or even death from sepsis. Post operative and post traumatic bacterial infections require prompt identification and treatment as they can be particularly aggressive. Microbiological analysis of tissue is of particular importance in cases of corneal ulceration or endophthalmitis.

With changing trends in world diseases (TB, AIDS, Sexually transmitted diseases), and the emergence of antimicrobial resistance, the clinician needs to be aware of the many different bacterial causes of eye infections.

References

[1] Acute bacterial conjunctivitis, Hovding G. Department of Clinical Medicine, Section of Ophthalmology, University of Bergen, and Haukeland University Hospital, Bergen, Norway. *Acta Ophthalmol.* 2008 Feb;86(1):5-17

[2] Blepharitis: current strategies for diagnosis and management – W. Bruce Jackson, *Canadian Journal of Ophthalmology* .–vol43:170-9, no2 2008

[3] Mills DM, Bodman MG, Meyer DR, Morton AD 3rd; ASOPRS Dacrocystitis Study Group. The microbiological spectrum of dacrocystitis:a national study of acute versus chronic infection Ophthalmic Plastic Reconstructive Surgery. 2007 Jul-Aug;23(4):302-6

[4] Acute bacterial conjunctivitis, Hovding G. Department of Clinical Medicine, Section of Ophthalmology, University of Bergen, and Haukeland University Hospital, Bergen, Norway. *Acta Ophthalmol.* 2008 Feb;86(1):5-17

[5] Acute bacterial conjunctivitis, Hovding G. Department of Clinical Medicine, Section of Ophthalmology, University of Bergen, and Haukeland University Hospital, Bergen, Norway. *Acta Ophthalmol.* 2008 Feb;86(1):5-17

[6] Infectious keratitis after laser in situ keratomileusis: results of an ASCRS survey. Solomon R, Donnenfeld ED, Azar DT, Holland EJ, Palmon FR, Pflugfelder SC, Rubenstein JB, *Journal of Cataract and Refractive Surgery.* 2003 October;29 (10): 2001-6

[7] Karp CL, Tuli SS, Yoo SH, Vroman DT, Alfonso EC, Huang AH, Pflugfelder SC, Culbertson WW. Infectious keratitis after LASIK, *Ophthalmology.* 2003 March;110(3) :503-510

[8] Lee Sao Bing, Oliver KM, Mohan SK, Slomovic AR, Fourth-generation fluoroquinolones in the treatment of mycobacterial infectious keratitis after laser-assisted in situ keratomileusis surgery. *Canadian Journal of Ophthalmology.* 2005 July;40:750-3

[9] Ocular manifestations of HIV infection. Cunningham ET Jr, Margolis TP. New *England Journal of Medicine.* 198;339:236-244

[10] Endophthalmitis Study Group, European Society of Cataract and Refractive Surgeons, *Journal of Cataract and Refractive Surgery.* 2007 June; 33(6):978-88

[11] Post-traumatic endophthalmitis.Essex RW, Yi Q, Charles PG, Allen PJ. *Ophthalmology*. 2004 Nov;111(11):2015-22

[12] Incidence and visual outcome of endophthalmitis associated with intraocular foreign bodies. Chaudry IA, Shamsi FA, Al-Harthi E, Al-Theeb A, Elzaridi E, Riley FC Graefes. *Arch. Clin. Exp. Ophthalmology.* 2008 Feb;246(2):181-6

[13] Okada AA, Johnson RP, Liles WC. Endogenous bacterial endophthalmitis: Report of a ten year retrospective study. *Ophthalmology.* 1994; 101: 832-8

[14] Ness T. Endogenous endophthalmitis. *Ophthalmologe.* (article in German) 2007 Nov;104(11):935-9

[15] Shanmuganathan VA, Armstrong M, Buller A, Tullo AB. External ocular infections due to methicillin-resistant Staphylococcus Aureus (MRSA). *Eye.* 2005 March;19(3):284-91

[16] Shanmuganathan VA, Armstrong M, Buller A, Tullo AB. External ocular infections due to methicillin-resistant Staphylococcus Aureus (MRSA). *Eye.* 2005 March;19(3):284-91

[17] Freidlin J, Acharya N, Lietman TM, Cevallos V, Whitcher JP, Margolis TP. *American Journal of Ophthalmology*. 2007 Aug;144(2):313-5

In: Eye Research Developments
Editor: Alan N. Westerhouse

ISBN: 978-1-60741-177-2

Short Communication B

Bacterial Flora on Slit Lamps

***Yew Chong Yap*[*1], *Alan Kosmin*[1], *Faye Barampouti*[1] *and Shyam Kodati*[1]**
Dept of Ophthalmology, Watford General Hospital,
Vicarage Road, Watford, WD18 0HB

Abstract

Purpose: To identify the bacteria flora on slit lamps in the clinic and the casualty of an Ophthalmology Department. In so doing we are able to determine the risk of transmission to patients.

Design: A cross sectional study of bacterial contamination of slit lamps in the ophthalmology clinics.

Setting: Ophthalmology clinics and the casualty of Watford General Hospital

Method: Swabs for culture were taken from 6 slit lamps(4 in the clinics, 1 in the urgent clinic and 1 from the A&E). These were performed at the beginning and at the end of the day in the clinic and nurses were told not to clean the slit lamp for the entire day. The swabs were taken from 3 areas the head support, chin rest and the joy stick. Two of the slit lamps in the clinics had disposable paper from the chin rest removed so as to assess the effectiveness of using them. 5 patients had their forehead and chin swabbed before and after using the slit lamp to find out the possibility of transmission during the consultation .

Results: The chin rest of slit lamps are the most contaminated area. Slit lamps that are most frequently used and those that are seldom cleaned are found to have heavy contamination. Coagulase negative staphylococci is the commonest organism isolated.

Conclusions: The slit lamp can be a source of cross infection in the clinic setting. Frequent cleaning of the slit lamp especially after treating infected cases can decrease the transmission of organisms

Introduction

The slit lamp plays an important role in ophthalmology practice as patients seen by the ophthalmologists are usually examined and have procedures performed through the use of the instrument. It is vital for the slit lamp to remain clean so as to reduce bacterial transmission

* Correspondence Dr Yap Yew Chong E mail: eyapyc@gmail.com

between patients. The areas of patients' skin contact with the slit lamp include the head and chin rests. Common skin commensals in these areas may be a source of cross infection. Nonpathogenic microorganisms found on normal healthy human skin include coagulase-negative staphylococci, diphtheroids, propionibacteria and Pityrosporum (Malassezia spp). Factors such as the age of patients and the environment- temperature, humidity and the amount of sebum secreted from the sebaceous glands will alter the density and distribution of bacterial flora[1].

Bacterial flora of clinically healthy conjunctiva were studied previously and mostly Gram positive cocci such as Staphylococcus Aureus were isolated[2,3] In the vitrectomy study Bannerman TL et al revealed that coagulase-negative staphylococci isolated from patients' periocular skin significantly contributed to the infections found in 225 cases of endophthalmits which implied that there is a need to reduce bacterial colonisations prior to eye procedures even if the organisms are non pathogenic[4]. In another study it was shown that cleaning the eyelids with 4% chlorhexidine followed by application of 10% povidone iodine was effective in decreasing the bacterial skin flora prior to cataract surgery from 90.2 % to 19.6% though the organisms were not completely eliminated[5]

Factors that determine the transfer of microorgamisms and cross contamination rates are the type of organisms, source and destination surfaces, moisture level and size of inoculums. During an outbreak of multidrug resistant Acinetobacte baumanni, strains from patients, healthcare workers' hands and the environment were identical. Corrective measures were undertaken to terminate the outbreak[6].

White coats of medical students have been found to contain *Staphylococcus Aureus* especially on areas such as the cuff and pocket in a study done by Loh W et al in 2000[7] and Wong et al in 1991 [8]. Frequent hand washing and a change of white coats were recommended in these studies.

There is at present no existing literature regarding bacterial flora on slit lamps. Our aim is to analyse the level and type of bacterial contamination on the different parts of slit lamps and also to determine whether pathogenic organisms can be isolated.

Materials and Methods

The slit lamps in the Ophthalmology unit that were studied consisted of 4 slit lamps in the consultation area, 1 in the urgent clinic and 1 in the emergency department. The slit lamps were manufactured by Haag Streit Model 900 of Switzerland. Samples were taken from the head rest, chin rest and the joy stick at 8am and 5.30pm.The sites on the slit lamp were first cleaned with sanicloth in the morning prior to being cultured. Doctors and nurses were told not to clean them between patients unless an infected case was being examined. Three of the slit lamps had the protective paper on the chin rests removed to assess their effectiveness in protection against bacterial contamination and in three others the protective paper were retained. The forehead and chin of 5 patients were swabbed before and after using the slit lamps so as to determine whether usage of the slit lamps had contributed to bacterial contamination. The eye cover used to occlude the patients' eyes while testing for visual acuity was also swabbed before and after usage at the end of the clinic.

5% Columbia blood agar plates were used as culture media. The plates were incubated aerobically for 48 hours at 37 Celsius and they were examined for the presence of Gram positive or Gram negative bacteria. A total bacterial count was also carried out. The two most frequently occurring colony types were gram stained and identified by standard microbiological methods. Staphylococci spp were confirmed as *Staphylococcus aureus* by the tube coagulase test. Antibiotic sensitivities were carried out on all isolates of *Staphylococcus Aureus* on Iso-sensitest agar without lysed blood (Oxoid, UK) by the disc- diffusion method in order to identify the presence of MRSA. Gram negative coliforms were identified using the commercially available biochemical tests ie API 20E (bioMerieux, France).

Results

A total of sixty- one patients were seen in the general clinic in the morning while 16 patients were seen in the urgent eye clinic. 45 patients were seen in the general clinic in the afternoon with a further 9 patients being seen in the urgent eye clinic. Varying degrees of bacterial contamination were detected at the 3 sites sampled on the slit lamp. The organisms were mostly normal skin commensals such as coagulase negative staphylococci and *Staphylococcus aureus*. One of the slit lamps had a scanty growth of Acinetobacter [9] and Enterobacter species. MRSA was detected on the head rest of one slit lamp and the forehead of one patient using a different slit lamp. Most organisms identified were environmental organisms not associated with significant infections such as coagulase negative Staphylococcus.

The chin rest is the commonest site of bacterial contamination followed by the head rest. Cultures from the joystick grew a scanty growth of organisms. The slit lamps that were frequently used throughout the day (for morning and afternoon sessions) yielded a heavy mixed growth of organisms. Sample taken from the accident and emergency slit lamp which was commonly used but seldom cleaned by the ophthalmology staff also produce a heavy growth of organisms especially from the chin rests. Samples from the head and chin rests of four patients showed a heavy mixed growth of coagulase negative Staphylococcus before and after using the slit lamps.

One of the slit lamps at the urgent clinic was cleaned at mid-day before the last sample was taken after it was used by a patient newly diagnosed with herpes zoster ophthalmicus. This may have reduced the bacteria load.

Slit lamps with protective disposable paper on the chin rests gave a lower yield of organisms compared to those without the paper protection which yield a heavy mixed growth of organisms. The eye cover grew a light mixed growth of predominantly coagulase negative staphylococci at the end of the day.

Discussion

The areas of frequent skin contact with the slit lamp such as the chin rest produced a higher yield of mixed growth of predominantly coagulase negative staphylococci. Chin rest can be a potential source of cross contamination and use of the disposable paper on the chin rest or wiping it clean after every usage can reduce the risk of transmission. The chin may be a region on the face that is difficult to clean especially for elderly patients compared to the forehead.

The head rest is closest to the eyes and cultures taken from it grew moderate mixed growth of organisms. This may be significant in cases of bacterial conjunctivitis or corneal ulcer. The need to clean the head rest after examining every infected patients or the use of disposable paper should be considered. Perhaps future slit lamps should have a narrower or disposable head rests to reduce the bacterial load for transmission of infection.

Joysticks on the slit lamps produced the lowest yield of organisms. The joystick is frequently touched by the ophthalmologist when examining patients. Infection can be reduced by handwashing, the use of alcohol rub after seeing infected patients or wearing of disposable gloves. It was also proposed that frequent handwashing can cause skin damage or a change in the operator's microbial flora, more skin shedding and risk of transmission of microorganisms [10]. In one study done by Mayo clinic it was found that alcohol rub is more effective as it causes less irritation to the skin and is less time consuming than hand washing [11]. Another study revealed that alcohol rub is also more cost effective than the traditional hand washing [12].

An observational study on hygiene practices among healthcare workers, hand hygiene adherence was strongly associated with duration of patient encounter: adherence was lowest (30%) after encounters lasting less than 1 minute and highest (65%) for encounters lasting more than 5 minutes [13].

Two specimens (1 from the head rest of the slit lamp and the other from the patient's forehead) yield MRSA but culture from the sites later did not reveal the presence of the organisms. In a retrospective analysis of 548 external ocular infections caused by S.aureus over a 44 month period in a British tertiary hospital 17(3%) of the isolates were MRSA. This figure of 3% is lower compare to a Japanese study of 64%. Conjunctivitis and keratitis are the commonest manifestations of MRSA infections. Most of the MRSA isolates are sensitive to gentamicin and chloramphrenicol. However the strain that affect older patients are resistant to ofloxacin and only 2 of the isolates which are from the younger age group were sensitive to ofloxacin [14].

A study on cross-infection by way of faces in which one hundred and seventy-eight MRSA isolates from 159 inpatients were studied. MRSA cross-infection was more frequent in the Department of Neurology compared to other departments and this could be due to fact that patients' faces were more often touched for examination of the cranial nerves than in the other departments [15].

Cultures taken from the patients' forehead and chin showed that there is no significant increase in the number and type of organisms isolated after using the slit lamp. Most of the skin cultures(4 out of 5 patients) produced a heavy mixed growth of coagulase negative staphylococci. As coagulase negative staphylococci are part of the skin flora it is difficult to quantify the level of skin contamination after the use of slit lamps.

The slit lamp is most often used in ophthalmology clinics across the different subspecialities. It is also an instrument with the most skin contact with patients and constitutes a potential for bacterial transmission to occur between patients. Better hygienic practices with the use of disposable paper at certain sites and frequent cleaning of the slit lamp can reduce the degree of cross contamination and transmission of infection between patients.

References

[1] Elsner P. Antimicrobials and the skin physiological and pathological flora. *Curr. Probl. Dermatol.* 2006; 33: 35-41

[2] Fukuda M, Ohashi H, Matsumoto C, Mishima S, Shimomura Y. Methicillin-resistant Staphylococcus aureus and methicillin-resistant coagulase-negative Staphylococcus ocular surface infection efficacy of chloramphenicol eye drops. *Cornea.* 2002 Oct;21(7 Suppl):S86-9.

[3] Watanabe K, Numata-Watanabe K, Hayasaka S. Methicillin-resistant staphylococci and ofloxacin-resistant bacteria from clinically healthy conjunctivas. *Ophthalmic Res.* 2001 May-Jun;33(3):136-9.

[4] Bannerman TL, Rhoden DL, McAllister SK, Miller JM, Wilson LA. The source of coagulase-negative staphylococci in the Endophthalmitis Vitrectomy Study. A comparison of eyelid and intraocular isolates using pulsed-field gel electrophoresis. *Arch. Ophthalmol.* 1997 Mar;115(3):357-61

[5] Rongrungruang Y, Tantaterdthum J, Tuntiwattanapibul Y, Sripalakij S, Danchaivijitr S. Bacterial flora--A potential source of endophthalmitis after cataract surgery . *J. Med. Assoc. Thai.* 2005 Dec;88 Suppl 10:S49-53

[6] Pittet D, Allegranzi B, Sax H, Dharan S, Pessoa-Silva CL, Donaldson L, Boyce JM; WHO Global Patient Safety Challenge, World Alliance for Patient Safety. Evidence-based model for hand transmission during patient care and the role of improved practices. *Lancet Infect. Dis.* 2006 Oct;6(10):641-52. Review

[7] Loh W, Ng VV, Holton J Bacterial flora on the white coats of medical students. *J. Hosp. Infect.* 2000 May;45(1):65-8.

[8] Wong D, Nye K, Hollis P.Microbial flora on doctors' white coats. *BMJ.* 1991 Dec 21-28;303(6817):1602-4.

[9] Fournier PE, Richet H The epidemiology and control of Acinetobacter baumannii in health care facilities . *Clin. Infect. Dis. Clin.* 006 Mar 1;42(5):692-9. Epub 2006 Jan 26

[10] Larson E. Skin hygiene and infection prevention: more of the same or different approaches? *Clin. Infect. Dis.* 1999 Nov:29(5): 1287-94

[11] Trampuz A, Widmer AF.Hand hygiene: a frequently missed lifesaving opportunity during patient care. *Mayo Clin. Proc.* 2004 Jan;79(1):109-16. Review

[12] Huber MA, Holton RH, Terezhalmy GT. Cost analysis of hand hygiene using antimicrobial soap and water versus an alcohol-based hand rub. *J. Contemp. Dent. Pract.* 2006 May 1;7(2):37-45.

[13] Dedrick RE, Sinkowitz-Cochran RL, Cunningham C, Muder RR, Perreiah P, Cardo DM, Jernigan JA. Hand hygiene practices after brief encounters with patients: an important opportunity for prevention. *Infect. Control Hosp. Epidemiol.* 2007 Mar;28(3):341-5. Epub 2007 Feb 20.

[14] Shanmuganathan VA, Armstrong M, Buller A, Tullo AB. External ocular infections due to methicillin-resistant Staphylococcus aureus (MRSA). *Eye.* 2005 Mar;19(3):284-91. Review.

[15] Kuramoto-Chikamatsu A, Honda T, Matsumoto T, Shiohara M, Kawakami Y, Yamauchi K, Kato Y. Transmission via the face is one route of methicillin-resistant Staphylococcus aureus cross-infection within a hospital. *Am. J. Infect. Control.* 2007 Mar;35(2):126-30

Index

A

B

C

D

E

F

G

H

I

J

K

L

M

N

O

P

Q

R

S

T

U

V

X

Y

Z